Diagnostic Meta-Analysis

Giuseppe Biondi-Zoccai
Editor

Diagnostic Meta-Analysis

A Useful Tool for Clinical Decision-Making

Springer

Editor
Giuseppe Biondi-Zoccai
Department of Medico-Surgical Sciences
Sapienza University of Rome
Latina
Italy

ISBN 978-3-030-07691-7 ISBN 978-3-319-78966-8 (eBook)
https://doi.org/10.1007/978-3-319-78966-8

Softcover re-print of the Hardcover 1st edition 2018

Printed on acid-free paper

This Springer imprint is published by the registered company Springer International Publishing AG part of Springer Nature.
The registered company address is: Gewerbestrasse 11, 6330 Cham, Switzerland

To Vincenzo, brother, friend, and father

Foreword

When they wake up in the morning in the third millennium medical students silently give thanks that they are no longer required to do diagnosis by tasting their patients' urine. Truly diagnosis has come a long way since then.

The growth of interest in the scientific study of diagnosis goes back many years and has its origins in a number of issues which emerged in the second half of the last century. The desire to compare the health not just of people within countries but also between countries gave rise to international classifications like that of the World Health Organization with its successive International Classification of Diseases. The regulation of medicinal products and their use gave rise to clinical trials of the new medicines and these trials triggered interest in precise and operationalizable diagnostic criteria. Finally researchers in various countries started international comparative studies of the causes and prognosis of disease and they needed to be sure that each team meant the same by each diagnostic label.

An interesting development in the last quarter of the last century was the realization that patients did not always present early in the course of their illness and so opportunities for effective intervention were being missed with resultant human suffering. In many cases this late presentation was perfectly understandable as the disease was often silent in its early stages. The technology of screening was rapidly developed but also revealed that the criteria for a successful screening test were very stringent as sensitivity and specificity needed to be very high. Low sensitivity would mean missing many true cases of disease which rather defeated the object of screening for it. Low specificity would mean, especially when the disease was of low community prevalence, that many true non-cases were erroneously identified and subject to both unnecessary follow-up investigations but also equally unnecessary anxiety and distress. Estimating the high values of both sensitivity and specificity was going to demand very large studies.

As interest in diagnosis began to grow for the reasons we have outlined it also became clear that many studies were far too small. There were many reasons for this. Researchers did not usually have as their primary interest the development and testing of their diagnostic tools and in their anxiety to proceed to the main part of their epidemiological study or clinical trial they understandably did a good job rather than an optimal one. Obtaining funding to develop diagnostic tools was difficult as such work often did not fit into the priorities of governments and charities.

Against all this background it is easy to see why researchers interested in diagnosis were attracted to the possibilities of taking some of the methods which their colleagues in clinical trials had been so keen to adopt to meta-analyze study results. It is the technology which diagnostic study meta-analysis requires which is both similar to but also subtly different from that for clinical trials that this book sets out.

King's College
London, UK

Michael Dewey

Preface

Kindness is the language which the deaf can hear and the blind can see

Mark Twain

What is the first goal that comes to my mind when conceiving the idea of a new book? Summarizing the evidence base on an intriguing topic? Leading an authoritative team of international experts? Forcing my personal agenda in shaping the present and future of scholarly endeavors? Actually, none of them. In all truth, I conceived the idea of this book devoted to diagnostic meta-analyses, my third opus on evidence synthesis after the others focusing on network meta-analyses and umbrella reviews [1–2], with a very personal goal. I wanted to thank and provide recognition to someone I have always felt very special to me: my brother, Vincenzo.

He has always been a father and a friend, on top of being a brother. He has always proved a formidable mentor, not simply a technical or knowledgeable one, but a true expert in empathy and affection. This holds even truer in these last years, which have been among the toughest for me and my sons, Attilio Nicola, Giuseppe Giulio, and Giovanni Vincenzo. Through his support, as well as the guidance of my mother, Giulia, my father, Gianni, and my sisters, Erica and Gina, I have been able to overcome several personal and professional hurdles, and luckily could complete the unique opportunity of editing this book.

On top of my family, I really wish to testify my gratitude to my friend and mentor, Antonio Abbate, who, despite the distance, has been as close as ever. Enrico Romagnoli, much closer in distance and as tight in friendship, has patiently listened to all my personal and professional complaints and has inspired me through his outstanding bearing as father and physician. Giacomo Frati, who has always believed in me and continues to do so in professional and personal terms, despite my ups and downs, is also to be thanked wholeheartedly for combining friendship and alliance for a common success. Last but not least, Laura Gatto lighted my recent path with her wholehearted, caring and forceful support.

Paradoxically, I also want to thank all those people who have criticized, debased, or challenged me professionally or personally in the last few years. They have been many and enthusiast in their ominous purpose, and this is one of the reasons I prefer to avoid identifying them. Despite often leaving marks and bruises, and occasionally scars, some quite profound, they have confirmed me that only our inner drive to sacrifice, success, and sharing can bring forward our very best.

Thinking about challenges, I often face people skeptical or derisive towards meta-analysis, who ask me why I have taken so much at heart and continue to focus attentively on a topic that many consider non-scientific at best. I have previously recounted my personal and professional journey into meta-analysis (now totaling more than 200 of them) [1–2]. Accordingly, I will be very brief: META-ANALYSIS IS FUN! Indeed, the best meta-analysis is a unique combination of clinical expertise, methodological insight, and communication skills, leading together towards a piece of original research that can guide researchers, clinicians, and patients, while also satisfying your ego and supporting your career [3]. No other type of research endeavor can timely combine these potent ingredients and eventually provide you an edible product.

Despite their fun, meta-analyses are facing several challenges in recent years [4]. The first obvious challenge is that, being relatively easy to plan and perform, at least in skilled hands, there are now several redundant if not copycat meta-analyses available [5]. In addition, in the information technology era, it is conceivable that meta-analyses as currently conducted will become obsolete and self-learning approaches will automatically provide comparable results in a fraction of a second [6]. Third, conversely, there is a booming literature on alternative methods for meta-analysis, which creates uncertainty on which method is best, and may also undermine the credibility of previously established methods [7]. As commonplace in research, "prediction is very difficult, especially about the future" [8]. However, we expect that some sort of expertise will always be required to conduct a meta-analysis, and, even in the worst-case scenario, to interpret and apply one correctly.

And this preamble brings forward the need for the present book, aiming at boosting methodological and operative knowledge in this field, with a specific focus on diagnostic tests. Indeed, most meta-analyses published today represent systematic reviews and pooled analyses at the study level of controlled clinical trials [1, 9, 10]. Other types of meta-analyses are available as well, but they are less prominent. One specific type of meta-analysis is the one focusing on diagnosis rather than therapy, i.e., a meta-analysis pooling diagnostic test accuracy studies [11]. While randomized trials of diagnostic strategies are also possible, they are quite uncommon, thus leaving the evidence on diagnostic decision making mainly relying on studies of diagnostic test accuracy [12].

As there is no book to date devoted to this interesting field of clinical and statistical research, we have aimed at filling such gap and provide clinicians and researchers with state-of-the-art guidance to conceive, design, conduct, report, and apply a meta-analysis of diagnostic test accuracy studies. Readers should be aware though that the Cochrane Library has put enormous efforts at improving the methodology of this type of research synthesis, and draft chapters of their upcoming book on this topic are available for free online [13]. Finally, diagnostic studies should best be viewed in the continuum of clinical practice, from prevention, to treatment, and rehabilitation. Accordingly, the best test of a diagnostic study remains, only apparently paradoxically, a randomized trial (or a set of randomized trials summarized in a dedicated meta-analysis) [14].

Despite these caveats, we hope people interested in evidence synthesis, clinical practice, and statistical methodology will find reading this book fruitful and enjoyable as much as we found editing it.

Because, in all truth, meta-analysis is fun!

Latina, Italy Giuseppe Biondi-Zoccai

References

1. Biondi-Zoccai G, editor. Network meta-analysis: evidence synthesis with mixed treatment comparison. Hauppauge, NY: Nova Science Publishers; 2014.
2. Biondi-Zoccai G, editor. Umbrella reviews. Evidence synthesis with overviews of reviews and meta-epidemiologic studies. Cham, Switzerland: Springer International; 2016.
3. Biondi-Zoccai G, Anderson LA. What is the purpose of launching World Journal of Meta-Analysis? World J Meta-Anal. 2013;1:1–4.
4. Fava GA. Evidence-based medicine was bound to fail: a report to Alvan Feinstein. J Clin Epidemiol. 2017;84:3–7.
5. Biondi-Zoccai GG, Lotrionte M, Abbate A, Testa L, Remigi E, Burzotta F, Valgimigli M, Romagnoli E, Crea F, Agostoni P. Compliance with QUOROM and quality of reporting of overlapping meta-analyses on the role of acetylcysteine in the prevention of contrast associated nephropathy: case study. BMJ. 2006;332:202–9.
6. Shekelle PG, Shetty K, Newberry S, Maglione M, Motala A. Machine learning versus standard techniques for updating searches for systematic reviews: a diagnostic accuracy study. Ann Intern Med. 2017;167:213–5.
7. Neupane B, Richer D, Bonner AJ, Kibret T, Beyene J. Network meta-analysis using R: a review of currently available automated packages. PLoS One. 2014;9:e115065.
8. Niels Bohr. https://en.wikiquote.org/wiki/Niels_Bohr. Last accessed 27 June 2018.
9. Borenstein M, Hedges LV, Higgins J, Rothstein HR. Introduction to meta-analysis. Hoboken, NJ: Wiley; 2009.
10. Higgins JPT, Green S. Cochrane handbook for systematic reviews of interventions. Hoboken, NJ: Wiley; 2008.
11. Gatsonis C, Paliwal P. Meta-analysis of diagnostic and screening test accuracy evaluations: methodologic primer. AJR Am J Roentgenol. 2006;187:271–81.
12. Nudi F, Lotrionte M, Biasucci LM, Peruzzi M, Marullo AG, Frati G, Valenti V, Giordano A, Biondi-Zoccai G. Comparative safety and effectiveness of coronary computed tomography: systematic review and meta-analysis including 11 randomized controlled trials and 19,957 patients. Int J Cardiol. 2016;222:352–8.

13. Cochrane methods—screening and diagnostic tests: handbook for DTA reviews. http://methods.cochrane.org/sdt/handbook-dta-reviews. Last accessed 27 June 2018.
14. Biondi-Zoccai GG, Agostoni P, Abbate A. Parallel hierarchy of scientific studies in cardiovascular medicine. Ital Heart J. 2003;4:819–20.

Contents

Contributors

Sousa Afonso Surgical Division, Gastroenterology Department, Clinics Hospital, University of Sao Paulo School of Medicine, Sao Paulo, Brazil

Eliana Al Haddad The Division of Cardiac Surgery, Department of Surgery, Columbia University, New York, NY, USA

Hutan Ashrafian The Department of Surgery and Cancer, Imperial College London, London, UK

Thanos Athanasiou The Department of Surgery and Cancer, Imperial College London, London, UK

Department of Cardiac Surgery, Imperial College Healthcare NHS Trust, London, UK

Umberto Benedetto Bristol Heart Institute, University of Bristol, Bristol, UK

Alessandra Bettiol Department of Neurosciences, Psychology, Drug Research and Child Health (NEUROFARBA), University of Florence, Florence, Italy

Giuseppe Biondi-Zoccai Department of Medico-Surgical Sciences and Biotechnologies, Sapienza University of Rome, Latina, Italy

Department of AngioCardioNeurology, IRCCS Neuromed, Pozzilli, Italy

Mario Bollati Department of Cardiology, IRCCS Pol. S. Donato, S. Donato Milanese, Milan, Italy

Alison Booth Department of Health Sciences, University of York, York, UK

Paul-Christian Bürkner Institute of Psychology, Faculty of Psychology and Sport Sciences, University of Münster, Münster, Germany

Yong Chen Department of Biostatistics, Epidemiology and Informatics, Perelman School of Medicine, University of Pennsylvania, Philadelphia, PA, USA

Salvatore De Masi Clinical Trial Office, University Hospital "Azienda Ospedaliero-Universitaria Meyer", Florence, Italy

Philipp Doebler Department of Statistics, TU Dortmund University, Dortmund, Germany

Konstantinos C. Fragkos University College London, London, UK

Giacomo Frati Department of Medico-Surgical Sciences and Biotechnologies, Sapienza University of Rome, Latina, Italy

Department of AngioCardioNeurology, IRCCS Neuromed, Pozzilli, Italy

Julie Glanville York Health Economics Consortium, University of York, York, UK

Su Golder Department of Health Sciences, University of York, York, UK

Julie Jones-Diette Centre for Reviews and Dissemination, University of York, York, UK

Bustamante-Lopez Leonardo Surgical Division, Gastroenterology Department, Clinics Hospital, University of Sao Paulo School of Medicine, Sao Paulo, Brazil

Isnard Elman Litvin Faculdade de Medicina, Universidade de Caxias do Sul (UCS), Caxias do Sul, Brazil

Yulun Liu Department of Biostatistics, Epidemiology and Informatics, Perelman School of Medicine, University of Pennsylvania, Philadelphia, PA, USA

Ersilia Lucenteforte Department of Clinical and Experimental Medicine, University of Pisa, Pisa, Italy

José Mauro Madi Faculdade de Medicina, Universidade de Caxias do Sul (UCS), Caxias do Sul, Brazil

Sulbaran Marianny Gastrointestinal Endoscopy Service, Gastroenterology Department, Clinics Hospital, University of Sao Paulo School of Medicine, Sao Paulo, Brazil

Simona Mastrangeli Superior School of Advanced Studies, Sapienza University of Rome, Rome, Italy

Colin Ng Singapore General Hospital, Singapore, Singapore

Machline Paim Paganella Laboratório de Pesquisa em HIV/AIDS, Universidade de Caxias do Sul (UCS), Caxias do Sul, Brazil

Mical Paul Rambam Heath Care Campus and The Ruth and Bruce Rappaport Faculty of Medicine, Technion—Israel Institute of Technology, Haifa, Israel

Valentina Pecoraro Laboratory of Toxicology, Department of Laboratory Medicine and Pathological Anatomy, Azienda USL of Modena, Modena, Italy

Mariangela Peruzzi Department of Medico-Surgical Sciences and Biotechnologies, Sapienza University of Rome, Latina, Italy

Bashar J. Qumseya Division of Gastroenterology and Hepatology, Archbold Medical Group/Florida State University, Thomasville, GA, USA

Gerta Rücker Faculty of Medicine, Institute for Medical Biometry and Statistics, Medical Center – University of Freiburg, Freiburg im Breisgau, Germany

Luca Testa Department of Cardiology, IRCCS Pol. S. Donato, S. Donato Milanese, Milan, Italy

Michail Tsagris Department of Computer Science, University of Crete, Heraklion, Greece

Gianni Virgili Department of Surgery and Translational Medicine (DCMT), University of Florence, Florence, Italy

Michael Wallace Division of Gastroenterology and Hepatology, Mayo Clinic, Jacksonville, FL, USA

Eliana Marcia Wendland Departamento de Saúde Coletiva, Universidade Federal de Ciências da Saúde de Porto Alegre (UFCSPA), Porto Alegre, Brazil

Kosma Wolinski Department of Endocrinology, Metabolism and Internal Medicine, Poznan University of Medical Sciences, Poznań, Poland

Antonia Zapf Department of Medical Statistics, University Medical Center Göttingen, Göttingen, Germany

Department of Medical Biometry and Epidemiology, University Medical Center Hamburg-Eppendorf, Hamburg, Germany

Part I

1 Introduction to Clinical Diagnosis

Giuseppe Biondi-Zoccai, Mariangela Peruzzi, Simona Mastrangeli, and Giacomo Frati

Art is long, life is short

Hippocrates

Since its initial formalizing attempts, medical practice has focused on the precise characterization of a patient's ailments and their cure. Whereas cure may often be beyond reach, no constructive management plan can be envisioned if the disease has not been identified and characterized in a formal and reproducible fashion, through the process of clinical diagnosis. Diagnosis, which has been formalized thousands of years ago in Ancient Greece, means indeed *knowing through* [1]. It is based on the iteratively approximating process of identifying the actual cause(s) of a complex maze of pathological signs and symptoms from beginning to late consequences, pinpointing management and providing an opportunity to improve health while minimizing the risk of adverse effects of clinical intervention [2].

Diagnostic practice, thus, is based on comparative analysis and probability concepts, in as much as a given diagnosis appears more likely than a competing one, eventually toppling in the practitioner's mind the less plausible alternatives, albeit using the falsification framework formalized by Karl Popper [3]. However, establishing a diagnosis requires the application of a rule or test, or set of them, that definitely or likely identify a given condition. Absolute certainty is not always

G. Biondi-Zoccai (✉) · G. Frati
Department of Medico-Surgical Sciences and Biotechnologies, Sapienza University of Rome, Latina, Italy

Department of AngioCardioNeurology, IRCCS Neuromed, Pozzilli, Italy
e-mail: giuseppe.biondizoccai@uniroma1.it

M. Peruzzi
Department of Medico-Surgical Sciences and Biotechnologies, Sapienza University of Rome, Latina, Italy

S. Mastrangeli
Superior School of Advanced Studies, Sapienza University of Rome, Rome, Italy

G. Biondi-Zoccai (ed.), *Diagnostic Meta-Analysis*,
https://doi.org/10.1007/978-3-319-78966-8_1

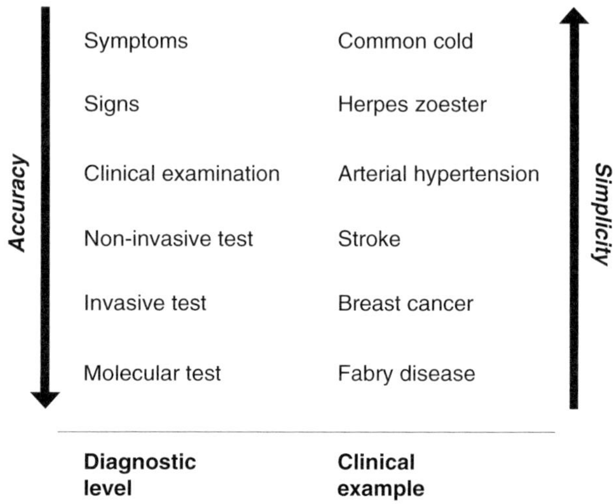

Fig. 1.1 Impact of different diagnostic levels in clinical practice, with suitable examples of clinical scenarios

required for clinical diagnosis, as a careful balance between efficiency and plausibility is always sought (Fig. 1.1) [4, 5]. In the absence of a pathological or post-mortem characterization, any diagnostic test requires comparative support from another test (typically called reference standard or gold standard), thus defining the peculiarity of studies appraising diagnostic tests [6, 7]. Once the features of the index and reference test have been defined and data collected, dimensions of comparative accuracy can be appraised quantitatively and their yield used to guide decision-making.

1.1 Index Test

The index test is the diagnostic test which is of interest to the clinician, as a novel diagnostic tool to identify a given condition. Several reasons may make it more appealing than the reference test. For instance, it may be less expensive, less invasive, and ultimately safer [8, 9]. Otherwise, it may be performed earlier than a reference test, and thus provide ampler means to prevent or treat the condition of interest [10]. Finally, it may serve as an add-on to refine diagnostic clustering after a preliminary test has been completed [11].

Typically, any diagnostic test, including thus the index test, provides a range of results, which may have a varying range of strengths of association with the condition of interest. There may be key exceptions to this paradigm (e.g., genetic tests aimed at identifying a specific mutation), but most tests used in clinical practice do not provide per se a yes or no answer. Accordingly, a diagnostic threshold is applied, such that test results lower than the threshold are considered negative and those higher than the threshold positive (Fig. 1.2) [12]. This continuum of possible

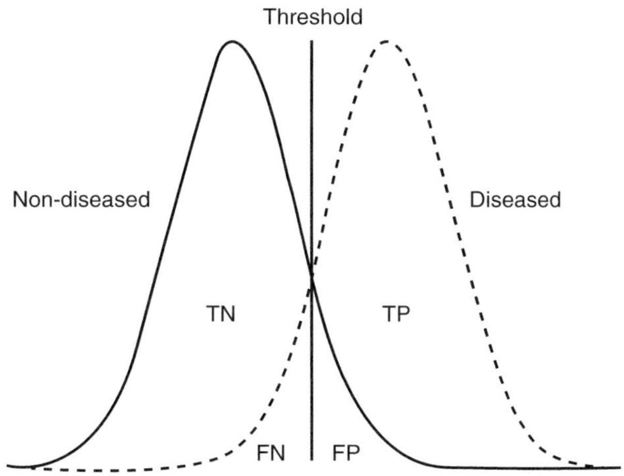

Fig. 1.2 Graphical representation of different results of the index test in non-diseased and diseased subjects (according to a dichotomous interpretation of the reference test), highlighting the choice of a threshold which balances sensitivity and specificity. *FN* false negatives, *FP* false positives, *TN* true negatives, *TP* true positives

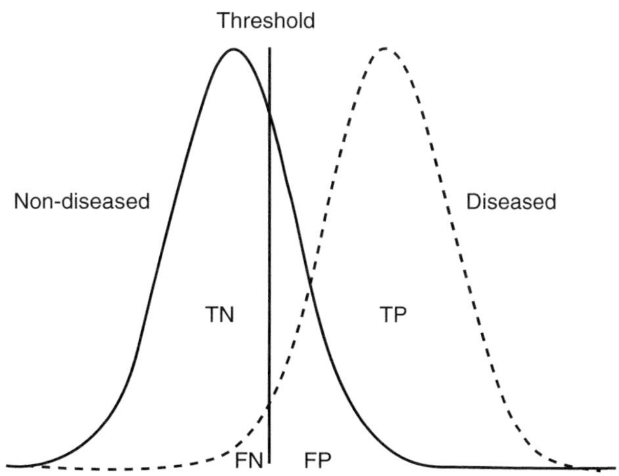

Fig. 1.3 Impact of a lower diagnostic threshold when interpreting different results of the index test in non-diseased and diseased subjects (according to a dichotomous interpretation of the reference test), highlighting the increase in sensitivity offset by a decrease in specificity (compared to the previous figure). *FN* false negatives, *FP* false positives, *TN* true negatives, *TP* true positives

diagnostic thresholds can be formally appraised in a comparative analysis with specific dimensions of diagnostic test accuracy [13]. Usually, there is indeed an obvious trade-off between a lower and a higher threshold. For instance, using a lower threshold to define the presence of diabetes based on fasting blood glucose testing will lead to more patients being considered diabetics (Fig. 1.3). This could result in more subjects being offered promising preventive means but could also increase the risk of side effects and inappropriate disability labeling. Conversely, using a higher threshold when interpreting the results of fine-needle aspiration biopsy for a breast lump might limit chemotherapy and radiotherapy to the few patients with large malignant masses but could also prevent other subjects with borderline lesions to receive timely and potentially life-saving treatment (Fig. 1.4).

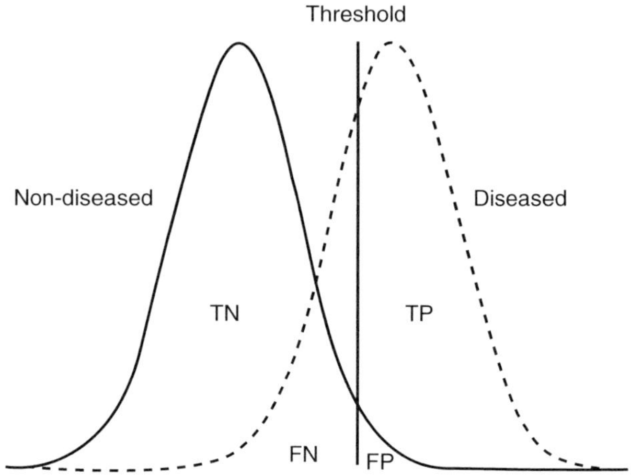

Fig. 1.4 Impact of a higher diagnostic threshold when interpreting different results of the index test in non-diseased and diseased subjects (according to a dichotomous interpretation of the reference test), highlighting the increase in specificity offset by a decrease in sensitivity (compared to the previous two figures). *FN* false negatives, *FP* false positives, *TN* true negatives, *TP* true positives

1.2 Reference Test

Any diagnostic test which is considered clinically established can be used as a reference test for a comparative diagnostic test accuracy study. In most clinical and research settings, a reference test is a testing procedure which is established and reliable, despite its inherent limitations. Obviously, in most cases, what is currently considered a reference test might well have been labeled in the past an index test requiring external validation. Thus, the arguments proposed beforehand to index tests may also apply to reference tests. Of course, in some cases the ultimate reference test is the self-evident clinical diagnosis itself, either considered clinically or appraised pathologically, e.g., post-mortem. Paradoxically, limitations in the accuracy of pathologic and post-mortem diagnosis can also apply. In any case, waiting for disease onset or even fatal disease is clinically inefficient and unethical, thus the need for more timely diagnosis. Typical reference tests can be considered, for instance, a diagnosis of myocardial infarction based on a complex set of symptoms, permanent electrocardiographic abnormalities, and changes in serum levels of cardiac biomarkers, or the pathognomonic features of brain magnetic resonance imaging shortly after and long after an ischemic stroke.

1.3 Dimensions of Diagnostic Accuracy

The comparison of two diagnostic tests, such as the index and the reference tests, can be considered as an appraisal of the consistency of the association between two variables [14]. The simplest scenario is when both provide a yes and no answer, leading to the creation of a two-by-two table with the accompanying measures of association (Tables 1.1 and 1.2). When one variable is continuous and the other dichotomous, different thresholds can be considered, or a continuous

Table 1.1 Appraisal of the diagnostic accuracy of an index test in comparison to a reference test (used to define disease status) using a 2×2 table

	Diseased	Non-diseased
Positive test	TP	FP
Negative test	FN	TN
Prevalence = (TP + FN)/(TP + FN + TN + FP)		
Sensitivity = TP/(TP + FP)		
Specificity = TN/(TN + FP)		

Other dimensions of diagnostic accuracy can be appraised formally using similar data, such as likelihood ratios, predictive values, and diagnostic odds ratios (see the Sect. 1.3)
FN false negatives, *FP* false positives, *TN* true negatives, *TP* true positives

Table 1.2 Example of the appraisal of the diagnostic accuracy of an index test in comparison to a reference test (used to define disease status) using a 2×2 table, assuming a total of 100 patients tested, with 50% diseased, sensitivity of 80%, and specificity of 90%

	Diseased	Non-diseased
Positive test	40	5
Negative test	10	45
Prevalence = 50%		
Sensitivity = 80%		
Specificity = 90%		

Other dimensions of diagnostic accuracy can be appraised formally using similar data, such as likelihood ratios, predictive values, and diagnostic odds ratios (see the Sect 1.3)
FN false negatives, *FP* false positives, *TN* true negatives, *TP* true positives

threshold approach can be used. If both variables are continuous, then different thresholds for both tests can be used. Otherwise, standard approaches to appraise correlation, regression, and bias (e.g., the Bland-Altman method) can be employed [15, 16].

The most common and clinically relevant scenario is however one in which both tests provide a yes and no answer, leading to the definition of four groups of patients: true negatives, false negatives, true positives, and false positives, with accompanying results for prevalence, sensitivity, and specificity.

Conclusion

Diagnosis is based on testing, and thus the precise purpose and context of the test must be borne in mind. Eventually, the test must be considered capable of improving patient health or, at the very minimum, provide societal utility, [17, 18] thus requiring proof of benefit from a randomized controlled trial [19]. More pragmatically, the applicability of the test, for screening, as an add-on, or a replacement of an existing test, impacts on its comprehensive evaluation and adoption [20].

Funding/Disclosure None.

References

1. Ackerknecht EH, Rosenberg CE, Hausshofer L. A short history of medicine. Baltimore, MD: Johns Hopkins University Press; 2016.
2. Adeleye GG, Acquah-Dadzie K, Dadzie KA, Sienkewicz TJ, McDonough JT. World dictionary of foreign expressions: a resource for readers and writers. Mundelein, IL: Bolchazy-Carducci; 1999.
3. Popper K. The logic of scientific discovery. London, UK: Routledge; 2002.
4. Montalescot G, Sechtem U, Achenbach S, Andreotti F, Arden C, Budaj A, Bugiardini R, Crea F, Cuisset T, Di Mario C, Ferreira JR, Gersh BJ, Gitt AK, Hulot JS, Marx N, Opie LH, Pfisterer M, Prescott E, Ruschitzka F, Sabaté M, Senior R, Taggart DP, van der Wall EE, Vrints CJ. 2013 ESC guidelines on the management of stable coronary artery disease: the task force on the management of stable coronary artery disease of the European Society of Cardiology. Eur Heart J. 2013;34:2949–3003.
5. Smith SC Jr, Allen J, Blair SN, Bonow RO, Brass LM, Fonarow GC, Grundy SM, Hiratzka L, Jones D, Krumholz HM, Mosca L, Pearson T, Pfeffer MA, Taubert KA, AHA; ACC; National Heart, Lung, and Blood Institute. AHA/ACC guidelines for secondary prevention for patients with coronary and other atherosclerotic vascular disease: 2006 update endorsed by the National Heart, Lung, and Blood Institute. J Am Coll Cardiol. 2006;47(10):2130–9.
6. Cochrane collaboration: handbook for diagnostic test accuracy reviews. http://methods.cochrane.org/sdt/handbook-dta-reviews. Accessed 27 June 2018.
7. EUnetHTA guideline: meta-analysis of diagnostic test accuracy studies. Available at: http://www.eunethta.eu/sites/default/files/sites/5026.fedimbo.belgium.be/files/Meta-analysis%20of%20Diagnostic%20Test%20Accuracy%20Studies_Guideline_Final%20Nov%202014.pdf. Accessed 27 June 2018.
8. Bossuyt PM, Irwig L, Craig J, Glasziou P. Comparative accuracy: assessing new tests against existing diagnostic pathways. BMJ. 2006;332:1089–92.
9. Nudi F, Iskandrian AE, Schillaci O, Peruzzi M, Frati G, Biondi-Zoccai G. Diagnostic accuracy of myocardial perfusion imaging with CZT technology: systemic review and meta-analysis of comparison with invasive coronary angiography. JACC Cardiovasc Imaging. 2017;10:787–94.
10. Pucci S, Bonanno E, Sesti F, Mazzarelli P, Mauriello A, Ricci F, Zoccai GB, Rulli F, Galatà G, Spagnoli LG. Clusterin in stool: a new biomarker for colon cancer screening? Am J Gastroenterol. 2009;104:2807–15.
11. D'Ascenzo F, Barbero U, Cerrato E, Lipinski MJ, Omedè P, Montefusco A, Taha S, Naganuma T, Reith S, Voros S, Latib A, Gonzalo N, Quadri G, Colombo A, Biondi-Zoccai G, Escaned J, Moretti C, Gaita F. Accuracy of intravascular ultrasound and optical coherence tomography in identifying functionally significant coronary stenosis according to vessel diameter: a meta-analysis of 2,581 patients and 2,807 lesions. Am Heart J. 2015;169:663–73.
12. Deeks JJ, Macaskill P, Irwig L. The performance of tests of publication bias and other sample size effects in systematic reviews of diagnostic test accuracy was assessed. J Clin Epidemiol. 2005;58:882–93.
13. Dinnes J, Deeks J, Kirby J, Roderick P. A methodological review of how heterogeneity has been examined in systematic reviews of diagnostic test accuracy. Health Technol Assess. 2005;9:1–113.
14. Irwig L, Tosteson AN, Gatsonis C, Lau J, Colditz G, Chalmers TC, Mosteller F. Guidelines for meta-analyses evaluating diagnostic tests. Ann Intern Med. 1994;120:667–76.
15. Garrone P, Biondi-Zoccai G, Salvetti I, Sina N, Sheiban I, Stella PR, Agostoni P. Quantitative coronary angiography in the current era: principles and applications. J Interv Cardiol. 2009;22:527–36.
16. Novara M, D'Ascenzo F, Gonella A, Bollati M, Biondi-Zoccai G, Moretti C, Omedè P, Sciuto F, Sheiban I, Gaita F. Changing of SYNTAX score performing fractional flow reserve in multivessel coronary artery disease. J Cardiovasc Med (Hagerstown). 2012;13:368–75.

17. Biondi-Zoccai G, editor. Network meta-analysis: evidence synthesis with mixed treatment comparison. Hauppauge, NY: Nova Science Publishers; 2014.
18. Biondi-Zoccai G. Umbrella reviews. Evidence synthesis with overviews of reviews and meta-epidemiologic studies. Springer International: Cham, Switzerland; 2016.
19. Nudi F, Lotrionte M, Biasucci LM, Peruzzi M, Marullo AG, Frati G, Valenti V, Giordano A, Biondi-Zoccai G. Comparative safety and effectiveness of coronary computed tomography: systematic review and meta-analysis including 11 randomized controlled trials and 19,957 patients. Int J Cardiol. 2016;222:352–8.
20. Siontis KC, Siontis GC, Contopoulos-Ioannidis DG, Ioannidis JP. Diagnostic tests often fail to lead to changes in patient outcomes. J Clin Epidemiol. 2014;67:612–21.

The Evidence Hierarchy

2

Mical Paul

Systematic reviews typically provide quantitative estimates of the pooled evidence. A crucial part of the systematic review is to appraise and report the quality of the evidence for the pooled estimates. This ranking then goes on to guideline panels and recommendation statements to support the strength of recommendations for or against an intervention or a test.

The classical evidence-based medicine hierarchy ranked evidence from systematic reviews of randomized controlled trials (RCTs) and randomized controlled trials at the top to cohort studies, followed by lower degrees of evidence and ending with expert opinion (Fig. 2.1) [1]. The underlying understanding was that unbiased comparisons can be achieved only through adequate, unbiased randomization. While this remains true, GRADE has taken a step further in appraising the evidence [2–5]. GRADE starts with the study design and the classical risk of bias assessment that appraises if and what internal biases exist in the studies and asks further:

1. Whether the evidence derived from different sources is consistent or not
2. Whether the evidence addresses directly the clinical question that was posed
3. The importance of the outcome assessed from the patient's perspective
4. How precise and how large the effect estimate is, considering the totality of the evidence
5. The existence of publication bias
6. Once again the risk of bias is addressed, specifically addressing plausible confounding
7. Whether a dose-response gradient exists that strengths our belief in the plausibility of an effect

M. Paul
Rambam Heath Care Campus and The Ruth and Bruce Rappaport Faculty of Medicine, Technion—Israel Institute of Technology, Haifa, Israel
e-mail: paulm@technion.ac.il

G. Biondi-Zoccai (ed.), *Diagnostic Meta-Analysis*,
https://doi.org/10.1007/978-3-319-78966-8_2

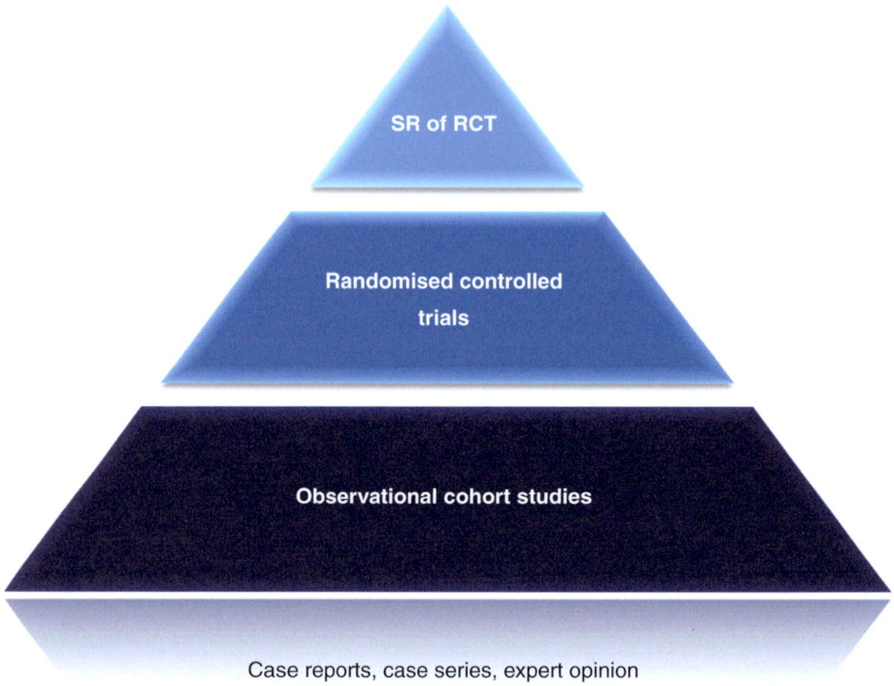

Fig. 2.1 The classical evidence hierarchy for intervention studies

Thus, GRADE expands risk of bias assessment of individual studies to an appraisal of the quality of the evidence for specific interventions, considering the totality of evidence, its relevance to the clinical scenario, its importance to patients, and its plausibility. Evidence is summarized in four grades from high to very low. GRADE has been largely accepted into evidence-based recommendations.

GRADE can be directly applied to diagnostic tests or strategies that were tested in RCTs. Such trials randomize patients to receive a new diagnostic test or strategy vs. the standard or older diagnostics and examine the impact of the test choice on patient-relevant outcomes. These constitute the real and only high-level evidence for diagnostic tests. A systematic survey of RCTs examining diagnostic tests published in MEDLINE up to December 2013 described a random sample of 103 such RCTs (out of an assumed total of 781 RCTs) [6]. Trials were rare prior to 2000, and since then their number seems to increase. Most trials (70%) assessed diagnostic imaging, and the leading fields were cardiology and general surgery. The review included only trials that examined at least one patient-important outcome. Of these, 41 (39.8%) reported on mortality, 63 (61.2%) on morbidities, and 14 (13.6%) on symptoms, quality of life, or functional status. A significant difference in patient outcomes was reported only in 12 (11.6%) RCTs. Similarly, diagnostic tests can be assessed in observational studies examining the association between diagnostic testing and patient outcomes. These can be evaluated by GRADE, receiving a priori lower quality of evidence due to unavoidable selection bias.

However, the large majority of the evidence on diagnostic tests relies on diagnostic studies examining test accuracy alone (sensitivity and specific, positive, and negative predictive values). A GRADing scheme has been devised to place such studies in the evidence hierarchy [7, 8]. The principle of this scheme is to proceed from the evaluation of the quality of diagnostic test accuracy studies to inferences regarding the effect of the test of patient-important outcomes, lacking clinical studies that have tested this. This is a multistage process. First, risk of bias of the diagnostic test accuracy study or studies in a systematic review is appraised using available tools such as the QUADAS-2 score (described in Chaps. 9 and 11) [9]. Then, assumptions have to be made regarding the effects that the diagnostic accuracy will have on patient outcomes. These outcomes should be defined. The effect on patient outcomes depends on the availability of treatment for the diagnosis and patients' prognosis with and without treatment. The consequnces of false positives and false negatives to the patient have to be considered; these include superfluous or missed treatment, further testing, and psychological consequences [10].

The same criteria used for GRADing interventions can be applied with slightly different definitions for diagnostic studies (Table 2.1) [7]:

Table 2.1 Quality of the evidence grading in systematic reviews of diagnostic test accuracy studies

N	Factors	GRADE classification[a]
1	Study design	Studies assessing consecutive representative patients and using an appropriate reference standard should be ranked as no serious bias
2	Risk of bias	Use the QUADAS-2 tool to perform quality assessment of the diagnostic studies included in the systematic review. Summarize the QUADAS-s score of studies included in the specific comparison to rank the overall risk of bias
3	Inconsistency	Inconsistency in sensitivity, specificity, or likelihood ratios. Very frequent in diagnostic systematic reviews
4	Indirectness	Deduct from results the presumed influences on patient-important outcomes, considering the implications of true and false positives and negatives and the potential complications of the test. Accuracy studies typically qualify as serious or very serious indirectness
5	Imprecision	Wide confidence intervals for estimates of test accuracy or true and false positive and negative rates results in serious to very serious risk. Consider the 95% confidence intervals of the hierarchical summary curve. Large confidence intervals typical in diagnostic systematic reviews
6	Other considerations	Consider the risk of publication bias
*	Importance	Consider the overall importance of the index test assessment, considering its applicability and potential implications to patient management given the assumed outcomes

[a]GRADE classifies each factor as not serious, serious, and very serious risk of bias. From factors 1–6, a single GRADE score is generated of high, moderate, low, or very low quality of the evidence. In addition, importance of the question on 1 (not important) to 9 (critical) scale. Guidance on classification is available at https://gradepro.org/

1. Study design: When comparing outcomes for patients undergoing different diagnostic tests (interventional diagnostic studies), RCTs will be graded highest followed by cohort studies. Diagnostic test accuracy studies are scored as no serious risk of bias if assessing an index test on consecutive and representative patients (i.e., those patients for whom the diagnostic test is relevant) and selecting a valid reference standard.
2. Risk of bias: The QUADAS-2 scoring system assesses four domains referring to the patient selection, index test, reference standard, and study flow [9]. A higher score is given to studies assessing the test among consecutive patients for which the test is intended (rather than case-control studies), when the index test and reference standard are evaluated independently of each other, when the reference standard adequately separates patients with and without the condition and does not define the condition, and when all patients undergo the index test and reference standard. RCTs and cohort studies are assessed using different domains. The most transparent strategy is that of The Cochrane Collaboration using the individual domain approach and available through the open access Cochrane Library.
3. Whether the evidence derived from different sources is consistent or not: Heterogeneity is very frequent in diagnostic meta-analyses, relating to different populations, tests, and reference standards. Even when assessing the same index tests and reference standard, local differences in test performance and interpretation may cause heterogeneity. Heterogeneity that can be explained by varying thresholds for test positivity is acceptable. Unfortunately, all too frequent threshold effects do not explain all heterogeneity, and the quality of the evidence must be downgraded for inconsistency.
4. Whether the evidence addresses directly the clinical question that was posed: Evidence that relies only on test accuracy studies is scored low on directness since the effects on patient-relevant outcomes were not measured but have to be inferred. Similarly, the directness of the patient population studied and testing is evaluated; was the relevant patient population included in the studies? Were the index test and reference standard applied in the studies as they would be applied in clinical practice? If competing index tests are evaluated, were they directly compared to each other?
5. How precise and how large the effect estimate is, considering the totality of the evidence: Similar to intervention effects, the confidence intervals surrounding test accuracy estimates determine the quality of evidence related to precision.
6. The existence of publication bias.

These six criteria are summarized to generate a GRADE score from high to very low quality of evidence. In addition to the quality of the evidence, the importance of the specific question addressed is ranked on a nine-point scale from critical to not important (Table 2.1) considering its impact from the patient's perspective. In clinical studies evaluating diagnostic strategy effects, the importance of the outcomes assessed in the studies can be appraised. In test accuracy studies, the overall importance of the index test assessment should be assessed, considering the need for the test, its applicability, and potential implications to patient management.

Clearly, the large majority of the evidence on diagnostic tests is ranked as low-quality evidence. When only studies evaluating sensitivity and specificity are available, evidence will be typically downgraded for heterogeneity, indirectness, and imprecision. The importance of ranking test accuracy studies as low-quality evidence in systematic reviews was demonstrated in a review of RCTs assessing the impact of different diagnostic tests on important patient outcomes, where only a small minority (12/103, 11%) of trials showed a significant difference in one or more of the outcomes [6]. Thus, excellent test performance should not be automatically assumed to change patients' outcomes.

GRADE has simplified the reporting of bias in systematic reviews, classifying the evidence on interventions or diagnostic tests into four simple categories: high, moderate, low, and very low quality of evidence. An open-access software (https://gradepro.org/) allows to perform evidence GRADing and provides guidance and easy creation of evidence tables. Many regulatory bodies, including the World Health Organization, have endorsed this strategy to summarize evidence for guidelines [11, 12]. GRADE simplifies reading through systematic reviews and guidelines. However, its disadvantage is common to risk of bias scores, where the final grade summarizes different domains that are not transparent. Thus, "low" quality evidence might derive from RCTs with risk of bias concerns (e.g., open trials), while "high" quality evidence can be derived from cohort studies that were considered to be well-conducted showing a large association and a dose-response gradient. The GRADE system has not undergone strict validation and the inter-reviewer agreement in scoring was not strong [12, 13]. Thus, systematic reviewers are encouraged to provide explicitly data on the study designs that have contributed to the final GRADE, their internal risk of bias, and the criteria that led to downgrading or upgrading the level of evidence. Readers are encouraged to look into the risk of bias assessment in systematic reviews further than the final GRADE, to better understand the quality of the evidence.

Evidence-based medicine places the patient at the center. At the top of the evidence hierarchy is research that is devoid of internal bias and assesses outcomes relevant to patients. The current understanding with regard to the evidence hierarchy is plotted in Fig. 2.2. Diagnostic test accuracy studies are rarely ranked as high-quality evidence, since the impact of patients' outcomes can only be assumed. Systematic reviews of diagnostic test accuracy most commonly will not result in higher quality evidence than the original studies because heterogeneity will preclude firm conclusions. Diagnostic systematic review has yet to find its place in the evidence hierarchy for diagnostic tests.

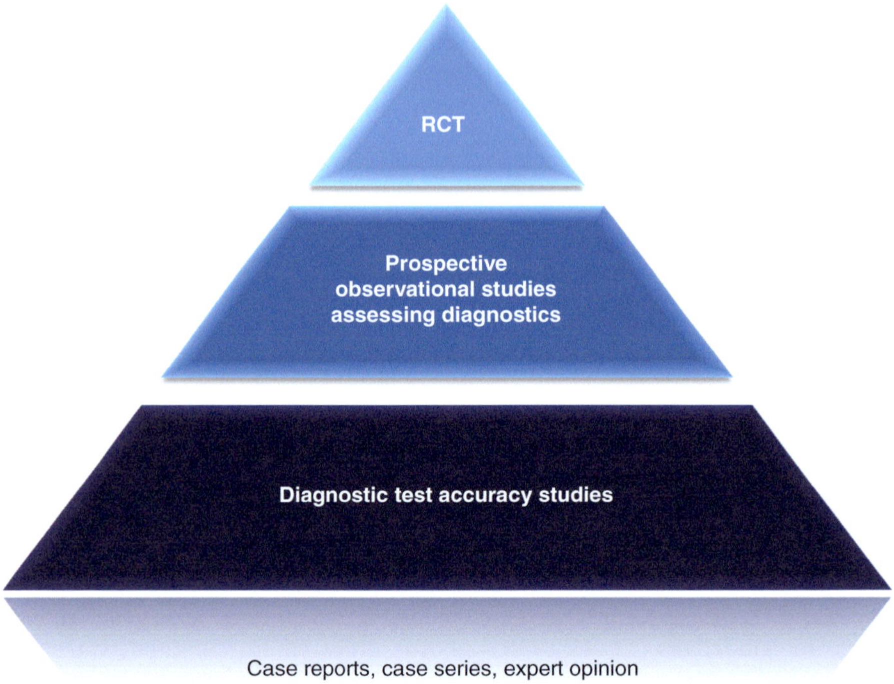

Fig. 2.2 The current evidence hierarchy for diagnostic studies, where at the top of the pyramid are randomized controlled trials assessing diagnostic tests/strategies

Conflicts of Interests None.
FundingNone.

References

1. Sackett DL, Rosenberg WM, Gray JA, Haynes RB, Richardson WS. Evidence based medicine: what it is and what it isn't. BMJ. 1996;312:71–2.
2. Alonso-Coello P, Schunemann HJ, Moberg J, Brignardello-Petersen R, Akl EA, Davoli M, et al. GRADE evidence to decision (EtD) frameworks: a systematic and transparent approach to making well informed healthcare choices. 1: introduction. BMJ. 2016;353:i2016.
3. Guyatt G, Oxman AD, Akl EA, Kunz R, Vist G, Brozek J, et al. GRADE guidelines: 1. Introduction-GRADE evidence profiles and summary of findings tables. J Clin Epidemiol. 2011;64:383–94.
4. Guyatt GH, Oxman AD, Vist GE, Kunz R, Falck-Ytter Y, Alonso-Coello P, et al. GRADE: an emerging consensus on rating quality of evidence and strength of recommendations. BMJ. 2008;336:924–6.
5. Jaeschke R, Guyatt GH, Dellinger P, Schunemann H, Levy MM, Kunz R, et al. Use of GRADE grid to reach decisions on clinical practice guidelines when consensus is elusive. BMJ. 2008;337:a744.

6. El Dib R, Tikkinen KA, Akl EA, Gomaa HA, Mustafa RA, Agarwal A, et al. Systematic survey of randomized trials evaluating the impact of alternative diagnostic strategies on patient-important outcomes. J Clin Epidemiol. 2017;84:61–9.
7. Schunemann HJ, Oxman AD, Brozek J, Glasziou P, Jaeschke R, Vist GE, et al. Grading quality of evidence and strength of recommendations for diagnostic tests and strategies. BMJ. 2008;336:1106–10.
8. Gopalakrishna G, Mustafa RA, Davenport C, Scholten RJ, Hyde C, Brozek J, et al. Applying grading of recommendations assessment, development and evaluation (GRADE) to diagnostic tests was challenging but doable. J Clin Epidemiol. 2014;67:760–8.
9. Whiting PF, Rutjes AW, Westwood ME, Mallett S, Deeks JJ, Reitsma JB, et al. QUADAS-2: a revised tool for the quality assessment of diagnostic accuracy studies. Ann Intern Med. 2011;155:529–36.
10. Schunemann HJ, Oxman AD, Brozek J, Glasziou P, Bossuyt P, Chang S, et al. GRADE: assessing the quality of evidence for diagnostic recommendations. Evid Based Med. 2008;13:162–3.
11. World Health Organization. WHO handbook for guideline development 2012. https://www.google.co.il/url?sa=t&rct=j&q=&esrc=s&source=web&cd=1&cad=rja&uact=8&ved=0ahUKEwjwiJLbrvHSAhUhI8AKHQIED2QQFggdMAA&url=http%3A%2F%2Fapps.who.int%2Firis%2Fbitstream%2F10665%2F75146%2F1%2F9789241548441_eng.pdf&usg=AFQjCNEpqjBi3ZIJ6REoEVwIn8jB5JJQqw&sig2=TJTmD1NM-o8WjD1ewlwArA. Accessed 28 June 2018.
12. Kavanagh BP. The GRADE system for rating clinical guidelines. PLoS Med. 2009;6:e1000094.
13. Berkman ND, Lohr KN, Morgan LC, Richmond E, Kuo TM, Morton S, et al. Reliability testing of the AHRQ EPC approach to grading the strength of evidence in comparative effectiveness reviews. Methods research report. (Prepared by RTI International–University of North Carolina Evidence-based Practice Center under contract No. 290-2007-10056-I.) AHRQ Publication No. 12-EHC067-EF. Rockville, MD: Agency for Healthcare Research and Quality. 2012.

Peculiarities of Diagnostic Test Accuracy Studies

3

Giuseppe Biondi-Zoccai, Simona Mastrangeli, Mariangela Peruzzi, and Giacomo Frati

The best physician is also a philosopher

Galen

3.1 Introduction

Given the unique goals and features of the diagnostic process, studies focusing on diagnostic tests are characterized by a set of specific methodological issues and sources of bias, as well as distinctive dimensions of accuracy [1, 2]. Of course, on top of such specificities, diagnostic test accuracy studies also share common methodological features and suitability for analysis with other types of clinical research endeavors [3]. This chapter highlights first the key methodological features of diagnostic test accuracy studies and then provides a synthetic overview of the main dimensions of diagnostic accuracy. Suitable examples are provided with the pertinent computing codes. Awareness of the premises and technicalities involved in the design, conduct, analysis, and reporting of a diagnostic test accuracy study remains a pivotal preliminary step before embarking in the qualitative and quantitative synthesis of a collection of several of such studies [4, 5].

G. Biondi-Zoccai (✉) · G. Frati
Department of Medico-Surgical Sciences and Biotechnologies,
Sapienza University of Rome, Latina, Italy

Department of AngioCardioNeurology, IRCCS Neuromed, Pozzilli, Italy
e-mail: giuseppe.biondizoccai@uniroma1.it

S. Mastrangeli
Superior School of Advanced Studies, Sapienza University of Rome, Rome, Italy

M. Peruzzi
Department of Medico-Surgical Sciences and Biotechnologies,
Sapienza University of Rome, Latina, Italy

G. Biondi-Zoccai (ed.), *Diagnostic Meta-Analysis*,
https://doi.org/10.1007/978-3-319-78966-8_3

3.2 Methodological Issues and Sources of Bias

The most important sources of bias for any clinical study include selection bias, performance bias, detection bias, attrition bias, and reporting bias [3]. There is ample literature on their features and impact, but in most cases elaborate discussions on these sources of bias focus on their impact in controlled studies [4, 5]. These types of bias can be better analyzed and expanded in a more analytical fashion for diagnostic test accuracy studies, focusing on the key features of this type of research endeavor, and on the different phases and steps in which such sources of bias can impact untowardly on the study and its impact for decision-making (Table 3.1) [6–13].

Table 3.1 Key methodological features and sources of bias of diagnostic test accuracy studies

Feature	Explanation
Availability of clinical information	The index and reference test should be performed based on similar preceding tests and data
Blinding	Readers of index test should be unaware of results of the reference test, and vice versa, to reduce confounding
Clinical review	Readers interpreting the reference test are aware of clinical features
Definition of the target condition	The target condition should be defined in the same fashion for the purpose of both index and reference test
Diagnostic uncertainty	Diagnosis should be uncertain before performing the index and the reference test to ensure internal validity
Differential verification	Parts of the results of the index test are compared to another reference test
Disease prevalence	Disease prevalence directly impacts on predictive values
Disease progression	Time lag between index and reference test may bias the comparison between the two, with subclinical disease inappropriately labeled by early tests as non-disease
Disease severity	Disease severity may impact on diagnostic performance of the index or reference test
Inappropriate reference standard	The reference test may be biased itself or imprecise
Incorporation	Results of the index test are actually used to define disease status
Observer variation	Variability in test interpretation between readers or by the same reader in different times may undermine the test internal validity
Partial verification	Only a subset of patients receiving the index test eventually receive the reference test
Prior testing	Tests conducted before the index or the reference test may impact on patient selection and study results
Reference standard data completeness	The reference standard should be performed in all suitable patients, and not only a subset of them
Rule-in performance	Capacity to establish the presence of disease among tested patients
Rule-out performance	Capacity to establish the non-diseased status among tested patients
Sample selection	Patients selected for the study are not representative of the whole population of at risk subjects

Table 3.1 (continued)

Feature	Explanation
Test execution	Details on how the index test is performed and reviewed are incompletely described
Test review	Readers interpreting the index test are aware of the results of the reference test
Test technology	Features of the index test change over time as result of experience or developments
Threshold selection	Diagnostic threshold should be chosen before analysis in order to avoid overoptimistic and non-replicable effect estimates
Treatment paradox	Treatment is initiated following the results of the index test, but before the reference test is administered
Withdrawals	Cases dropping out from the study before receiving either the index or the reference test, or both

In extreme synthesis, the first general feature that must be appraised is whether the study design and scope is coherent with the ultimate goal of the index test, which can be categorized as screening, replacement, or add-on. Most importantly, patient selection and attrition are subject to precise scrutiny. Patients should be representative of the actual population which will be the subject of the test. The index test and the reference test should be interpreted as eventually used in clinical practice, but each should be read independently from each other, which is often not the case in clinical outcome and observational research. The choice of threshold is also important. In most cases the threshold to define an abnormal test result is not pre-specified, yielding potentially overoptimistic effect estimates. It remains utmost difficult to conduct a diagnostic test accuracy study devoid of any risk of bias. Thus in most cases common sense and judgment must be applied, and reasonable robustness can be assumed unless the threat of bias is evident. Eventually, only a pairwise or network meta-analysis of diagnostic test accuracy studies can pinpoint and establish the presence of major bias, for instance, small study bias or confounding.

3.3 Dimensions of Diagnostic Accuracy

The appraisal of diagnostic tests is typically based on one or more index tests being compared to a reference test [1, 2, 14, 15]. The most common scenario is an index test providing a continuous result, which is interpreted dichotomously applying a specific threshold, to define abnormal versus normal test results, indicating diseased versus non-diseased status. Other scenarios are possible, such as an index and a reference test both providing dichotomous or otherwise categorical (usually hierarchically) results. In other less common scenarios, both tests provide continuous results. A sample dataset is provided to familiarize the reader to the above three types of subdatasets (Tables 3.2 and 3.3). In keeping with definitions provided in the Introduction to diagnosis chapter, we may thus introduce the most important

Table 3.2 Sample dataset for a study comparing a diagnostic index test with continuous results with a reference test (both tests are considered abnormal if ≥50)

ID	Index test dichotomous	Index test continuous	Reference test dichotomous	Reference test continuous
1	1	89	1	88
2	1	84	1	89
3	1	71	1	70
4	1	67	1	66
5	1	61	1	60
6	1	59	1	61
7	1	59	1	58
8	1	55	1	51
9	1	53	1	53
10	1	51	1	51
11	0	47	1	52
12	0	34	1	52
13	0	29	1	53
14	0	19	1	51
15	1	52	0	44
16	1	64	0	29
17	1	53	0	44
18	1	51	0	49
19	0	34	0	24
20	0	32	0	31
21	0	31	0	33
22	0	30	0	41
23	0	28	0	25
24	0	26	0	26
25	0	25	0	24
26	0	23	0	31
27	0	22	0	21
28	0	17	0	17
29	0	16	0	14
30	0	9	0	11

Table 3.3 Summary contingency table for a study comparing a diagnostic index test with continuous results with a reference test (using a 50 cutoff to define an abnormal index test)

		Index test		
		Positive	Negative	Subtotal
Reference test	Abnormal	10 (34%)	4 (13%)	14 (47%)
	Normal	4 (13%)	12 (40%)	16 (53%)
	Subtotal	14 (47%)	16 (53%)	30 (100%)

Table 3.4 Dimension of diagnostic test accuracy

Feature	Explanation	Elaboration
Sensitivity	TP/(TP + FN)	Capacity of a test of labeling as abnormal a diseased patient
Specificity	TN/(TN + FP)	Capacity of a test of labeling as normal a non-diseased patient
Positive predictive value	TP/(TP + FP)	Prevalence-dependent capacity of an abnormal test of recognizing a diseased patient
Negative predictive value	TN/(TN + FN)	Prevalence-dependent capacity of a normal test of recognizing a non-diseased patient
Positive likelihood ratio	Sensitivity/(100 − specificity)	Prevalence-independent capacity of a test of increasing the probability of diseased status in a patient with abnormal test
Negative likelihood ratio	(100 − sensitivity)/specificity	Prevalence-independent capacity of a test of decreasing the probability of diseased status in a patient with normal test
Diagnostic odds ratio	(TP/FN)/(FP/TN)	Prevalence-independent ratio of the odds of an abnormal test among diseased against the odds of an abnormal test among diseased
Diagnostic accuracy	(TP + TN)/(TP + FP + FN + TN)	Summary of the correct diagnostic yield of the index test
Youden index	Sensitivity + specificity − 1	Estimate of the comprehensive diagnostic accuracy of a test

FN false negatives, *FP* false positives, *TN* true negative, *TP* true positives

Table 3.5 Analysis for a study comparing a diagnostic index test with dichotomous results with a reference test

Feature	Point estimate	95% confidence interval
Prevalence	47.0%	28.0–65.7%
Sensitivity	71.4%	41.9–91.6%
Specificity	75.0%	47.6–92.7%
Positive likelihood ratio	2.86	1.15–7.11
Negative likelihood ratio	0.38	0.16–0.91
Positive predictive value	71.4%	41.9–91.6%
Negative predictive value	75.0%	47.6–92.7%
Diagnostic odds ratio	7.50	1.55–36.40

dimensions of diagnostic accuracy (Table 3.4), with accompanying analytical results (Table 3.5).

Briefly, prevalence is the proportion of diseased patients in the whole study and may be considered as the pretest probability. Indeed, when results of a given diagnostic test accuracy study are applied to other patient groups, more or less informal estimates of pretest probability of disease are always assumed. Sensitivity and specificity define the accuracy of the index test in recognizing diseased patients and in correctly identifying non-diseased subjects, respectively. Of course, sensitivity and specificity vary inversely changing the diagnostic threshold, with their overall coverage being potentially maximized in keeping with the maximum value of the

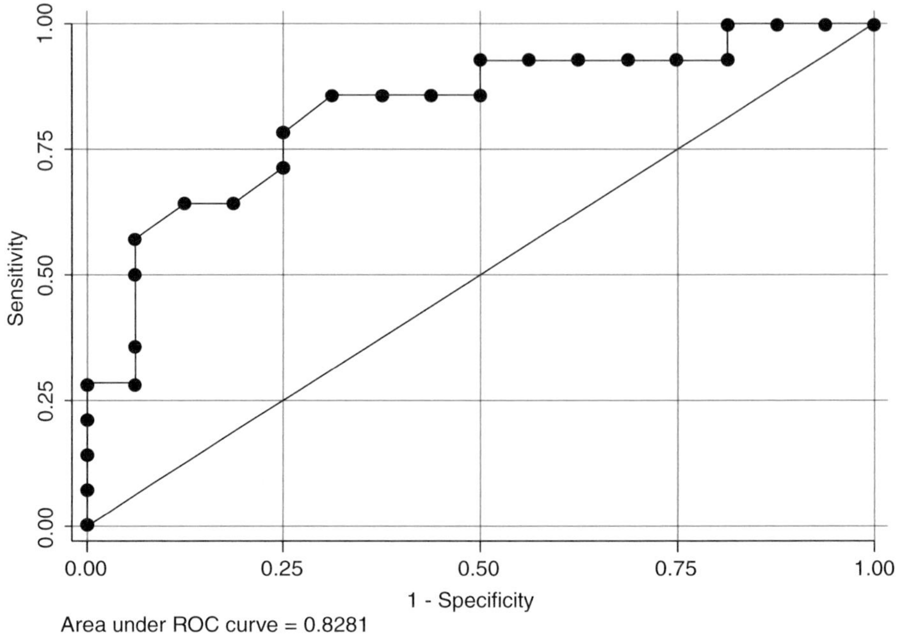

Fig. 3.1 Receiver operating characteristic (ROC) curve and corresponding area under the curve (AUC) for a diagnostic index test with continuous results compared with a reference test, using a nonparametric method

Youden index. In addition, sensitivity and specificity may be best appraised together with the area under the curve of the receiver operating curve, with coin tossing assuming a 50% prevalence having a 0.50 value and a perfect test with a 1 value (Fig. 3.1).

In the past it was commonplace to consider predictive values as useful measures of diagnostic accuracy. They represent the probability of a patient with an abnormal test to actually be diseased (positive predictive value) and that of a subject with a normal test to actually be non-diseased (negative predictive value). Despite their clinical soundness in a specific practice scenario, they are not prevalence-independent and thus cannot be used to compare different studies on the same index test or on alternative ones.

Likelihood ratios are instead prevalence-independent and can be immediately used given an estimate of pretest probability of disease to provide estimates of post-test probability of disease. The application to specific prevalence scenarios are clearly illustrated by means of the Fagan plot (Fig. 3.2) [16]. In particular, it has been argued that positive likelihood ratio > 10 is required to reliably rule in the disease, whereas a negative likelihood ratio <0.1 is required to reliably rule out the disease [17]. Less accurate tests may still be informative, especially with an intermediate pretest probability of disease (Fig. 3.2), but they may end up less useful when disease prevalence is low (Fig. 3.3) or high (Fig. 3.4). Finally, the diagnostic

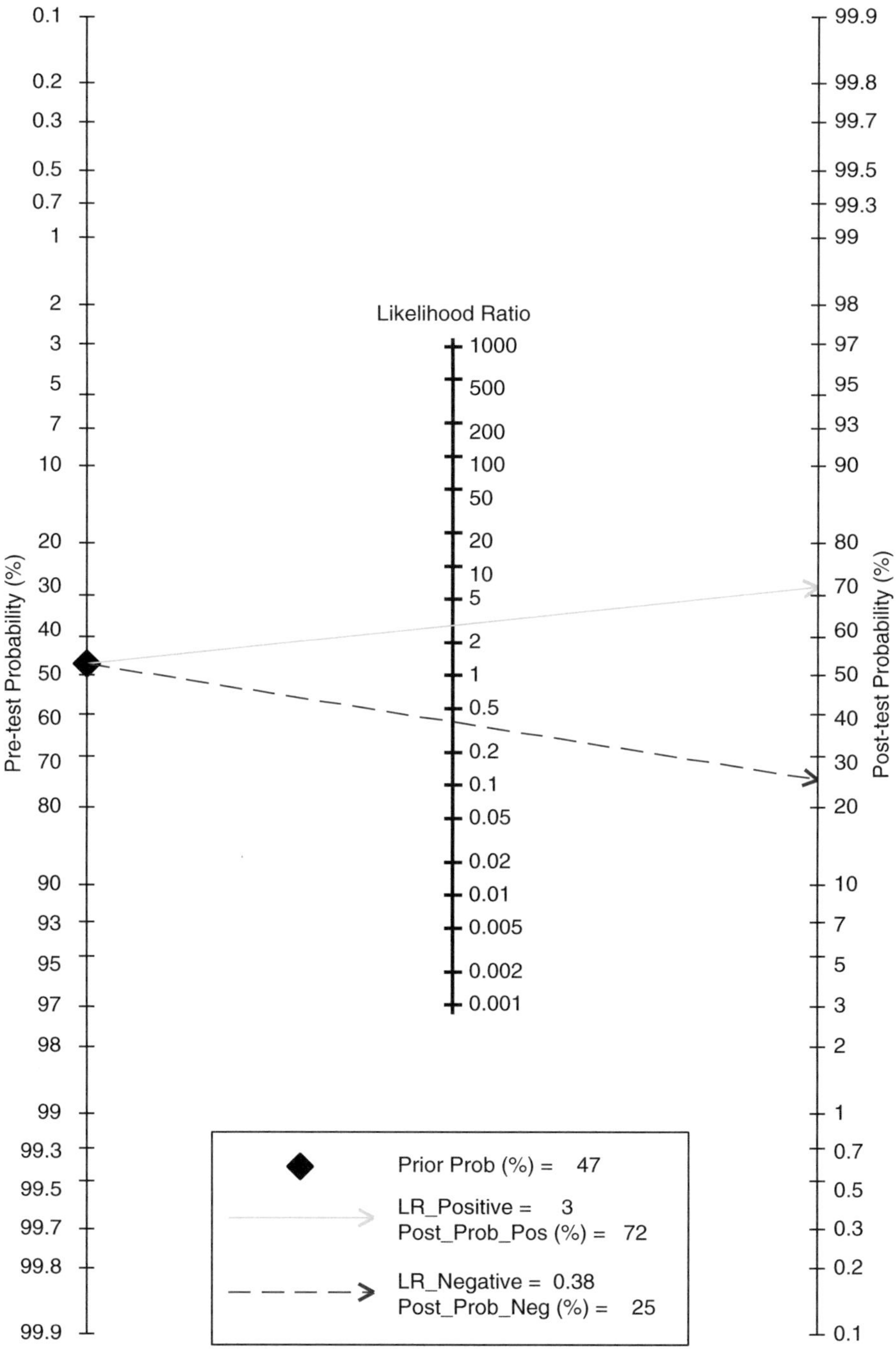

Fig. 3.2 Fagan plot highlighting the impact of prevalence and likelihood ratios on posttest probabilities of disease status, assuming a 47% prior probability of disease

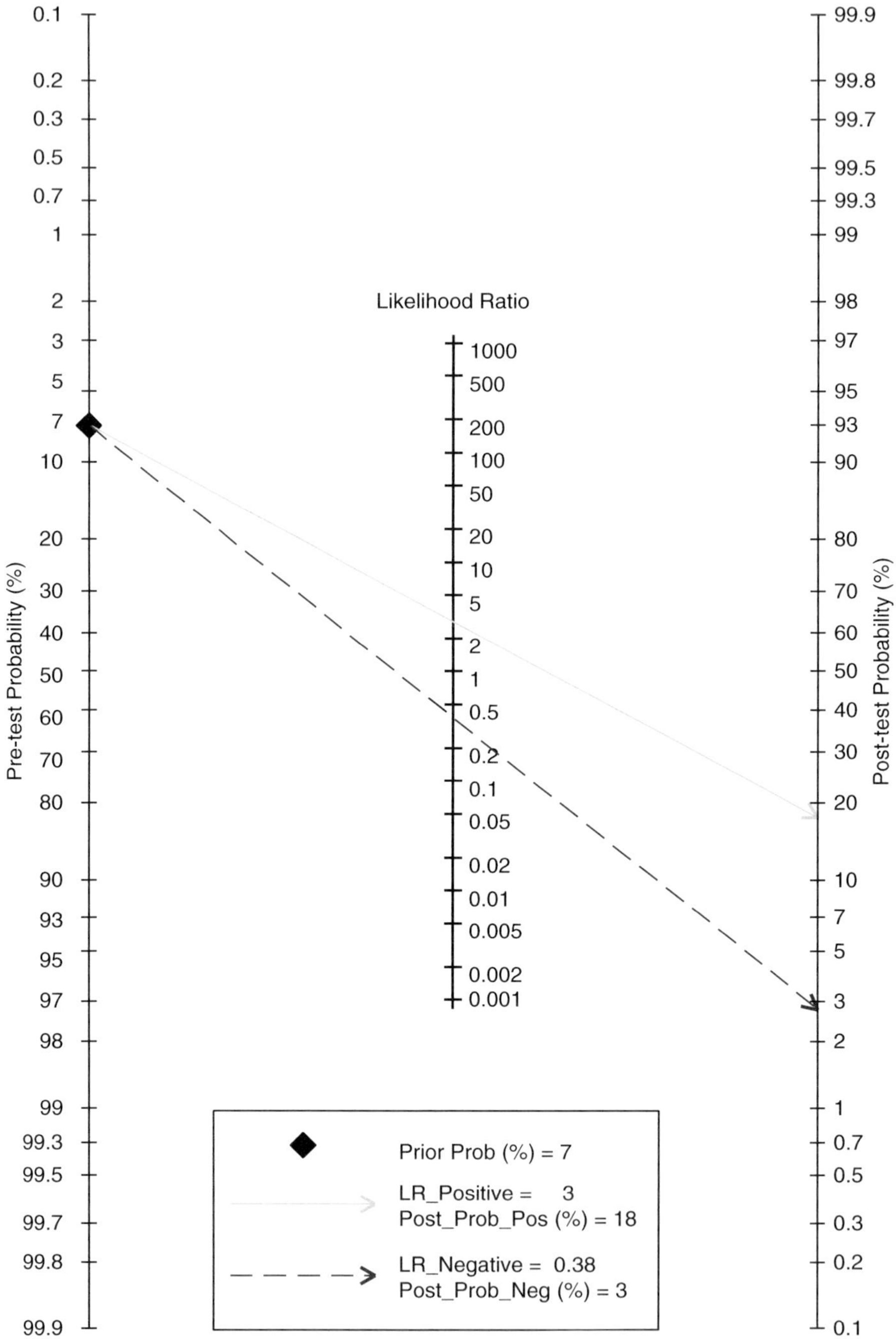

Fig. 3.3 Fagan plot highlighting the impact of prevalence and likelihood ratios on posttest probabilities of disease status, assuming a 7% prior probability of disease

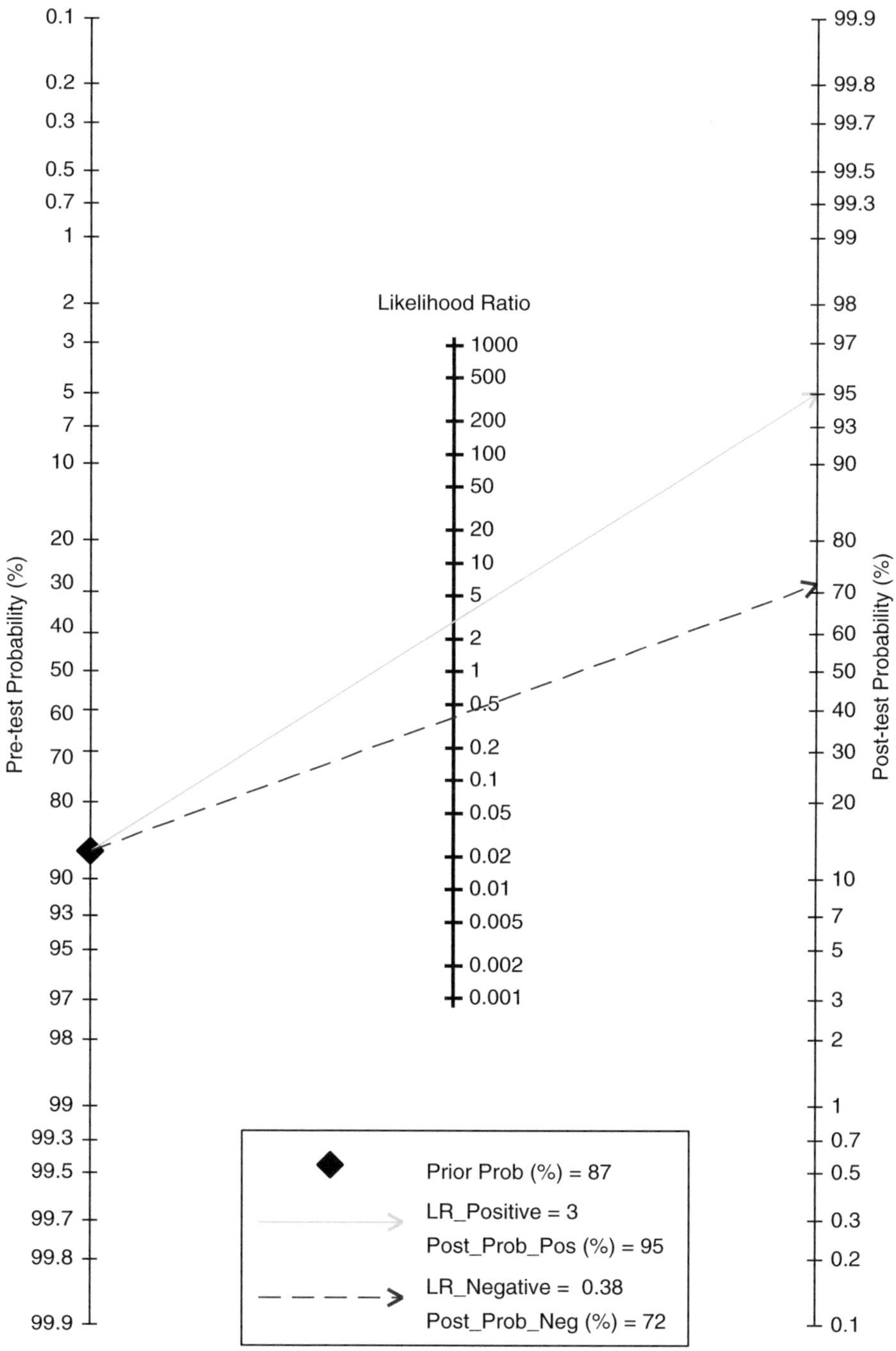

Fig. 3.4 Fagan plot highlighting the impact of prevalence and likelihood ratios on post-test probabilities of disease status, assuming a 87% prior probability of disease

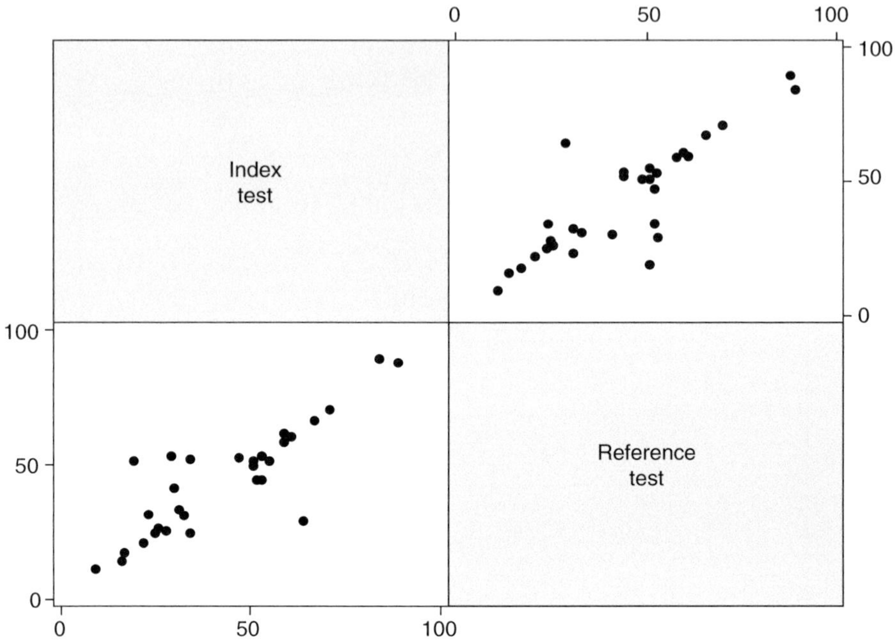

Fig. 3.5 Scatterplot for a diagnostic index test with continuous results compared with a reference test with continuous results (Pearson $r = 0.850$, Spearman rho = 0.799)

odds ratio remains a useful individual summary of diagnostic test accuracy, given its efficiency and prevalence-independency [18].

At odds with scenarios in which the reference test is categorical or dichotomous, other methods of analysis are required when both index and reference tests are continuous. Such cases resemble those in which the goal is to appraise the association between continuous variables, thus requiring correlation and regression methods (Fig. 3.5) [1–3]. More poignantly, the Bland-Altman method should be routinely employed in such cases to obtain effect estimates of average bias between the two tests at hand (Fig. 3.6) [19, 20].

Conclusion

Detailed knowledge of the methodological subtleties, key sources of bias, and dimensions of accuracy are crucial to thoroughly understand and optimally exploit diagnostic test accuracy studies for evidence synthesis. While the enterprise of seamlessly completing a diagnostic study which is free of bias and meticulously analyzed may appear overwhelming, robustness often overcomes limitations, supporting the inclusion of most diagnostic test accuracy studies in a systematic review and meta-analysis. Nonetheless, careful readers must remain aware that the ultimate and most rigorous proof of the internal and

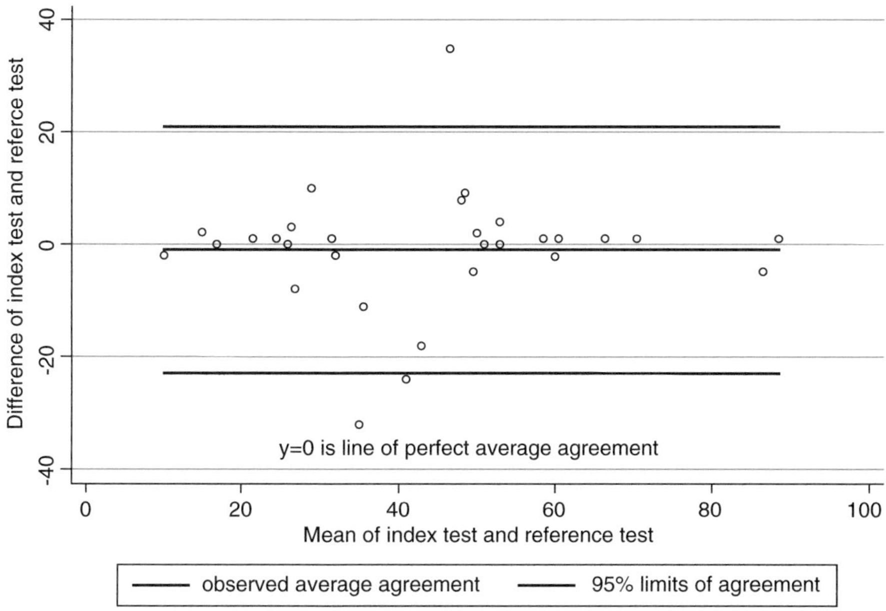

Fig. 3.6 Bland-Altman plot for a diagnostic index test with continuous results compared with a reference test with continuous results (mean bias = −0.933)

external validity of a diagnostic test remains a pragmatic randomized trial, as well as the eventual inclusion of a set of such studies in an ad hoc meta-analysis [4, 5, 21].

Funding/Disclosure None.

Appendix

Stata code to repeat all the analyses and graphs reported in this chapter:

```
diagt Referencetestdichotomous Indextestdichotomous
roctab Referencetestdichotomous Indextestcontinuous, table graph
summary
fagani 0.47 2.86 0.38, scheme(s2mono)
fagani 0.07 2.86 0.38, scheme(s2mono)
fagani 0.87 2.86 0.38, scheme(s2mono)
graph matrix Indextestcontinuous Referencetestcontinuous
ci2 Indextestcontinuous Referencetestcontinuous, corr
spearman Indextestcontinuous Referencetestcontinuous
concord Indextestcontinuous Referencetestcontinuous, summary loa
```

References

1. Cochrane collaboration: handbook for diagnostic test accuracy reviews. http://methods.cochrane.org/sdt/handbook-dta-reviews. Accessed 28 June 2018.
2. EUnetHTA guideline: meta-analysis of diagnostic test accuracy studies. http://www.eunethta.eu/sites/default/files/sites/5026.fedimbo.belgium.be/files/Meta-analysis%20of%20Diagnostic%20Test%20Accuracy%20Studies_Guideline_Final%20Nov%202014.pdf. Accessed 28 June 2018.
3. Guyatt G, Rennie D, Meade MO, Cook DJ. Users' guides to the medical literature: a manual for evidence-based clinical practice. New York, NY: McGraw-Hill Education; 2014.
4. Biondi-Zoccai G, editor. Network meta-analysis: evidence synthesis with mixed treatment comparison. Hauppauge, NY: Nova Science Publishers; 2014.
5. Biondi-Zoccai G. Umbrella reviews. Evidence synthesis with overviews of reviews and meta-epidemiologic studies. Springer International: Cham, Switzerland; 2016.
6. Bossuyt PM, Irwig L, Craig J, Glasziou P. Comparative accuracy: assessing new tests against existing diagnostic pathways. BMJ. 2006;332:1089–92.
7. Deeks JJ, Macaskill P, Irwig L. The performance of tests of publication bias and other sample size effects in systematic reviews of diagnostic test accuracy was assessed. J Clin Epidemiol. 2005;58:882–93.
8. Dinnes J, Deeks J, Kirby J, Roderick P. A methodological review of how heterogeneity has been examined in systematic reviews of diagnostic test accuracy. Health Technol Assess. 2005;9:1–113.
9. Irwig L, Tosteson AN, Gatsonis C, Lau J, Colditz G, Chalmers TC, Mosteller F. Guidelines for meta-analyses evaluating diagnostic tests. Ann Intern Med. 1994;120:667–76.
10. Siontis KC, Siontis GC, Contopoulos-Ioannidis DG, Ioannidis JP. Diagnostic tests often fail to lead to changes in patient outcomes. J Clin Epidemiol. 2014;67:612–21.
11. Whiting PF, Rutjes AW, Westwood ME, Mallett S, QUADAS-2 Steering Group. A systematic review classifies sources of bias and variation in diagnostic test accuracy studies. J Clin Epidemiol. 2013;66:1093–104.
12. Jarvik JG. The research framework. AJR Am J Roentgenol. 2001;176:873–8.
13. Krupinski EA, Jiang Y. Anniversary paper: evaluation of medical imaging systems. Med Phys. 2008;35:645–59.
14. Thornbury JR. Eugene W. Caldwell lecture. Clinical efficacy of diagnostic imaging: love it or leave it. AJR Am J Roentgenol. 1994;162:1–8.
15. Kim KW, Lee J, Choi SH, Huh J, Park SH. Systematic review and meta-analysis of studies evaluating diagnostic test accuracy: a practical review for clinical researchers-part I. General guidance and tips. Korean J Radiol. 2015;16:1175–87.
16. Lins S, Icks A, Meyer G. Understanding, comprehensibility and acceptance of an evidence-based consumer information brochure on fall prevention in old age: a focus group study. BMC Geriatr. 2011;11:26.
17. Spencer-Bonilla G, Singh Ospina N, Rodriguez-Gutierrez R, Brito JP, Iñiguez-Ariza N, Tamhane S, Erwin PJ, Murad MH, Montori VM. Systematic reviews of diagnostic tests in endocrinology: an audit of methods, reporting, and performance. Endocrine. 2017;57:18–34.
18. Pewsner D, Battaglia M, Minder C, Marx A, Bucher HC, Egger M. Ruling a diagnosis in or out with "SpPIn" and "SnNOut": a note of caution. BMJ. 2004;329:209–13.
19. Bland JM, Altman DG. Statistical methods for assessing agreement between two methods of clinical measurement. Lancet. 1986;1:307–10.
20. Novara M, D'Ascenzo F, Gonella A, Bollati M, Biondi-Zoccai G, Moretti C, Omedè P, Sciuto F, Sheiban I, Gaita F. Changing of SYNTAX score performing fractional flow reserve in multivessel coronary artery disease. J Cardiovasc Med (Hagerstown). 2012;13:368–75.
21. Nudi F, Lotrionte M, Biasucci LM, Peruzzi M, Marullo AG, Frati G, Valenti V, Giordano A, Biondi-Zoccai G. Comparative safety and effectiveness of coronary computed tomography: systematic review and meta-analysis including 11 randomized controlled trials and 19,957 patients. Int J Cardiol. 2016;222:352–8.

4 Meta-Analyses of Clinical Trials Versus Diagnostic Test Accuracy Studies

Michail Tsagris and Konstantinos C. Fragkos

4.1 Introduction

Meta-analysis has become an important part of modern research. Meta-analysis was traditionally applied in the context of synthesising results from studies that had a form of intervention (e.g. a clinical trial). However, it is moved to include other outcomes as well and other types of studies. In healthcare, meta-analysis is being readily applied to diagnostic accuracy study which is a type of study examining performance of test measures. Hence, in the present chapter, we initially discuss meta-analysis of clinical trials followed by meta-analysis of diagnostic accuracy studies and conclude with their comparison.

4.2 Meta-Analysis of Clinical Trials

Prior to discussing about meta-analysis, it would be convenient to give a short definition or description of clinical trials first. These are experiments applied in humans or animals in order to see the efficacy of a new intervention (e.g. drug). They usually involve two comparison groups, and the design is ideally a double-blind, randomised, placebo-controlled study. In their simplest form, the one group receives a treatment, and the other group receives placebo. None of the patients is aware of their type of treatment. The aim is to examine whether the treatment's effect is not statistically but also clinically or scientifically significant. The allocation to each group is usually random and ideally double blind. Many steps and protocols have to be adhered to; hence the amount of time and money required is usually large.

M. Tsagris (✉)
Department of Computer Science, University of Crete, Heraklion, Greece

K. C. Fragkos
University College London, London, UK

G. Biondi-Zoccai (ed.), *Diagnostic Meta-Analysis*,
https://doi.org/10.1007/978-3-319-78966-8_4

Meta-analysis of clinical trials can include many types and variations (e.g. network meta-analysis, meta-epidemiology, umbrella reviews, overviews of reviews, etc.) (see Tsagris and Fragkos [1] for more information). It is a statistical method, and the aim of a meta-analysis is to combine all different and previous studies in an efficient and valid way in order to make broader conclusions than by looking at each study separately.

4.2.1 Fixed and Random Effects Models

The main models of analysis in meta-analysis are through a fixed or random effects model [2–4]. Let us assume, without loss of generality, that the odds ratio (OR) is of interest and information has been gathered from many different clinical trials. If we assume that there is no variability between the different clinical trials, we can apply a fixed model and estimate the combined odds ratio as

$$\mathrm{OR}_c = \frac{\sum_{i=1}^{k} w_i \mathrm{OR}_i}{\sum_{i=1}^{k} w_i},$$

where $w_i = \frac{1}{Var\left(\widehat{OR}_i\right)} = \frac{1}{\sigma_i^2}$. If on the other hand we assume that there is heterogeneity between the different studies, the weights become $w_i = \frac{1}{\sigma_i^2 + \tau^2}$, where τ^2 denotes this heterogeneity. The latter leads to what is called random (or mixed in general) effects model. Numerical (iterative) methods are employed to estimate τ^2.

The random effects model in general is expressed as $y_i = \mu_i + \varepsilon_i$, where $\mu \sim N(\mu, \tau^2)$ and $\varepsilon_i \sim N\left(0, \sigma_i^2\right)$. If $\tau^2 = 0$ then $\mu_i = \mu$ and we end up with the fixed effects model. An advantage of meta-analyses is that the random effects model can capture the variation satisfactorily. The form of the covariance matrix necessary to capture the between variation in the mixed effects models is a really difficult and in some cases impossible (at the present) task to do.

The assumption of homogeneity ($\tau^2 = 0$) between the estimated odds ratios of many clinical studies can be assessed using the Cochran-Mantel-Haenszel test [5–7]. This tests whether the fixed model type of weights can be used. It does not give an estimate of τ^2 in the heterogeneous case.

The assumption of no heterogeneity can lead to false conclusions. On the other hand, an estimate close to 0, i.e. nonsignificant heterogeneity, is not that impactful. DerSimonian and Laird [3] were the first to suggest the mixed effects model for this purpose. More recently they published an update of that paper [4]. Prior to that, DerSimonian and Kacker [2] reviewed iterative and closed form formulae for estimating τ^2.

DerSimonian and Kacker [2] suggested the use of the Paule and Mandel [8] estimate of τ^2 as being more robust than the asymptotic method of DerSimonian and Laird [3]. The Paule and Mandel estimate does not assume normality, but when this assumption holds, the method is statistically optimal. This does not come by surprise, since under the normality assumption, their estimate is the restricted maximum likelihood (REML) estimate of τ^2 which is known to be unbiased.

4.2.2 Funnel Plot

An important part of meta-analysis is examining the presence of publication bias which is most frequently performed with a funnel plot [9, 10]. A funnel plot is a scatter plot of the effect estimates from individual studies against some measure of each study's effect or precision [11]. The inverse of the standard error of the estimates is usually chosen to be the effect. Other effects can be the variance or the inverse of the standard deviation or the variance [12]. Figure 4.1 presents a funnel plot created using the R package metaphor [13].

As for the shape of the funnel plot, that is a triangle,[1] where the middle is located at the combined estimate and the two bottom vertices of the triangle are the plus/minus 1.96 (or the 1-α/2 percentile of the standard normal distribution in general) standard errors. In the absence of bias and heterogeneity, the 95% of the estimates is expected to lie within the triangle region.

Another characteristic of the funnel plot is asymmetry. There can be many reasons for this to occur, and Sterne et al. [11] summarise a few. They suggest that the author of a systematic review or a meta-analysis (not only in clinical trials) should

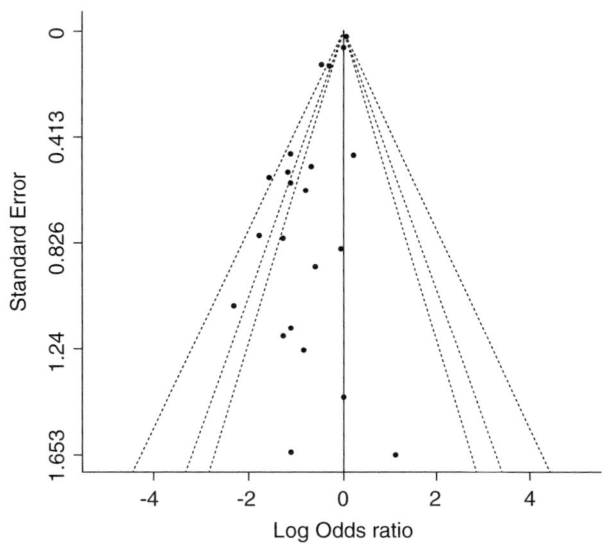

Fig. 4.1 Example funnel plot. The lines, moving from zero outwards correspond to 90%, 95%, and 99% confidence level

[1] This is true in the case of the vertical axis being the standard error. See Sterne and Egger [12] for more options and shapes.

know or at least investigate in detail the collected studies because this will help identify some of these reasons. In Fig. 4.1, we can clearly observe that most of the log odds ratio estimates are gathered on the left side of the plot, indicating asymmetry. The presence of asymmetry traditionally indicates the presence of publication bias.

Sterne et al. [11] correctly points out that statistical tests devised for testing the symmetry assumption of a funnel plot are not unbiased. One reason is the lack of knowledge of the mechanism that created these numbers. Sterne et al. [11] suggest some guidelines, but again, they are predominantly rules of thumb. Bootstrap methodology is something that could perhaps be examined more [14, 15]. Closing our brief mention to funnel plots, we must say that mixed models are also suggested in this case [11].

4.2.3 Sources of Heterogeneity in Meta-Analyses of Clinical Trials

When dealing with many clinical trials in order to estimate a pooled effect, the researcher must take into consideration the different sources of variations or heterogeneities often present in clinical trials. Statistical heterogeneity is the assumption that the effect is not different from study to study. This can be a strict assumption and violation of this can lead to serious flaws.

Clinical heterogeneity refers to different features of characteristics measured between among the studies. The effect or the variable of interest is the same, but the means to achieve can be different among the studies. Finally, an example of methodological heterogeneity is when the studies have not followed the same methods or the standard methods.

4.2.4 Network Meta-Analysis

Network meta-analysis is a rather new technique in the field. It is a meta-analysis in which multiple treatments (three or more) are being compared using both direct comparisons of interventions within randomised controlled trials and indirect comparisons across trials based on a common comparator [16]. Figure 4.2 shows an example of a network created using the R package netmeta [17].

A disadvantage of the classical meta-analysis is the fact that one can only compare pairs of treatments. Network meta-analysis can provide a global estimate of efficacy or safety of multiple experimental treatments that have not before been directly compared with adequate precision, or at all [18].

A key feature is its ability to combine direct and indirect evidence; for example, the comparison of treatments A and B is performed both using studies that directly compare A with B (direct evidence) and using studies that compare A with C and B with C (indirect evidence) [19]. Another important advantage of network meta-analysis is its visualisation.

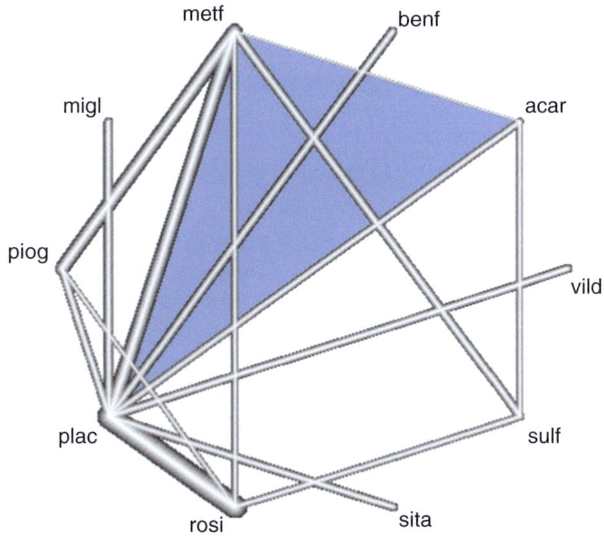

Fig. 4.2 Example graph of network meta-analysis. No directed arcs exist in this one

In White [19] there are no directed arrows, whereas in Elliott and Meyer [20] there are. In Elliott and Meyer [20] the directions indicate the class of drugs with higher risk of incident diabetes. However, caution must be taken as these graphs should not be confused with Bayesian networks [21] which are also directed graphs, but with additional assumptions and conditions. It is also worthy to mention the popularity of the mixed models, as Madden et al. [22] and White [19] suggest the usual random effects models for network meta-analysis.

We briefly described meta-analysis for clinical trials, and we next move on to meta-analysis of diagnostic accuracy studies.

4.3 Meta-Analysis of Diagnostic Test Accuracy Studies

Ever since the advent of meta-analysis in the post 1970 period [23], a new research area started to appear in which meta-analysis of the measures of test performance (sensitivity and specificity) was trialled [24]. Diagnostic test accuracy studies aim at measuring the ability of a new test, called index test, to detect the presence or absence of a specific disease or condition. The presence of this disease or condition is defined using a reference standard [25].

Although the methods for meta-analysis for clinical trials clarified after the random effects model suggested by DerSimonian and Laird [3], the meta-analysis of test performance measures made it slightly more difficult to approach, with specific issues that of the bivariate nature of these measures and their intercorrelation [25–27]. The following models are described for meta-analysis of diagnostic accuracy data [28]: simple pooling, separate random effects meta-analysis of sensitivity and specificity, separate meta-analysis of positive and negative likelihood ratios, Litteberg-Moses summary receiver operating characteristic (ROC) curve, and bivariate random effects meta-analysis/hierarchical summary ROC curve (HSROC) analysis. Harbord et al. [29] found that the bivariate random effects meta-analysis and HSROC models are closely related and even equivalent in the absence of covariates.

4.3.1 Types of Data and of Measures of Test Accuracy

Test results may be expressed as measurements (counts or continuous) or classifications (binary or ordered categories). Standard methods for computing test accuracy demand binary classification of the results of the index test and the reference standard, usually depending on a predefined cutoff level [27]. Test performance measures are either paired or single (global) indicators of test performance. The paired measures – sensitivity and specificity [the most commonly reported [28]], positive and negative predictive values, and positive and negative likelihood ratios – separately describe the performance of a test for ascertaining first the presence and then the absence of the target condition [25, 27, 30–33]. A ROC curve plot is used to show how as the test threshold decreases sensitivity increases while specificity decreases, and vice versa. The position of the ROC curve depends on the discriminatory ability of the test; the more accurate the test is, the closer the curve to the upper left hand corner of the ROC plot.

The most common global measures are the diagnostic OR (DOR) and the area under the curve (AUC). These measures summarise the accuracy of the test across all possible thresholds but are not helpful in clinical practice because they do not provide information on the error rates in the diseased (false negative) and non-diseased groups (false positives). In meta-analysis, the DOR can be a useful measure when comparing tests or subgroups, particularly if there is no preference for either superior sensitivity or specificity, and interest is in global performance [25].

4.3.2 Models

The following models are currently in use for meta-analysis of diagnostic accuracy data.

Simple pooling. This approach derives a single-summary two-by-two table by adding the numbers of true positives, false positives, true negatives, and false negatives across all studies [28, 29]. Test sensitivity and specificity can then be estimated as though all the data came from a single study. This is a form of fixed-effect meta-analysis of sensitivity and specificity, ignoring any correlation between them and assuming no between-study heterogeneity [34].

Separate random effects meta-analysis of sensitivity and specificity based on their logit transforms. This allows for between-study heterogeneity in sensitivity and specificity but again ignores their correlation. Logit (log odds) transforms of sensitivity and specificity are used, as the assumption of a normal distribution between studies is more reasonable on the logit scale. In addition to summary points and confidence intervals for these points, a summary ROC curve can be obtained from this method using the ratio of the estimated between-study variances [28, 29].

Separate meta-analysis of positive and negative likelihood ratios. Likelihood ratios are ratios of probabilities so positive and negative likelihood ratios can be meta-analysed separately using the same methods as risk ratios based on either fixed effect or random effects models. This ignores the correlation between positive and negative likelihood ratios [24, 34].

Littenberg-Moses summary ROC curve [35, 36]. This approach again uses the logit transforms of sensitivity and specificity and is based on simple linear regression of their sum (the log of the diagnostic odds ratio) on their difference. A summary ROC curve can be derived from the fitted regression line. This method allows for the correlation between sensitivity and specificity but is not statistically rigorous, as the assumptions of linear regression (constant variance, covariate measured without error) do not hold [29].

Bivariate random effects meta-analysis [37]. This approach can be considered an extension of separate random effects meta-analyses of logit-transformed sensitivity and specificity but allows for the negative correlation between sensitivity and specificity. In addition to summary estimates of average sensitivity and specificity across studies, it can be used to provide a confidence region for this summary point and a prediction region within which we may expect the true sensitivity and specificity of a future study to lie. Let $\mu_{A,i}$ be the logit-transformed sensitivity in study i and $\mu_{B,i}$ as the logit-transformed specificity. Then, the bivariate random effects model is

$$\begin{pmatrix} \mu_{A,i} \\ \mu_{B,i} \end{pmatrix} \sim N\left(\begin{pmatrix} \mu_A \\ \mu_B \end{pmatrix}, \Sigma \right) \quad \text{with} \quad \Sigma = \begin{pmatrix} \sigma_A^2 & \sigma_{AB} \\ \sigma_{AB} & \sigma_B^2 \end{pmatrix}$$

where Σ is the correlation/covariance matrix.

Hierarchical summary ROC curve analysis [38]. In this approach, the relationship between logit-transformed sensitivity and specificity in each study is expressed in terms of key test characteristics: accuracy (quantified by the log of the diagnostic odds ratio) and threshold. The method allows for between-study variation in each of these quantities, as well as for a parameter that determines the shape of the summary ROC curve. The results of this type of analysis are usually expressed as a summary ROC curve.

Overall the parameters computed from the two most used techniques are show in Table 4.1. Common sources of heterogeneity in meta-analysis of diagnostic accuracy are the different cutoff levels of the test under investigation and design conditions (sample sizes, sample characteristics, etc.).

Table 4.1 Parameters computed from HSROC and bivariate model

HSROC model	Bivariate model
Mean accuracy	Mean logit sensitivity
Mean threshold	Mean logit specificity
Variance of random effects for accuracy	Variance of random effects for logit sensitivity
Variance of random effects for threshold	Variance of random effects for logit specificity
Shape of SROC curve	Correlation between the logits of sensitivity and logits of specificity

Table 4.2 Characteristics of each type of meta-analysis

	Clinical trials	Diagnostic accuracy studies
Studies	Usually randomised control studies Can also be case control studies or case series	Studies need to investigate a test (index) against a reference test
Models	Random effects and fixed effects model	Simple pooling, separate random effects meta-analysis of sensitivity and specificity, separate meta-analysis of positive and negative likelihood ratios, Litteberg-Moses summary receiver operating characteristic (ROC) curve, bivariate random effects meta-analysis/hierarchical summary ROC curve (HSROC) analysis
Outcomes	Odds ratio, risk ratio, risk difference, mean difference, standardised mean difference, proportion, correlation coefficient	Sensitivity and specificity, positive and negative predictive values, positive and negative likelihood ratios, diagnostic odds ratio, AUC
Heterogeneity sources	Design, sample size	Cutoff levels, reference standard, design, sample size
Software	Software readily available (e.g. Stata, R, Comprehensive meta-analysis, RevMan, other written packages)	Meta-DiSc, Metandi (Stata), many currently developed but still not as many as for meta-analysis of clinical trials

Conclusion

The differences and similarities between the two types of meta-analysis are shown in Table 4.2. Researchers need to be aware of each type of meta-analysis and the particular characteristics each one entails. Sources of heterogeneity are always important to investigate since they could be significantly enough to obscure results and consequent interpretation.

References

1. Tsagris M, Fragkos KC. Umbrella reviews, overviews of reviews, and meta-epidemiologic studies: similarities and differences. In: Biondi-Zoccai G, editor. Umbrella reviews: evidence synthesis with overviews of reviews and meta-epidemiologic studies. Cham: Springer International Publishing; 2016. p. 43–54.
2. DerSimonian R, Kacker R. Random-effects model for meta-analysis of clinical trials: an update. Contemp Clin Trials. 2007;28:105–14.
3. DerSimonian R, Laird N. Meta-analysis in clinical trials. Control Clin Trials. 1986;7:177–88.
4. DerSimonian R, Laird N. Meta-analysis in clinical trials revisited. Contemp Clin Trials. 2015;45:139–45.
5. Cochran WG. Some methods for strengthening the common χ^2 tests. Biometrics. 1954;10:417–51.

6. Mantel N. Chi-Square tests with one degree of freedom; extensions of the mantel- Haenszel procedure. J Am Stat Assoc. 1963;58:690–700.
7. Mantel N, Haenszel W. Statistical aspects of the analysis of data from retrospective studies of disease. J Natl Cancer Inst. 1959;22:719–48.
8. Paule RC, Mandel J. Consensus values and weighting factors. J Res Natl Bur Stand. 1982;87:377–85.
9. Fragkos KC, Tsagris M, Frangos CC. Publication Bias in meta-analysis: confidence intervals for Rosenthal's fail-safe number. Int Sch Res Notices. 2014;2014:17.
10. Fragkos KC, Tsagris M, Frangos CC. Exploring the distribution for the estimator of Rosenthal's 'fail-safe' number of unpublished studies in meta-analysis. Commun Stat Theory Methods. 2017;46:5672–84.
11. Sterne JA, Sutton AJ, Ioannidis JP, Terrin N, Jones DR, Lau J, Carpenter J, Rucker G, Harbord RM, Schmid CH, Tetzlaff J, Deeks JJ, Peters J, Macaskill P, Schwarzer G, Duval S, Altman DG, Moher D, Higgins JP. Recommendations for examining and interpreting funnel plot asymmetry in meta-analyses of randomised controlled trials. BMJ. 2011;343:d4002.
12. Sterne JA, Egger M. Funnel plots for detecting bias in meta-analysis: guidelines on choice of axis. J Clin Epidemiol. 2001;54:1046–55.
13. Viechtbauer W. Conducting meta-analyses in R with the metafor package. J Stat Softw. 2010;36:1–48.
14. Frangos CC. An updated bibliography on the jackknife method. Commun Stat Theory Methods. 1987;16:1543–84.
15. Tsagris M, Elmatzoglou I, Frangos CC. The assessment of performance of correlation estimates in discrete bivariate distributions using bootstrap methodology. Commun Stat Theory Methods. 2012;41:138–52.
16. Li T, Puhan MA, Vedula SS, Singh S, Dickersin K, Ad Hoc Network Meta-analysis Methods Meeting Working G. Network meta-analysis-highly attractive but more methodological research is needed. BMC Med. 2011;9:79.
17. Rücker G. Network meta-analysis, electrical networks and graph theory. Res Synth Methods. 2012;3:312–24.
18. Greco T, Biondi-Zoccai G, Saleh O, Pasin L, Cabrini L, Zangrillo A, Landoni G. The attractiveness of network meta-analysis: a comprehensive systematic and narrative review. Heart Lung Vessel. 2015;7:133–42.
19. White IR. Network meta-analysis. Stata J. 2015;15:951–85.
20. Elliott WJ, Meyer PM. Incident diabetes in clinical trials of antihypertensive drugs: a network meta-analysis. Lancet. 2007;369:201–7.
21. Neapolitan RE. Learning Bayesian networks. Harlow: Prentice Hall; 2004.
22. Madden LV, Piepho HP, Paul PA. Statistical models and methods for network meta-analysis. Phytopathology. 2016;106:792–806.
23. Glass GV. Primary, secondary, and meta-analysis of research. Educ Res. 1976;5:3–8.
24. Irwig L, Macaskill P, Glasziou P, Fahey M. Meta-analytic methods for diagnostic test accuracy. J Clin Epidemiol. 1995;48:119–30.
25. Virgili G, Conti AA, Murro V, Gensini GF, Gusinu R. Systematic reviews of diagnostic test accuracy and the Cochrane collaboration. Intern Emerg Med. 2009;4:255–8.
26. Moreno GG, Pantoja CT. Systematic reviews of studies of diagnostic test accuracy. Rev Med Chil. 2009;137:303–7.
27. Takwoingi Y, Riley RD, Deeks JJ. Meta-analysis of diagnostic accuracy studies in mental health. Evid Based Ment Health. 2015;18:103–9.
28. Harbord RM, Whiting P, Sterne JA, Egger M, Deeks JJ, Shang A, Bachmann LM. An empirical comparison of methods for meta-analysis of diagnostic accuracy showed hierarchical models are necessary. J Clin Epidemiol. 2008;61:1095–103.
29. Harbord RM, Deeks JJ, Egger M, Whiting P, Sterne JA. A unification of models for meta-analysis of diagnostic accuracy studies. Biostatistics. 2007;8:239–51.
30. Begg CB. Meta-analysis methods for diagnostic accuracy. J Clin Epidemiol. 2008;61:1081–2.

31. Chen Y, Liu Y, Chu H, Ting Lee ML, Schmid CH. A simple and robust method for multivariate meta-analysis of diagnostic test accuracy. Stat Med. 2017;36:105–21.
32. Dukic V, Gatsonis C. Meta-analysis of diagnostic test accuracy assessment studies with varying number of thresholds. Biometrics. 2003;59:936–46.
33. Leeflang MM. Systematic reviews and meta-analyses of diagnostic test accuracy. Clin Microbiol Infect. 2014;20:105–13.
34. Deeks JJ. Systematic reviews of evaluations of diagnostic and screening tests. In: Egger M, Davey Smith G, Altman DG, editors. Systematic reviews in health care. London: BMJ Publishing Group; 2008. pp 248–282.
35. Littenberg B, Moses LE. Estimating diagnostic accuracy from multiple conflicting reports: a new meta-analytic method. Med Decis Mak. 1993;13:313–21.
36. Moses LE, Shapiro D, Littenberg B. Combining independent studies of a diagnostic test into a summary ROC curve: data-analytic approaches and some additional considerations. Stat Med. 1993;12:1293–316.
37. Reitsma JB, Glas AS, Rutjes AW, Scholten RJ, Bossuyt PM, Zwinderman AH. Bivariate analysis of sensitivity and specificity produces informative summary measures in diagnostic reviews. J Clin Epidemiol. 2005;58:982–90.
38. Rutter CM, Gatsonis CA. A hierarchical regression approach to meta-analysis of diagnostic test accuracy evaluations. Stat Med. 2001;20:2865–84.

Part II

Designing the Review

5

José Mauro Madi, Machline Paim Paganella,
Isnard Elman Litvin, and Eliana Marcia Wendland

5.1 Chapter Introduction

Evidence-based medicine (EBM) or practice is the integration of the best research evidence with clinical experience and client values [1]. Decision-making is the process of making a selective intellectual judgement when presented with several complex alternatives that consist of several variables, and it usually defines a course of action or an idea (PubMed MeSH—Medical Subject Headings). Clinical decision-making requires the synthesis of an often complex evidence base; in this context, systematic reviews (SRs) are at the heart of EBM [2]. These literature reviews are performed in a systematic and transparent way and are explicit about where their information comes from and how the included references were selected [3]. SRs also allow us to establish whether findings are consistent and can be generalized in various situations [4].

To perform a systematic review (SR), the authors or investigators typically follow steps as follows: define the research team; write and develop a protocol; frame an answerable research question; perform the search; evaluate the risk of bias; conduct a qualitative synthesis and, when applicable, conduct a meta-analysis; publish the SR; and update it as necessary.

J. M. Madi (✉) · I. E. Litvin
Faculdade de Medicina, Universidade de Caxias do Sul (UCS), Caxias do Sul, Brazil
e-mail: jmmadi@ucs.br; ielitvin@ucs.br

M. P. Paganella
Laboratório de Pesquisa em HIV/AIDS, Universidade de Caxias do Sul (UCS),
Caxias do Sul, Brazil
e-mail: mppagane@ucs.br

E. M. Wendland
Departamento de Saúde Coletiva, Universidade Federal de Ciências da Saúde de Porto Alegre
(UFCSPA), Porto Alegre, Brazil

G. Biondi-Zoccai (ed.), *Diagnostic Meta-Analysis*,
https://doi.org/10.1007/978-3-319-78966-8_5

Diagnostic tests are used to aid health professionals in the diagnosis or detection of a disease. Generally, diagnostic test studies are performed on small samples, especially when the disease is rare and they provide imprecise estimates. In these cases, meta-analysis can help investigate the consistency of test performance between various study designs and in different population profiles, or it can help define the best test to use when various diagnostic approaches exist for a specific disease. SRs of diagnostic test accuracy often aim to compare the accuracy of two different tests or to establish the accuracy of a single test [5].

An SR protocol is a key process in designing a review, and it is essential for anticipating potential problems and avoiding bias during the review process. Registration and publication of the protocol allow others to compare a protocol to the complete review, which can reduce duplicate publications.

Similar to SRs and meta-analyses of other study designs, the protocol of an accuracy test review describes the methods used in the review. Decisions about the review question, inclusion criteria, search strategy, study selection, data extraction, quality assessment, and data synthesis and plans for dissemination should be addressed, as specifying the methods in advance reduces the risk of introducing bias into the review [6]. Therefore, the success of an SR and meta-analysis depends on planning a standardized protocol that encompasses all phases of the review and guarantees its reproducibility; the protocol should be established and documented in advance.

The objective of this chapter is to present the main concepts needed to design and register a protocol for an SR of diagnostic test accuracy using simple language for healthcare professionals.

5.1.1 Body of the Protocol

The protocol for a diagnostic test accuracy review may include the suggested topics listed in the box below:

Title
- **Author's information**
- **Background**
- **Objectives**
- **Methodology**
  - Registration
  - PIRO (Population, Index test, Standard test, Outcome) Question
    - Description of the population
    - Description of the target condition
    - Description of the index test
    - Description of the standard test
    - Description of the outcomes

Search Methods Plan
Databases
Other resources
Eligibility Criteria
Type of studies
Participants
Target condition
Index test: technical aspects
Reference test: technical aspects
Data Collection Plan
Tables
Risk of Bias Assessment Plan
Quality Assessment Plan
Statistical Analysis Plan

Results
Results of the search
Findings

Discussion
Summary of the results
Limitations
Applications

Conclusion
Implication for practice
Implication for research

References

Adapted from (Source): Chapter 4: Guide to the contents of a Cochrane Diagnostic Test Accuracy Protocol. Cochrane Handbook for Systematic Reviews of Diagnostic Test Accuracy Version 1.0.0 [7].

The format may also include acknowledgments, a conflict of interest declaration, support sources, sponsorships, appendices and, of course, the references used so far. Additionally, the structure of the content may vary if the authors intend to publish the protocol in a scientific journal that includes protocols, such as *Systematic Reviews Journal* from BioMed Central. If the investigators intend to develop a Cochrane review, the protocol can be designed in a software package called RevMan® that is offered by the collaboration. The Cochrane collaboration is the largest organization that produces and publishes systematic reviews. It has a Cochrane Screening and Diagnostic Tests Methods Group (SDTM) that provides resources and information and establishes the standards for the Cochrane systematic reviews of diagnostic test accuracy (http://methods.cochrane.org/sdt/welcome).

5.1.2 Title

As in any primary study or SR, the title should be as clear as possible. The title of an SR in diagnostic test accuracy often includes the structure of "PIRO (population, index test, reference test and outcome) question" (further described). For instance: "Accuracy of (index test) compared with (reference test) in the diagnostic of (outcome or target condition) in (population): *a protocol for systematic review (and meta-analysis)*". For example: Accuracy of p57KIP2 compared with genotyping for the diagnosis of complete hydatidiform mole: protocol for a systematic review and meta-analysis [8].

5.2 Background of the Systematic Review

The background section of the protocol should provide a brief definition of the healthcare problem or target condition and its prevalence, along with a description of the diagnostic tests available (including the index and reference tests) and their rationale for use. It should communicate the main elements of the review question. The background also should explain why the SR is required, justifying what this review adds to the existing evidence.

This section can address how the index test may be incorporated in practice (replacing or being used in combination with an existing test) and if it benefits the population (as a less invasive or a less expensive technique) while explaining the choice of tests that are considered in the review [6].

5.3 Objectives

The review objectives should be clearly stated. The primary objective of a diagnostic test accuracy SR is focused, and it is related to the accuracy of the index test(s) for the target condition, as verified by the reference standard. The Cochrane Handbook for Systematic Reviews of Diagnostic Test Accuracy presents the following formula to frame an objective:

> "To determine the diagnostic accuracy of (index test) for detecting (target condition) in (participant description)".

The objective should also communicate the proposed role of the index test(s), if it is known. In a typical SR, a Cochrane review usually compares one test with another, rather than simply evaluating the accuracy of a single test. All comparisons between tests should be listed as objectives. The review can also include secondary objectives that are broader; however, these secondary objectives also need to be explicitly listed to try to answer the research question [7].

5.4 Methodology

5.4.1 Registration

The protocol should be established and documented in advance. Registering the protocol reduces the risk of multiple reviews addressing the same question by establishing that a group is already performing the review.

Additionally, besides reducing the potential for duplication, the publication of a protocol prior to knowledge of the available studies reduces the impact of review authors' biases, promotes the transparency of methods and processes, and enables a peer review of the planned methods [7].

For instance, some of the available platforms to register an SR are as follows:

- **Cochrane Collaboration**—An international organization that produces and disseminates systematic reviews of healthcare interventions (http://www.cochrane.org/)
- **PROSPERO**—An international prospective register of systematic reviews (https://www.crd.york.ac.uk/PROSPERO/)
- **Campbell Collaboration**—A collaboration that produces systematic reviews of the effects of social interventions (https://www.campbellcollaboration.org/)

5.4.2 PIRO Question

As in all types of research, framing the research question is perhaps the most important introductory step, as it leads to a hypothesis and guides the methods and processes of the review. The protocol should clearly state the research question; the research question is a key component of any SR, and it should be objective and answerable.

Systematic reviews of randomized clinical trials have the established acronym PICO (Population, Intervention, Control, and Outcome). This framework may vary according to the authors' needs. In terms of diagnostic test accuracy review, the **PIRO** framework is a tool for breaking the question into its components and restructuring them in a way that makes it easy to design the review question:

- **P** = Population/target condition
- **I** = Index test
- **R** = Reference test
- **O** = Outcome

5.4.2.1 Description of the Population

Diagnostic tests have different results based on the patient population. In this context, authors should describe the population characteristics (such as sex, age, etc.)

that may influence the test's performance and results. In other words, the population should be appropriate for the review objectives, and it should reflect who will undergo the diagnostic test in clinical practice [9].

In primary studies, a restricted study population may limit bias and increase the internal validity of the study; however, this approach will limit the external validity of the study and, thus, the generalizability of the findings to practical clinical settings. Conversely, a broadly defined study population and inclusion criteria may be representative of practical clinical practice, but it may increase bias and reduce the internal validity of the study [10]. In terms of an SR, a restricted study population directly affects the number of eligible studies, so its justification should be explained in the protocol.

5.4.2.2 Description of the Target Condition

The protocol must describe a target condition that corresponds to a health outcome that the tests (index and standard) can detect. The tests diagnose the current stage or condition, so the protocol must consider and describe the clinical context, including a diagnostic dilemma that considers many possible categories, such as severity.

5.4.2.3 Description of the Index Test

Diagnostic test accuracy refers to the ability of a test to distinguish between patients with disease (or more generally, a specified target condition) and those without the disease. In such a test accuracy study, the results of the test under evaluation, or the "index test", are compared with those of the reference standard, as determined in the same patients [11].

It is important to clearly state the purpose of the tests (index or reference) that are being compared, such as whether they are used to measure the response of an intervention or are used for screening, diagnosis, monitoring, disease staging, predisposition, or surveillance [12]. Usually, diagnosis test accuracy reviews evaluate the accuracy of tests used for diagnosis or staging. The index test is the test under study; its performance is being evaluated. The index test may be an alternative to or a less invasive technology than the reference test.

5.4.2.4 Description of the Standard Test

The reference standard is the best currently available method for identifying patients who have the target condition; it also called the gold standard. The reference test will be compared with the index test. The reference standard is a critical validation point for an accuracy study, as it is used to define the target condition; the underlying assumption is that the reference test reflects the truth [4, 11].

5.4.2.5 Description of the Outcomes

The protocol should briefly state the outcomes of interest while considering the clinical context. For diagnostic test accuracy SRs, the outcomes may be written in terms of true positives, false positives, true negatives, false negatives, sensitivity and specificity, as well as other related outcomes.

5.4.3 Search Methods

The authors must design strategies for searching the literature, and the protocol should present at least one detailed search strategy (the strategy must be replicable) for one of the main databases.

To build the strategy, a good starting point is to break the PIRO framework into its components, then identify and list the MeSH terms (in case of MEDLINE) and text words for each component. The next step is build the strategy using the Boolean operators "OR" for the synonym(s) and "AND" between the PIRO components. For instance:

(Population **OR** synonym(s)) **AND** (Index test **OR** synonym(s)) **AND** (Reference test **OR** Synonym(s)) **AND** (Outcome **OR** synonym(s)).

Usually, the databases automatically help to create the search by identifying and adding terms. The database shows the terms and indicates their corresponding field tags, such as text words (tw), title and abstract (tiab), date (dp), and all fields (all) in MEDLINE/PubMed. The field tags can be managed to narrow the search strategy.

In addition to synonyms, the authors should pay attention to variations in spelling, as well as plurals and abbreviations. The use of any restrictions is not suggested (for example, restricting languages or dates); however, when restrictions are applied, it is necessary to justify them. For example, a search may be limited by date, depending on the specific year that the test was introduced. The constructed search strategy must be adapted to various databases.

The intended search period also needs to be outlined. For example, it should be stated whether the search will be updated. The use of reference managing software is strongly recommended, and the software, along with its version, must be previously stated in the protocol.

5.4.3.1 Databases

The databases should be chosen according to the topic of the review or the study population. There are multi-subject databases as well as databases in specific areas of healthcare. For example, PsycInfo is specific to the American Psychological Association. Some of the major databases are the following:

- **MEDLINE/PubMed**—Medical Literature Analysis and Retrieval System Online (https://www.ncbi.nlm.nih.gov/pubmed/)
- **EMBASE**—Excerpta Medica Database (https://www.elsevier.com/solutions/embase-biomedical-research)
- **Cochrane Library**—(http://www.cochranelibrary.com/)
- **Web of Science**—(http://www.webofknowledge.com/)
- **DARE**—The Database of Abstracts of Reviews of Effects (https://www.crd.york.ac.uk/crdweb/HomePage.asp)

- **LILACS**—Latin American and Caribbean Health Sciences Literature (http://lilacs.bvsalud.org/en/)
- **CINHAL**—The Cumulative Index to Nursing and Allied Health Literature (https://health.ebsco.com/products/the-cinahl-database)

The protocol should also state if a manual search strategy will be used, including snowballing (checking the reference list of the selected articles).

5.4.3.2 Other Resources

Other sources, such as "grey literature", should be searched in order to retrieve data for nonacademic purposes or unpublished evidence. Some examples of websites/databases to search for grey literature are as follows:

- **The Grey Literature Report** (http://www.greylit.org/)
- **Open Grey** (http://www.opengrey.eu/)
- **The OAIster Database** (http://www.oclc.org/en/oaister.html)

In addition, the protocol must state if the referenced authors will be personally contacted, if needed.

5.4.4 Eligibility Criteria

Predetermined criteria related to the research question must be stated in the protocol.

5.4.4.1 Type of Studies

The protocol must describe the type of studies that will be included in the review. Generally, diagnostic test studies include observationally designed studies, such as cross-sectional studies; however, they may also include case-control studies.

Identifiable design features of the eligible studies must be stated. Review authors should describe the design as well as provide a design name, as there is no universal terminology for diagnostic study designs. Key aspects include a statement on whether the protocol will include only prospective studies or both prospective and retrospective studies, a description of how and where participants were recruited (e.g. as a consecutive series of new presentations in primary care), and a statement on whether the study was cross-sectional or if it included longitudinal assessment as the reference standard. Authors should always state whether they included or excluded diagnostic case-control studies and the strategy used to make this decision. Any restrictions based on a minimal quality standard, minimal sample sizes, or the number of diseased cases should be stated, but there is no clear guidance on how these limitations should be determined [7].

5.4.4.2 Participants

As one of the objectives of an SR is to provide a decision-making process regarding a specific condition and tests, the population is a key component. The protocol must describe the population for whom the test is suitable, including any restrictions on diagnoses, age groups, and settings [7].

5.4.4.3 Target Condition

The target condition is a health condition or a particular disease, in a current stage, that the index test is intended to identify. Some reviews may evaluate the ability of tests to differentiate between several target conditions—if this is the case, all of the target conditions should be listed [7].

5.4.4.4 Index Test: Technical Aspects

A description of the test index and its characteristics and technical aspects should be included. The test may be based on samples, a physiological measure, an imaging test, or a physical examination. For example, if the test is based on samples, the protocol should describe the type of assay kit and the criteria used to declare a positive test result (including the normal ranges that may vary across population groups, such as age). For example, the index test of a meta-analysis was an immunohistochemistry test of the antigen p57 to diagnose the complete hydatidiform mole [8].

5.4.4.5 Reference or Standard Test

Similar to the index test, the protocol should describe the reference test, its characteristics, and technical aspects, including the criteria used to declare a positive test result. For example, in the previously mentioned meta-analysis, the standard test was the genotyping technique (short tandem repeat) to diagnose the complete hydatidiform mole in pregnant women [8].

5.4.5 Data Collection Plan

The planned method of data extraction should be clearly stated. It is typically recommended that at least two reviewers independently select and evaluate the studies and extract their data. The protocol should also state the steps of the study selection based on the eligibility criteria. For example:

- **Step 1**: title review
- **Step 2**: abstract review (in cases where the titles indicated that a study might be of relevance)
- **Step 3**: identification of the eligible studies based on their full text

As indicated in the Guide to the contents of a Cochrane Diagnostic Test Accuracy Protocol version 1.1, this section should indicate the rigour of the selection and data extraction processes by describing the processes used for duplicate selection and extraction decisions, the method for resolving discrepancies, and the method for checking (and double checking) key data [7].

The type of data that will be extracted should have been previously described in the protocol. The information that will be extracted from each study should be listed, and this description should state the possibility of adding more information during the extraction process, when appropriate. The tables and tools that will be used to extract the data can be included in the protocol. For example, the extraction tools may include the following:

- Study characteristics, such as title, author, country, design, language of publication, year of publication, sample size, and number of centres
- Population characteristics, such as total number of patients, number of patients in groups for comparison, and age of the patients
- Index test information, such as type of test and diagnostic criteria
- Standard test information, such as the type of test and diagnostic criteria
- Outcomes: number of true positives, false positives, true negatives, false negatives, sensitivity and specificity, negative predictive value (NPV) and positive predictive value (PPV), and the positive likelihood ratio (LR+) and negative likelihood ratio (LR−) [8]

Articles do not typically present all the information regarding the outcome measures of interest; in this case, it is better to use a broad tool to collect all types of outcome measures so that the authors can conduct calculations and transformations to reach the measure of interest. Some articles may present data from the test results (standard and index), including sensitivity and specificity; in this case, the authors can perform calculations to obtain results, such as true positives, false positives, true negatives, and false negatives. These measures than can be used to create a 2×2 contingency table, especially if the article followed the STARD—list of essential items for reporting diagnostic accuracy studies, 2015. The objective of the STARD initiative is to improve the completeness and transparency of reports of diagnostic accuracy studies so that readers can assess the potential for bias in the study (internal validity) and evaluate its generalizability (external validity) [13].

If the authors will use a software or web-based program to retrieve the data, it should be outlined in the protocol. Another aspect that must be approached in the protocol is how the authors will treat missing data. If there are any missing or insufficient data in the included studies, the protocol should state whether the reviewers will contact the corresponding authors, and the way the contact will occur (e.g. via email) to obtain the additional or missing information.

5.4.5.1 Tables

The protocol should present the developed and standardized tools that will be used to extract the data from the retrieved articles. Usually, the tables and tools are presented in the appendices of the protocol.

5.4.6 Risk of Bias and Quality Assessment

More variability is expected in the results of a diagnostic accuracy study compared to other study designs, such as randomized controlled trials. This variability may occur due to chance, as many diagnostic studies have small sample sizes. Heterogeneity may be due to differences in the study populations, but differences in the study methods are also likely to result in differences in accuracy estimates. Additionally, as in any other type of study, test accuracy studies with design deficiencies can produce biased results.

Quality assessment of the individual studies included in an SR is a crucial step to identifying potential sources of bias and to limiting the effects of these biases on the estimates and the conclusions of the review [11].

It is thereby recommended that the protocol indicates what methodology will be used for quality assessment. For an SR of diagnostic test accuracy, the Quality Assessment of Diagnostic Accuracy Studies (QUADAS-2) is recommended. QUADAS-2 consist of four key domains: patient selection, index test, reference standard, and flow and timing. Each domain is assessed in terms of its risk of bias, while the first three domains are assessed in terms of concerns regarding applicability. Signalling questions are included to assist in judgements about the risk of bias [14].

The protocol should describe the anticipated methods for assessing the risk of bias in individual studies, including whether this assessment will be done at the outcome, study level, or both. The protocol should also state how this information will be used in data synthesis [15].

Although it may be difficult to use Grades of Recommendation, Assessment, Development and Evaluation (GRADE) in diagnostic test accuracy reviews, the reviewers should consider using GRADE to assess the body of evidence (even though a GRADE rating may not be provided). As the quality of the methodology differs from the quality of the evidence, GRADE not only considers the risk of bias across studies, but it also considers inconsistency, imprecision, indirectness, publication bias, and factors that increase the confidence in an effect [16].

Another interesting source of information for review design is the Enhancing the Quality and Transparency of Health Research (EQUATOR) Network website. The EQUATOR Network is an international initiative that seeks to improve the reliability and value of published health research literature by promoting transparent and accurate reporting and a wider use of robust reporting guidelines. It attempts to tackle the problems of inadequate reporting systematically and on a global scale; it advances the work done by individual groups over the last 15 years (https://www.equator-network.org/).

5.4.7 Statistical Analysis Plan

Although some decisions can only be made after data extraction, the authors may briefly describe the statistical analysis plan in the protocol. The planned strategy may consider the possibility of performing a meta-analysis with heterogeneity and sensitivity analysis (subgroup analysis) or any additional analysis. However, the plan may change during the development of the SR, depending on the data that is obtained from the selected studies.

Meta-analysis is the process of combining the quantitative results of similar individual studies (retrieved in an SR) by formal statistical methods in order to increase the precision of the estimated treatment effect. The protocol should mention the type of model that will be used.

Diagnostic test studies often report measures such as sensitivity and specificity, positive and negative predictive values, likelihood ratios for the respective test results, and the receiver operating characteristic (ROC) curve.

Two forest plots are usually presented: one for sensitivity and the other for specificity. Thus, these graphs show the means and confidence intervals for sensitivity/specificity in each of the selected primary studies [9].

The summary of the different ROC curves is called the summary receiver operating characteristic (SROC) curve. SROC is used to represent the performance of a specific diagnostic test. It uses a linear regression model proposed by Moses and Littenberg that is based on bivariate data and the inverse correlation between sensitivity and specificity. This model is limited because it does not appropriately account for the imprecision in individual study estimates or in estimates of heterogeneity between studies (random effects); it underestimates test accuracy due to zero-cell corrections and bias in the weights [17, 18].

To obtain better estimates of diagnostic accuracy, mixed models have been recommended. The bivariate random effects model summarizes a pooled estimate for sensitivity and specificity, and the hierarchical summary ROC (HSROC) models the parameters of the summary ROC curve [4]. Both models are mathematically equivalent in the absence of covariables.

The protocol should present a method for publication bias assessment. As the funnel plot method is not suitable for diagnostic test accuracy reviews, the authors can consider a regression of lnDOR and the effective sample size (ESS) based on the methods described by Deeks et al. [19]. Finally, the software that the authors intend to use, along with its version, must be stated in the protocol.

5.5 Results

The protocol should describe how the results will be presented, combined, and reported. Test accuracy is most often expressed as test sensitivity (the proportion of those patients who are positive to the reference standard and who are also positive to the index test) and specificity (the proportion of those patients who are negative to the reference standard and who are also negative to the index test), but many alternative measures have been proposed and are in use [11].

As mentioned in the statistical analysis plan, a meta-analysis of diagnostic test accuracy generally presents forest plots for sensitivity and specificity, along with the corresponding confidence intervals and the ROC curve.

5.5.1 Search Results

The protocol should state how the search results will be documented. The search results are usually presented as a flow diagram that indicates the identified studies, included and excluded, and the reasons for exclusion. The PRISMA statement guidelines have developed a flow diagram template that depicts the flow of information through the different phases of an SR (Fig. 5.1). This tool is currently incorporated into most SRs, and it is a well-established method for presenting the results [15].

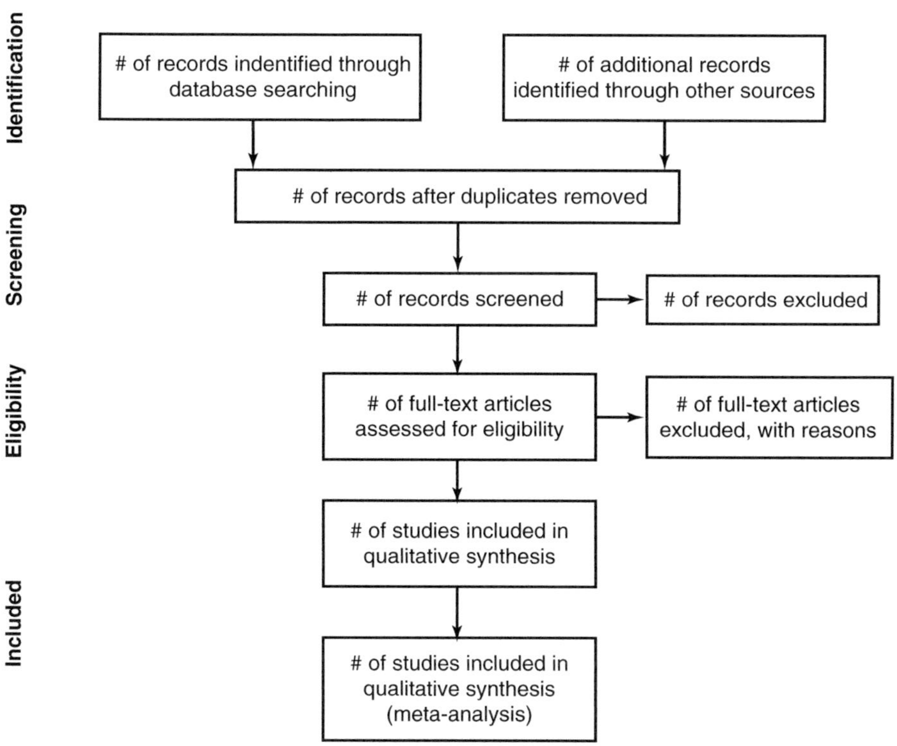

Fig. 5.1 Flow of information through the different phases of a systematic review [15]

5.5.2 Findings

The protocol may mention how the results will be interpreted in order to reach the conclusions of the review.

5.6 Discussion

5.6.1 Summary of the Results

As SRs should be accompanied by a summary of findings table, the protocol should mention it. Usually, the summary table includes the question, the accuracy estimates, the number of studies and participants, the quality of the evidence, and the practical implications. The GRADE working group developed a tool named GRADEpro GDT that can be used to build the summary of results table (https://gradepro.org/).

5.6.2 Limitations

As with all research, the value of an SR depends on what was done, what was found, and the clarity of reporting. As with other publications, the reporting quality of an SR varies, limiting the readers' ability to assess the strengths and weaknesses of those reviews [15, 20].

Limitations also apply to SRs of diagnostic test accuracy; however, knowledge of these limitations allows the authors to design a rigorous protocol in attempt to minimize them. In this way, a final SR is the result of a well-established protocol, and it can at least present well-described limitations, allowing the readers to take them into account during their decision-making.

5.6.3 Applications

The authors may briefly mention the applications of the results in the protocol.

5.7 Conclusion

5.7.1 Implication for Practice

Test accuracy is not a permanent property of the diagnostic tests. In this context, authors may indicate the expected implications of the design review in practice. The authors can anticipate the advantages of the index test beyond its accuracy evaluation at this point in the review design. In practice, the diagnostic test under review (index test) may be more accurate, less invasive, easier to perform, less risky, less uncomfortable for patients, quicker to yield results, technically less challenging, or more easily interpreted than the standard test [21].

In fact, the index test may have three possible roles as a new test: replacement, triage, or add-on [21]. If a new test is to replace an existing test, then comparing the accuracy of both tests on the same population and with the same reference standard provides the most direct evidence. In triage, the new test is used before the existing test or existing testing pathway, and only patients with a particular result on the triage test continue on the testing pathway. When a test is needed to rule out disease in patients who do not need further testing, one will be looking for a test that minimizes the proportion of false negatives and thus has a relatively high sensitivity. Triage tests may be less accurate than existing tests, but they have other advantages, such as simplicity or low cost. A third possible role of a new test is add-on. The new test is positioned after the existing testing pathway; its aim is to identify false positives or false negatives after the existing pathway. The review should provide data to assess the incremental change in accuracy that results from adding the new test. According to Leeflang et al. (2008), the review authors should at least consider whether the test of interest would be mainly used in general practice or in a secondary or even a tertiary setting [11].

5.7.2 Implication for Research

Similar to the implications for practice, the protocol should indicate the expected implications for research in its field, identifying gaps in the literature or pointing out the best available evidence on a specific research question.

References

1. Sackett DL, Straus SE, Richardson WS, Rosenberg W, Haynes RB. Evidence-based medicine: how to practice and teach EBM. 2nd ed. Edinburgh: Churchill Livingstone; 2000.
2. Biondi-Zoccai G, Abbate A, Benedetto U, Palmerini T, Ascenzo FD, Frati G. Network meta-analysis for evidence synthesis: what is it and why is it posed to dominate cardiovascular decision making? Int. J. Cardiol. 2015;182:309–14.
3. Mulrow CD. Systematic reviews rationale for systematic reviews. BMJ. 1994;309:597–9.
4. MMG L. Systematic reviews and meta-analyses of diagnostic test accuracy. Clin. Microbiol. Infect. 2013;20:105–13.
5. Diretrizes Metodológicas: Elaboração de Revisão Sistemática e Metanálise de Estudos de Acurácia Diagnóstica [Internet]. Ministério. Brasília, DF: Ministério da Saúde, Secretaria de Ciência, Tenologia e Insumos Estratégicos, Departamento de Ciência e Tecnologia; 2014. http://bvsms.saude.gov.br/bvs/ct/PDF/diretrizes_metodologicas_revisao_sistematica_metanalise_de_estudos.pdf. Accessed 28 June 2018.
6. Centre for Reviews and Dissemination. Systematic reviews: CRD's guidance for undertaking reviews in healthcare. Centre for Reviews and Dissemination, editor. Centre for Reviews and Dissemination; 2009.
7. Deeks JJ, Wisniewski S, Davenport C. Chapter 4: guide to the contents of a Cochrane diagnostic test accuracy protocol. In: Deeks JJ, Bossuyt PM, Gatsonis C, editors. Cochrane handbook systematic reviews of diagnostic test accuracy version 1.0.0: The Cochrane Collaboration; 2013. p. 1–15. srdta.cochrane.org. Accessed 28 June 2018.

8. Madi JM, Braga AR, Paganella MP, Litvin IE, Da Ros Wendland EM. Accuracy of p57KIP2 compared with genotyping for the diagnosis of complete hydatidiform mole: protocol for a systematic review and meta-analysis. Syst Rev. 2016;5:169.
9. Campbell JM, Klugar M, Ding S, Carmody DP, Hakonsen SJ, Jadotte YT, White S, Munn Z. Chapter 9: diagnostic test accuracy systematic reviews. In: Aromataris E, Munn Z, editors. The systematic review of studies of diagnostic test accuracy. Adelaide, SA, Australia: The Joanna Briggs Institute Reviewers' Manual; 2015.
10. Farrugia P, Petrisor BA, Farrokhyar F, Bhandari M. Research questions, hypotheses and objectives. Can J Surg. 2010;53:278–81.
11. Leeflang MMG, Deeks JJ, Gatsonis C, Bossuyt PMM. Systematic reviews of diagnostic test accuracy. Ann Intern Med. 2008;149:889–97.
12. Deeks JJ, Takwoingi Y, Leeflang MM, Davenport C. Use of medical tests. Lesson 1.1: Cochrane collaboration DTA online learning materials. The Cochrane Collaboration. 2014.
13. Bossuyt PM, Reitsma JB, Bruns DE, Gatsonis CA, Paul P, Irwig L, et al. Research methods & reporting STARD 2015: an updated list of essential items for. BMJ. 2015;5527:1–9.
14. Whiting PF, Rutjes AWS, Westwood ME, Mallet S, Deeks JJ, Reitsma JB, et al. Research and reporting methods accuracy studies. Ann Intern Med. 2011;155:529–36.
15. Moher D, Liberati A, Tetzlaff J, Altman DG, Group TP. Preferred reporting items for systematic reviews and Meta-analyses: the PRISMA statement. PLoS Med. 2009;6:e1000097.
16. Guyatt GH. GRADE: an emerging consensus on rating quality of evidence and strength of recommendations. BMJ. 2008;336:924–6.
17. Littenberg B, Moses LE. Estimating diagnostic accuracy from multiple conflicting reports: a new meta-analytic method. Med Decis Mak. 1993;13:313–21.
18. Moses LE, Shapiro D. Combining independent studies of a diagnostic test into a summary ROC curve: data-analytic approaches and some additional considerations. Stat Med. 1993;12:1293–316.
19. Deeks JJ, Macaskill P, Irwig L. The performance of tests of publication bias and other sample size effects in systematic reviews of diagnostic test accuracy was assessed. J Clin Epidemiol. 2006;58:882–93.
20. Gopalakrishnan S, Ganeshkumar P. Systematic reviews and meta-analysis: understanding the best evidence in primary healthcare. J Family Med Prim Care. 2013;2:9–14.
21. Bossuyt PM, Irwig L, Craig J, Glasziou P. Comparative accuracy: assessing new tests against existing diagnostic pathways. BMJ. 2006;332:1089–92.

Registering the Review 6

Alison Booth and Julie Jones-Diette

6.1 Introduction

Systematic reviews of any type of evidence should involve a consistent, transparent and reproducible approach to identifying, evaluating and summarising the evidence on a topic. To achieve this, development of a protocol, a plan of how the review will be carried out, is essential; and registration of the protocol can provide transparency.

This chapter explains the principles and purpose of protocol registration and presents PROSPERO a key example of a purpose built, open register of systematic review protocols. The requirements for prospective registration of reviews of diagnostic test accuracy studies are illustrated with examples of protocols registered in PROSPERO. This chapter is based on information provided on the PROSPERO website and is included here by kind permission of the Centre for Reviews and Dissemination (CRD) who produce the register [1].

6.2 The Need for Registration

Mandatory trial registration was introduced following methodological research that confirmed what systematic reviewers suspected: that there were publication and outcome reporting biases in trials [2, 3]. A similar problem was later found in the conduct and reporting of systematic reviews. Of 47 Cochrane review publications

A. Booth (✉)
Department of Health Sciences, University of York, York, UK
e-mail: alison.booth@york.ac.uk

J. Jones-Diette
Centre for Reviews and Dissemination, University of York, York, UK
e-mail: julie.jones-diette@york.ac.uk

G. Biondi-Zoccai (ed.), *Diagnostic Meta-Analysis*,
https://doi.org/10.1007/978-3-319-78966-8_6

examined, 43 reported outcomes not consistent with that described in the associated protocol [4]. However, poor reporting in the reviews meant it was not clear if this finding was the result of some form of bias or justifiable but undocumented changes made as the review methods were developed. A review in 2007 found the quality of reporting of 300 published systematic reviews to be disappointing [5]. Problems identified included the absence of fundamental details such as risk of bias assessment of the included studies in about a third of the reviews; and only a quarter reported undertaking any analysis to look for publication bias in the included studies. Only 11% of the non-Cochrane reviews examined mentioned having a protocol. It may be that a protocol had been produced and followed but not reported or one had not been prepared. Whether through poor reporting or total absence, the lack of a protocol raises concerns about the effect of a range of biases on the findings and the rigour of the conduct of the review. Most of the reporting failures were in non-Cochrane reviews: a reflection of the value of inclusion of the production and publication of a protocol as an integral part of the Cochrane process.

In recognition of the need to improve the standard of reporting, the Quality of Reporting of Meta-analyses (QUOROM) guideline was published in 1999 [6]. This was revised and replaced by the Preferred Reporting Items for Systematic Review and Meta-analysis (PRISMA) guideline in 2009 [7, 8]. PRISMA identified access to the protocol and a registration number as desirable. At the time the PRISMA statement was published, access to systematic review protocols was limited to the outputs of individual organisations such as the Cochrane and Campbell Collaborations and the Joanna Briggs Institute [9–11]. There were also limited options for publishing protocols in journals. Recognising this situation, the Centre for Reviews and Dissemination at the University of York, UK, launched PROSPERO in February 2011. One year later the first journal dedicated to publishing systematic reviews and protocols was added to the BioMed Central portfolio: *Systematic Reviews* [12]. In 2015 PRISMA guidance specifically for reporting protocols (PRISMA-P) was published [13, 14]. PRISMA-P was developed using information from the consultation exercise that identified the PROSPERO registration fields. As a result PRISMA-P provides a framework for developing a protocol that will coincide with PROSPERO requirements and in a reporting format for submission for publication in a journal.

PRISMA-P aims to help improve the reporting of protocols in the same way as STARD made modest improvements over time in the reporting of diagnostic studies [15]. As with all guidelines, the most appropriate tool for the job should be selected, for example, STARDdem for cognitive disorders [16]. The EQUATOR Network website (http://www.equator-network.org/) provides free, comprehensive access to current reporting guidelines.

Concerns about biases in the systematic review process also drove the realisation that review protocol registration was needed. The prevalence of outcome reporting bias in randomised controlled trials (RCTs) and the impact of those biases on 288 Cochrane reviews were examined in 2010 by Kirkham et al. [17]. In comparing the protocol with the final published review, 22% were found to have discrepancies in at least one outcome measure, 75% of which were in the primary outcome. Potential bias from changes being made after seeing the results from individual trials was found in 29% (8/28) of these reviews. Of the 64 reviews with an outcome discrepancy, only 6% explained the reason for the change in the report of the review. Kirkham et al. also found that outcomes promoted from secondary in the protocol to primary in the review report were more likely to be significant than if there was no discrepancy (relative risk 1.66 95% CI (1.10–2.49), $p = 0.02$).

In 2014 Page et al. published a Cochrane methodological review of empirical studies that examined selective inclusion and/or reporting of outcomes in systematic reviews of RCTs [18]. The review found that at least one outcome had been added, omitted, upgraded or downgraded between the protocol and final report in 38% of the systematic reviews included in four empirical studies. However, the association between statistical significance and discrepancies in reporting of outcomes was unclear. The reason for discrepancies was rarely reported, and it was also unclear whether the decision to make these changes was related to the significance of the treatment effect for that outcome. There was evidence that 32% of the systematic reviews did not report all of the outcomes in the abstract of the review. Outcomes with more statistically convincing results were more likely to be completely reported in the abstract than other outcomes. PRISMA for abstracts was published in 2013, after the studies included in Page et al.'s review, to provide guidelines for writing abstracts for systematic reviews in journals and for conferences [19].

Bias in research can arise from a variety of sources [20] and is still occurring in trials [21, 22]. Even the most rigorous approach to undertaking a systematic review cannot eliminate bias. But it is possible to minimise some of the risks and add transparency in the process allowing the reader to assess the remaining potential risk and influence of bias on the findings of the review. Making key details of the protocol publicly available through registration can provide such transparency if the appropriate information is provided. Simply registering a protocol is not the whole answer, as Tricco et al. found in their 2016 study comparing outcome reporting between PROSPERO records and their published review reports [23]. Of the 96 reviews identified, just over a third did not explicitly state their primary outcome; just under a third had a discrepancy between the primary outcome in the protocol and final report, and 6% of primary outcomes were omitted from the review report. No significant increased risk was found from adding/upgrading (RR 2.14, 95% CI 0.53–8.63) or decreased risk of downgrading (RR 0.76, 0.27–2.17) an outcome when the meta-analysis result was favourable and statistically significant. Likewise, there was no significant increased risk of adding/upgrading (RR 0.89, 0.31–2.53) or decreased risk of downgrading (RR 0.56, 0.29–1.08) an outcome when the conclusion was positive. Registration has facilitated such research, which in turn supports further efforts to provide transparency and improve reporting in the systematic review process.

Another major driver for prospective registration of systematic review protocols is to help avoid unplanned duplication. Minimising waste is high on research agendas around the world [24]. There are justifiable reasons for repeating or undertaking complementary systematic reviews, but these should be planned and undertaken in the full knowledge of existing and ongoing reviews [25, 26]. Siontis et al. found that 49 out of 73 (67%) meta-analyses included in their study had overlapping meta-analyses on the same topic. They concluded that while some independent replication can be justified, the study findings indicate that some research resources are being wasted [27].

A database of ongoing reviews provides reviewers, funders and commissioners with searchable access to details of what is already being addressed and when the results are likely to be available. This helps to avoid unplanned duplication and has the potential to promote collaborations. As part of a wider movement to improve the transparency of methods and quality of reporting research, journals that publish systematic reviews are increasingly requiring details of protocol registration as part of the submission process. Major publishers, such as BioMed Central, BMJ, BMJ Open and PLoS, have endorsed prospective registration of systematic reviews and ask for the PROSPERO registration number to be included in submissions of final reports [28]. PLoS Journals also make registry details and protocols available to editors and reviewers and include them alongside published papers for readers [29]. Both journals of the RSNA *Radiology* and the *British Journal of Radiology* request authors follow the PRISMA checklist for systematic review manuscripts, which includes reporting details of protocol registration.

6.3 Options for Registration

Many of the major funders of reviews such as the US Agency for Healthcare Research and Quality (AHRQ) and the UK National Institute for Health Research (NIHR) make protocols for research they fund available on their websites. Likewise organisations such as the Cochrane and Campbell Collaborations and the Joanna Briggs Institute publish protocols for their reviews on their organisation's database or website [9–11]. The Cochrane Collaboration and the Joanna Briggs Institute both include protocols for reviews of diagnostic studies. While not the same as registration, more journals now publish protocols, for example, PLoS ONE and BMC *Systematic Reviews*. Publication puts the protocol in the public domain but can take time and usually still requires details of registration to be reported.

Some clinical trial registers have accepted registration of systematic review protocols. However, the information required for a protocol of a trial is significantly different to that of a review. A study in 2011 found that the anticipated benefits of trial registration were being undermined by deficiencies in the provision of key information: a potential problem for all registers [30]. It is also counter-intuitive to look in trial registers when searching for protocols of systematic reviews.

The Open Science Framework (OFS) is an example of an initiative arising from the broader calls for transparency in research processes and data [31]. OSF is a free, open source service that facilitates project management, including permanent, data stamped versions of all documentation such as protocols. However, a dedicated register of systematic review protocols provides a single site to search for ongoing reviews and avoids the need to find and search a range of places.

Funded by the NIHR, PROSPERO was launched in February 2011, as the first free, open access international prospective register of systematic reviews [28]. The PROSPERO dataset was agreed through an international consensus exercise specifically for the registration of systematic review protocols [32, 33]. In addition to registrations from individual review teams around the world, protocols from the major organisations producing reviews such as the Cochrane Collaboration and the Joanna Briggs Institute are included in PROSPERO. The UK NIHR mandate registration of all the reviews they fund which meet PROSPERO inclusion criteria. Other major funders such as the Canadian Institute for Health Research (CIHR) also strongly encourage protocol registration.

Register content has grown rapidly with 10,000 registrations in November 2015, doubling to 20,000 records in just over a year. PROSPERO offers international exposure as registrations come from 107 countries, and during 2016 there were 364,806 visits to the website from 210 countries and territories worldwide.

In addition to providing a single site for searching, PROSPERO records are permanent. This ensures that even if the findings of a registered review are never published and/or referenced in the registration record, details of the review team are available for users to contact.

6.4 Reviews of Diagnostic Accuracy Studies in PROSPERO

Participants in the international Delphi consultation to establish the dataset for registration comprised a range of experts from around the world in systematic reviewing, methodology, commissioning and guideline development in health and social care, as well as journal editors, including those specialising in diagnostic accuracy reviews [33].

The focus for registration was initially on reviews of the effects of interventions; this was then expanded to include any systematic review with a health-related outcome in the broadest sense [34, 35]. The consensus panel included experts in reviewing diagnostic test accuracy studies, but it was agreed no guidance specific to DTA was necessary. Registrants proved to be capable of adapting the form to their particular review and from launch submissions accepted included: reviews of diagnostic, prognostic, prevention, service delivery, adverse effect, epidemiology, prevalence and risk studies [36]. Methodological reviews are only included if there is an outcome of direct patient or clinical relevance. So a review comparing the reporting of studies of diagnostic tools for a condition could be included, as long as there was an element of assessment of the value of the tools that would help a clinician decide on a tool in a given situation.

At the end of February 2017, there were 166 reviews with "diagnostic and accuracy" in their title registered in PROSPERO, including four Cochrane reviews. The results of a year-by-year search of Ovid MEDLINE and PROSPERO for records with diagnostic and accuracy in the title are shown in Fig. 6.1. This demonstrates the need to further promote an understanding of both the value and availability of protocol registration to those undertaking diagnostic reviews.

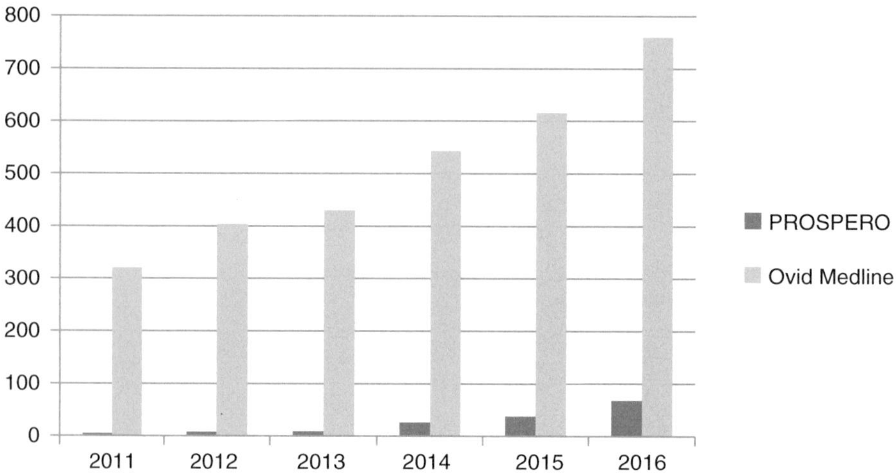

Fig. 6.1 Reviews with diagnostic accuracy in the title entered in PROSPERO and Ovid MEDLINE

The records in PROSPERO can provide a useful learning tool; however, submissions are not peer reviewed, only checked to ensure they meet the inclusion criteria, so should be critically assessed for methodological validity and, as with all research, should not be taken at face value. A periodic reminder is sent by the PROSPERO administration team, but it is the responsibility of the named contact on the registration to update the status of a review; therefore, if this is not updated, an ongoing study that has passed its anticipated completion date may have been completed and/or published or even abandoned.

6.5 Registering a Review of Diagnostic Accuracy Studies on PROSPERO

Registration on PROSPERO involves the prospective and permanent publication of key information about the design and conduct of a systematic review. Registration is free of charge. Registrants are responsible for the information entered in the registration form and, by submitting this, agree to be accountable for the accuracy and timeliness of the record and its content. The person submitting the completed form, known as the *Named contact*, is also expected to keep the record up to date, including provision of a citation and a link to the report or publication on completion of the review.

Prospective registration is essential for the comparison of what was planned with what is reported on completion, so retrospective registrations are not accepted. It is not possible to account for all potential biases, so from a practical perspective, the earliest point in the review process where bias may potentially be accounted for is during screening against eligibility criteria. For this reason registration forms should be completed and submitted before screening commences.

Protocols are iterative documents, and during the course of a review, amendments may become necessary. PROSPERO facilitates the documentation of revisions and updates on progress, so transparency can be maintained throughout the review. It is important to justify any changes and to be clear when in the review process they have been made, as changes should not be made after commencing data extraction.

Submissions must be in English for practical reasons related to record management (CRD is UK based), but search strategies and protocols attached to a record may be in any language.

In developing and writing a protocol and the subsequent final report, it is important to pay attention to all of the information provided. A qualitative study requested clinicians, researchers and policy makers unfamiliar with the design and methodology to read three Cochrane diagnostic test accuracy reviews. The participants found the reviews largely inaccessible and had a range of difficulties with understanding related to the level of explanation provided in the text [37]. In striving to meet the requirements of guidelines or registration templates, context and user-friendly language to facilitate accessibility should not be forgotten.

6.5.1 Administrative Fields

The PROSPERO dataset contains 22 required items and 18 optional items (Table 6.1). The more administrative fields are common to all types of reviews and are fairly self-explanatory. Of particular importance though is specifying the stage of the review at the time of submission which, as discussed above, may be taken as an indicator of whether selection bias may have occurred. The stage of review at registration can be seen in relation to the anticipated start and completion dates.

Although many items are optional, registrants are encouraged to provide as much information as possible. The data in PROSPERO offer the opportunity for methodological research, to hopefully provide a better understanding of issues with planning and undertaking reviews. For example, Borah et al. (2017) used the data on start and completion dates from 195 registered and published reviews in PROSPERO to look at how long reviews are taking [38]. They found the mean estimated time to complete the project and publish the review was 67.3 weeks. Funded reviews took significantly longer (mean 42 vs. 26 weeks, $p < 0.001$) and involved more authors and team members (mean = 6.8 vs. 4.8 people, $p < 0.001$) than those that did not report funding.

6.5.2 Methods Fields

In preparing your protocol and prior to registration, it is worth considering the areas of methodological weakness identified in the Cochrane diagnostic test accuracy editorial process [39]. Common methodological issues with Cochrane diagnostic test

Table 6.1 The PROSPERO dataset

Review title and time scale
1. Review title[a]
2. Original language title
3. Anticipated or actual start date[a]
4. Anticipated completion date[a]
5. Stage of review at time of this submission[a]
Review team details
6. Named contact[a]
7. Named contact email[a]
8. Named contact address
9. Named contact phone number
10. Organisational affiliation of the review[a]
11. Review team members and their organisational affiliations
12. Funding sources/sponsors[a]
13. Conflicts of interest[a]
14. Collaborators
Review methods
15. Review question(s)[a]
16. Searches[a]
17. URL to search strategy
18. Condition or domain being studied[a]
19. Participants/population[a]
20. Intervention(s), exposure(s)[a]
21. Comparator(s)/control[a]
22. Types of study to be included[a]
23. Context
24. Primary outcome(s)[a]
25. Secondary outcomes[a]
26. Data extraction (selection and coding)
27. Risk of bias (quality) assessment[a]
28. Strategy for data synthesis[a]
29. Analysis of subgroups or subsets[a]
General information
30. Type of review
31. Language
32. Country
33. Other registration details
34. Reference and/or URL for published protocol
35. Dissemination plans
36. Keywords
37. Details of any existing review of the same topic by the same authors
38. Current review status[a]
39. Any other information
40. Details of final report/publication(s)

[a]Indicates a required field

accuracy protocols include definition of the research question (in particular alternative diagnostic pathways), choice of reference standard, design of the search strategy, quality assessment of the included studies and the statistical methods for meta-analysis.

6.5.2.1 Review Question and Title

The title for a review of diagnostic test accuracy studies should state the test and the condition being diagnosed; for example, "Anion gap as a diagnostic tool to screen for elevated lactate levels in patients admitted to an acute care setting: protocol of a diagnostic test accuracy review", (CRD42015016470). Or where tests are being compared, the index test(s) and reference test and what they aim to diagnose should be included; for example, "The accuracy of Quantitative interim PET compared to Qualitative interim PET in prognosis of Hodgkin lymphoma: a systematic review protocol of diagnostic test accuracy" (CRD42016027953).

Including "protocol for a systematic review" and "diagnostic test accuracy" in the title helps users and search engines find the review protocol, identify study design and distinguish it from a completed review.

The review question should clearly state the index test or tests that are to be assessed for accuracy, which is the reference test or comparator, details of the condition being diagnosed and/or the subgroup of those with the condition and the circumstances and method of use of the test(s). The title may also specify the measure of accuracy to be used (e.g. sensitivity, specificity; positive and negative likelihood ratios; area under the curve) and the types of studies to be included.

6.5.2.2 Searches

Details of the sources to be searched and any restrictions should be provided. The full search strategy is not required but may be supplied as a link or attachment.

Remembering that what is included in the registration of the protocol is the plan you should follow, choice and range of electronic databases to be searched should take into account the volume of literature that may be found. Borah et al. found the number of studies identified from literature searches registered in PROSPERO ranged from 27 to 92,020, the mean yield rate of included studies was 2.94% (IQR = 2.5) and the mean number of authors per review was 5, $SD = 3$ [38]. It is always worth reviewing methodological papers when planning a review, for example, three studies suggest that limiting searching to MEDLINE may be appropriate for reviews of diagnostic test accuracy [40–42].

Plans to search for unpublished literature should also be documented. Leeflang et al. (2013) note that not much is known about publication bias in diagnostic research and promotes the development of an equivalent to www.alltrials.net for the publication of all diagnostic studies. In the meantime they encourage every effort to search for unpublished works [43]. A study of handsearching suggests efforts may best be focussed on identifying relevant journals as diagnostic imaging studies are published in a wide variety of places [44].

In the future we expect to see search strategies include repositories of data such as OSF and the Systematic Reviews Data Register (SRDR) [31, 45]. The SRDR platform facilitates the extraction and management of data for systematic reviews and meta-analyses, creating a central database that can be critiqued, updated and augmented on an ongoing basis.

6.5.2.3 Condition, PICO, Context

PROSPERO is structured for the PICO items, population, intervention, comparator, outcomes and the condition or domain being studied, which are all required fields for any systematic review. Generally, for diagnostic test accuracy reviews, the intervention will be the index test being assessed, and the comparator will be the standard test against which it is being compared. For example, Barbic et al. (2015) listed their intervention as "Point-of-care ultrasonography for the differentiation of cellulitis and abscess", and for their comparator, "Computed tomography, results from incision and drainage, or final diagnosis from clinical follow-up will be accepted as reference standards" [46]. Selection and definition of reference tests need careful consideration as they frequently have inherent challenges to their validity and often there is no one perfect way of measuring something.

Ideally, sufficient details of the tests to be included should be given to enable reproduction, for example, stating where in the patient pathway the test would be undertaken, details of the setting, skills of those undertaking the test and those interpreting the results and the manufacturer of the test.

Outcomes are the measures of diagnostic accuracy to be used, and as with any systematic review, the primary or most important outcome should be clearly stated, separately from any secondary, additional outcomes. Where there is no generally agreed value or range of values, studies are likely to report different thresholds, it is worth considering and stating how you will handle these.

Barbic et al.'s (2015) primary outcome is the diagnosis of abscess versus cellulitis, and secondary outcome is time to conduct point-of-care ultrasonography [46]. It is essential to give clear and accurate details about outcomes in the registration form as it is this record of a priori decisions that will be compared with what is reported in the final publication.

6.5.2.4 Data Extraction

You should set out the procedure you will use for selecting studies for inclusion and extracting data. For study selection make it clear how many stages will be involved and describe the rigour of the selection process.

For data extraction, this should include a list of the data to be extracted and information such as the number of researchers that will be involved, whether extraction will be done independently, how key data will be checked for accuracy or how discrepancies will be resolved.

For example, in their review of magnetic resonance imaging for diagnosing rotator cuff tears, Smith et al. (2011) state that for data extraction:

> All data will be independently extracted by one reviewer (HD) and independently verified by a second (JG). Disagreements in data collected between the reviewers will be resolved through discussion. The data extracted will include: sample size, cohort gender, average age, MRI and surgical procedure, the frequency of true positive, true negatives, false posi-

> tives and false negatives for the index to reference test analysis. When insufficient data is available, attempts will be made to calculate this using summary estimates. If not possible, corresponding authors will be contacted to obtain this data. [47]

6.5.2.5 Quality Assessment

Diagnostic test accuracy studies tend to be less well funded than randomised controlled trials and as a result are often poorly conducted and/or reported [48–50]. This section should include a statement of how quality assessment or risk of bias will be undertaken, for example, independently by two reviewers, or assessed by one and checked by a second. How discrepancies will be resolved should also be stated, for example, through discussion or referral to a third party. Also state the risk assessment tool that will be used; for diagnostic accuracy studies, this will most likely be the QUADAS-2 tool [51], though the Joanna Briggs Institute also have a checklist for diagnostic test accuracy studies [52]. Tools relevant to other study designs to be included should be stated.

You should also state whether and how this assessment will influence your planned synthesis. Reitsma et al. (2012) provide the following plans for using their assessment of risk of bias:

> The results of the quality assessment will be used for descriptive purposes to provide an evaluation of the overall quality of the included studies and to provide a transparent method of recommendation for design of any future studies. In addition, if enough data are available from the included studies, each of the quality components will be included as explanatory variables in a meta-regression analysis to investigate the association of each of these components with study results as a way of explaining possible heterogeneity. Based on the findings of the quality assessment, recommendations will be made for the conduct of future studies. [53]

6.5.2.6 Data Synthesis and Subgroup Analyses

Plans for data synthesis may have to change depending on the data identified as meeting the inclusion criteria; however prespecification of intent is an essential part of a protocol and required for registration in PROSPERO. The planned general approach is asked for, and for reviews of diagnostic accuracy studies, this should include definitions for test results and the analysis for comparing tests. The outline of presentation for a descriptive estimate of diagnostic accuracy should be given, to include tables and graphs as appropriate. The circumstances under which a meta-analysis will be undertaken should be stated, such as the type of statistical model(s) to be used or the basis for selection of a model. Also include how heterogeneity will be investigated and the statistical tests that will address any issues. Any sensitivity analyses such as subgroups or subsets within the review should also be planned and stated in the registration form. It is good practice to indicate the statistical package that will be used, being clear it has the capacity to undertake the planned analysis, for example, Stata, R or SAS.

In their review of MRI for rotator cuff tears, Smith et al. (2012) planned to use two-by-two tables detailing true-positive, false-positive, false-negative and true-negative values to calculate sensitivity and specificity with 95% confidence intervals for each study, presenting the results in a forest plot [47]. They go on to describe how heterogeneity will be assessed and how the assessment will influence the planned meta-analysis: with homogeneity demonstrated in a summary Receiver Operating Characteristic (ROC) plot. Finally, they intended to construct pooled sensitivity and specificity values. Smith et al. also planned subgroup analysis of MRI field strengths and of differences in outcomes of partial- to full-thickness rotator cuff tears [47]. The matching results can be seen in the published paper [54].

Your data synthesis plan should also include any tests for publication bias. A study of analyses of publication bias in reviews of diagnostic test accuracy studies found that while authors frequently investigated publication bias, the test used was suboptimal [55]. Van Enst et al. (2014) compared the Begg, Egger and Deeks tests [56–58] and as they gave different results concluded they are not interchangeable; the Deeks test was the authors' preferred choice.

6.5.3 Dissemination

Although this is an optional field, dissemination is an essential part of any research project, and brief details of plans for communicating essential messages from the review to the appropriate audiences should be given. Every effort should be made to publish a report, irrespective of the findings. When writing reports, authors should adhere to the PRISMA guidelines for reporting a systematic review; this will also help in ensuring your final report is in line with your planned methods. On completion and publication of the review, the status should be updated in PROSPERO, and details of, and links to, final publications of any type can be added to the record at any time.

Depending on the findings and their importance to practice and policy, dissemination should include other activities, for example, presentation at scientific meetings, production of a lay summary distributed to relevant audiences such as Royal Colleges and charities and organisation of a workshop for all relevant stakeholders.

6.6 Practicalities of Registration

To register any review, including a review of diagnostic test accuracy studies, users "Join" to create a username and password, so they can "Sign in" as a registered user. This allows access to create a new record and/or to view existing records for updating or amending. The dataset has four sections, Review title and timescale, Review team details, Review methods and Review general information. Required fields are marked with a red asterisk and must be completed before the final document can be submitted. The form can be saved and exited at any time and revisited at a later date to add or edit information prior to submission, but once submitted any subsequent changes require resubmission to ensure an audit trail of amendments. Personal information can be updated and PROSPERO passwords changed in "*My details*".

Forms can be printed or saved in portable document format (pdf) or as a word processing document to enable sharing and collaboration on development of the submission. However, only one member of the review team can submit the registration and make future updates and amendments via their personal log in. Fields can be completed by cutting and pasting information from a prepared protocol. The PROSPERO form has also been used as a template for developing the review protocol [35]. Records need to be fully searchable, so information needs to be entered in the specified fields: it is not sufficient to refer to an attached protocol or publication. Brief guidance is given for each field, and further information and examples can be accessed via a link to "more" or downloaded as a pdf [28].

When all the required fields have been completed, the "*Submit*" button becomes active, and the form can be sent to the PROSPERO administrators. Access to your record is suspended during the administrative process. Receipt of submissions is acknowledged in an automated email sent to the named contact. Application forms are checked against the inclusion criteria for PROSPERO and for clarity of content, and Medical Subject Heading (MESH) indexing terms are added to the record to assist the search function. The record is then approved and published on the register, returned for clarification or rejected. Submissions are processed and a response given, usually within 5 working days of receipt.

Once published on the register, the record becomes accessible again in the "*My records*" section of the registrants account. This then allows amendments and updates within the record to be performed by the named contact. On submitting changes you will be prompted to give brief details in a revision note of the changes made. The information entered here will appear in the public record and should inform users of the register about the nature of the changes made (e.g. removed one of the outcome measures; changed the anticipated completion date as data extraction is taking longer than anticipated). All submitted edits and changes to a PROSPERO record are recorded, dated and made available within the public record audit trail. The most recent version appears, and previous versions are accessible from dated archive links in the record together with the revision notes.

Records remain permanently on PROSPERO. Once the review is completed, the status should be updated in the record and the anticipated publication date given. Once available, the bibliographic reference and electronic links to final publications should be added to the record. In the absence of a publication, details of availability of the review's unpublished results, or reasons for the termination of the review, may be documented.

When it comes to updating a completed review that has already been registered on PROSPERO, details should be added to the existing record by selecting the "*Update of a review*" status option and resubmitting. This ensures that the history and previous versions are all linked and available in the same record using the unique identification number of the records.

Conclusion

It takes a considerable amount of time and effort to design, plan and agree a systematic review protocol, and registration may feel like an additional burden. However the value of a sound protocol and transparency in methods should never be underestimated. Good design and a well-thought through protocol provide the essential basis for a high-quality review. Making detailed planned methods publicly available via an open register such as PROSPERO provides transparency in the process and helps avoid unplanned duplication. Registration is best practice and demonstrates that sound, reproducible methods have been used, giving journal editors, peer reviewers and readers confidence in the reliability of the findings.

Acknowledgements The authors would like to thank the Centre for Reviews and Dissemination, the producers of PROSPERO, for permission to base this chapter on information provided on the register website. We are also grateful to Dr. Nick Meader for his advice and peer comments on the draft.

References

1. Centre for reviews and dissemination. University of York. 2017. https://www.york.ac.uk/crd/. Accessed 28 June 2018.
2. Chan AW, Hrobjartsson A, Haahr MT, Gotzsche PC, Altman DG. Empirical evidence for selective reporting of outcomes in randomized trials: comparison of protocols to published articles. JAMA. 2004;291:2457–65.
3. Dwan K, Altman DG, Arnaiz JA, Bloom J, Chan A-W, Cronin E, et al. Systematic review of the empirical evidence of study publication Bias and outcome reporting Bias. PLoS One. 2008;3:e3081.
4. Silagy CA, Middleton P, Hopewell S. Publishing protocols of systematic reviews: comparing what was done to what was planned. JAMA. 2002;287:2831–4.
5. Moher D, Tetzlaff J, Tricco AC, Sampson M, Altman DG. Epidemiology and reporting characteristics of systematic reviews. PLoS Med. 2007;4:e78.
6. Moher D, Cook DJ, Eastwood S, Olkin I, Rennie D, Stroup DF. Improving the quality of reports of meta-analyses of randomised controlled trials: the QUOROM statement. Quality of reporting of meta-analyses. Lancet (Lond Engl). 1999;354:1896–900.
7. Liberati A, Altman DG, Tetzlaff J, Mulrow C, Gotzsche PC, Ioannidis JP, et al. The PRISMA statement for reporting systematic reviews and meta-analyses of studies that evaluate health care interventions: explanation and elaboration. PLoS Med. 2009;6:e1000100.
8. Moher D, Liberati A, Tetzlaff J, Altman DG. Preferred reporting items for systematic reviews and meta-analyses: the PRISMA statement. BMJ. 2009;339:b2535.
9. Joanna Briggs Institute. The Joanna Briggs Institute. 2017. http://joannabriggs.org/. Accessed 28 June 2018.
10. The Campbell Collaboration. Campbell collaboration: better evidence for a better world. 2017. https://www.campbellcollaboration.org/. Accessed 28 June 2018.
11. The Cochrane Collaboration. Cochrane. 2017. http://www.cochrane.org/. Accessed 28 June 2018.
12. Moher D, Stewart L, Shekelle P. Establishing a new journal for systematic review products. Syst Rev. 2012;1:1.

13. Moher D, Shamseer L, Clarke M, Ghersi D, Liberati A, Petticrew M, et al. Preferred reporting items for systematic review and meta-analysis protocols (PRISMA-P) 2015 statement. Syst Rev. 2015;4:1–9.
14. Shamseer L, Moher D, Clarke M, Ghersi D, Liberati A, Petticrew M, et al. Preferred reporting items for systematic review and meta-analysis protocols (PRISMA-P) 2015: elaboration & explanation. BMJ. 2015;349:g7647.
15. Smidt N, Rutjes AWS, Van der Windt D, Ostelo R, Bossuyt PM, Reitsma JB, et al. The quality of diagnostic accuracy studies since the STARD statement: has it improved? Neurology. 2006;67:792–7.
16. Noel-Storr AH, McCleery JM, Richard E, Ritchie CW, Flicker L, Cullum SJ, et al. Reporting standards for studies of diagnostic test accuracy in dementia: the STARDdem initiative. Neurology. 2014;83:364–73.
17. Kirkham JJ, Altman DG, Williamson PR. Bias due to changes in specified outcomes during the systematic review process. PLoS One. 2010;5:e9810.
18. Page MJ, McKenzie JE, Kirkham J, Dwan K, Kramer S, Green S, et al. Bias due to selective inclusion and reporting of outcomes and analyses in systematic reviews of randomised trials of healthcare interventions. Cochrane Database Syst Rev. 2014;(10):MR000035. https://doi.org/10.1002/14651858.MR000035.pub2. Accessed 28 June 2018.
19. Beller EM, Glasziou PP, Altman DG, Hopewell S, Bastian H, Chalmers I, et al. PRISMA for abstracts: reporting systematic reviews in journal and conference abstracts. PLoS Med. 2013;10:e1001419.
20. Tricco AC, Pham B, Brehaut J, Tetroe J, Cappelli M, Hopewell S, et al. An international survey indicated that unpublished systematic reviews exist. J Clin Epidemiol. 2009;62:617–23.e5.
21. Dwan K, Altman DG, Clarke M, Gamble C, Higgins JP, Sterne JA, et al. Evidence for the selective reporting of analyses and discrepancies in clinical trials: a systematic review of cohort studies of clinical trials. PLoS Med. 2014;11:e1001666.
22. Dwan K, Gamble C, Williamson PR, Kirkham JJ. Systematic review of the empirical evidence of study publication bias and outcome reporting bias—an updated review. PLoS One. 2013;8:e66844.
23. Tricco AC, Cogo E, Page MJ, Polisena J, Booth A, Dwan K, et al. A third of systematic reviews changed or did not specify the primary outcome: a PROSPERO register study. J Clin Epidemiol. 2016;79:46–54.
24. Ioannidis JPA, Greenland S, Hlatky MA, Khoury MJ, Macleod MR, Moher D, et al. Increasing value and reducing waste in research design, conduct, and analysis. Lancet. 2014;383:166–75.
25. Moher D. The problem of duplicate systematic reviews. BMJ. 2013;347:f5040.
26. Moher D, Booth A, Stewart L. How to reduce unnecessary duplication: use PROSPERO. BJOG. 2014;121:784–6.
27. Siontis KC, Hernandez-Boussard T, Ioannidis JPA. Overlapping meta-analyses on the same topic: survey of published studies. BMJ. 2013;347:f4501.
28. Centre for Reviews and Dissemination. PROSPERO International prospective register of systematic reviews. 2017. https://www.crd.york.ac.uk/PROSPERO/. Accessed 28 June 2018.
29. The PME. Best practice in systematic reviews: the importance of protocols and registration. PLoS Med. 2011;8:e1001009.
30. Viergever RF, Ghersi D. The quality of registration of clinical trials. PLoS One. 2011;6:e14701.
31. Centre for Open Science. Open science framework. 2017. https://osf.io/jsznk/register/565fb3678c5e4a66b5582f67. Accessed 28 June 2018.
32. Booth A, Clarke M, Ghersi D, Moher D, Petticrew M, Stewart L. An international registry of systematic-review protocols. The Lancet. 2011;377:108–9.
33. Booth A, Clarke M, Ghersi D, Moher D, Petticrew M, Stewart L. Establishing a minimum dataset for prospective registration of systematic reviews: an international consultation. PLoS One. 2011;6:e27319.
34. Booth A. PROSPERO's progress and activities 2012/13. Syst Rev. 2013;2:111.

35. Booth A, Clarke M, Dooley G, Ghersi D, Moher D, Petticrew M, et al. PROSPERO at one year: an evaluation of its utility. Syst Rev. 2013;2:4.
36. Booth A, Clarke M, Dooley G, Ghersi D, Moher D, Petticrew M, et al. The nuts and bolts of PROSPERO: an international prospective register of systematic reviews. Syst Rev. 2012;1:2.
37. Zhelev Z, Garside R, Hyde C. A qualitative study into the difficulties experienced by healthcare decision makers when reading a Cochrane diagnostic test accuracy review. Syst Rev. 2013;2:32.
38. Borah R, Brown AW, Capers PL, Kaiser KA. Analysis of the time and workers needed to conduct systematic reviews of medical interventions using data from the PROSPERO registry. BMJ Open. 2017;7:e012545.
39. Pennant M, Wisniewski S, Hyde C, Davenport C, Deeks JJ, Cochrane Diagnostic Test Accuracy Editorial T, editors. A tool to improve efficiency and quality in the production of protocols for Cochrane Reviews of Diagnostic Test Accuracy. 19th Cochrane Colloquium; 2011; Madrid, Spain.
40. van Enst WA, Scholten RJ, Whiting P, Zwinderman AH, Hooft L. Meta-epidemiologic analysis indicates that MEDLINE searches are sufficient for diagnostic test accuracy systematic reviews. J Clin Epidemiol. 2014;67:1192–9.
41. Rice DB, Kloda LA, Levis B, Qi B, Kingsland E, Thombs BD. Are MEDLINE searches sufficient for systematic reviews and meta-analyses of the diagnostic accuracy of depression screening tools? A review of meta-analyses. J Psychosom Res. 2016;87:7–13.
42. Preston L, Carroll C, Gardois P, Paisley S, Kaltenthaler E. Improving search efficiency for systematic reviews of diagnostic test accuracy: an exploratory study to assess the viability of limiting to MEDLINE, EMBASE and reference checking. Syst Rev. 2015;4:82.
43. Leeflang MM, Deeks JJ, Takwoingi Y, Macaskill P. Cochrane diagnostic test accuracy reviews. Syst Rev. 2013;2:82.
44. Glanville J, Cikalo M, Crawford F, Dozier M, McIntosh H. Handsearching did not yield additional unique FDG-PET diagnostic test accuracy studies compared with electronic searches: a preliminary investigation. Res Synth Methods. 2012;3:202–13.
45. Agency for Healthcare Research and Quality. Systematic reviews data register (SRDR). 2017. https://srdr.ahrq.gov/. Accessed 28 June 2018.
46. Barbic D, Chenkin J, Cho D, Jelic T. Point-of-care ultrasonography for the diagnosis of abscess in patients presenting with skin and soft tissue infections to the emergency department. PROSPERO 2015 CRD42015017115. www.crd.york.ac.uk/PROSPERO/display_record.php?ID=CRD42015017115. Accessed 28 June 2018.
47. Smith T, Daniell A, Geere J, Toms A, Hing C. The diagnostic accuracy of MRI for rotator cuff tears: a systematic review and meta-analysis. PROSPERO. 2011;CRD42011001283. www.crd.york.ac.uk/PROSPERO/display_record.php?ID=CRD42011001283. Accessed 28 June 2018.
48. Centre for Reviews and Dissemination. Clinical tests. In: Systematic reviews: CRD's guidance for undertaking reviews in health care. York: University of York; 2009. www.york.ac.uk/inst/crd/index_guidance.htm. Accessed 28 June 2018.
49. Deeks JJ. Systematic reviews of evaluations of diagnostic and screening tests. BMJ. 2001;323:157–62.
50. Deeks JJ, Bossuyt PM, Gatsonis C, editors. Cochrane handbook for systematic reviews of diagnostic test accuracy Version 1.0.0. The Cochrane Collaboration; 2013. srdta.cochrane.org. Accessed 28 June 2018.
51. Whiting PF, Rutjes AW, Westwood ME, Mallett S, Deeks JJ, Reitsma JB, et al. QUADAS-2: a revised tool for the quality assessment of diagnostic accuracy studies. Ann Intern Med. 2011;155:529–36.
52. The Joanna Briggs Institute critical appraisal tools for use in JBI systematic reviews: checklist for diagnostic test accuracy studies. 2016. http://joannabriggs.org/research/critical-appraisal-tools.html. Accessed 28 June 2018.
53. Riemsma R, Al M, Deshpande S, Ramos IC, Armstrong N, Lee Y-C, et al. A systematic review and economic evaluation of SeHCAT (Tauroselcholic [75Selenium] acid) for the

investigation of bile acid malabsorption (BAM) and measurement of bile acid pool loss. PROSPERO. 2012:CRD42012001911. www.crd.york.ac.uk/PROSPERO/display_record.php?ID=CRD42012001911. Accessed 28 June 2018.

54. Smith TO, Daniell H, Geere J-A, Toms AP, Hing CB. The diagnostic accuracy of MRI for the detection of partial- and full-thickness rotator cuff tears in adults. Magn Reson Imaging. 2012;30:336–46.
55. van Enst W, Ochodo E, Scholten RJ, Hooft L, Leeflang MM. Investigation of publication bias in meta-analyses of diagnostic test accuracy: a meta-epidemiological study. BMC Med Res Methodol. 2014;14:70.
56. Begg CB, Mazumdar M. Operating characteristics of a rank correlation test for publication bias. Biometrics. 1994;50:1088–101.
57. Deeks JJ, Macaskill P, Irwig L. The performance of tests of publication bias and other sample size effects in systematic reviews of diagnostic test accuracy was assessed. J Clin Epidemiol. 2005;58:882–93.
58. Egger M, Davey Smith G, Schneider M, Minder C. Bias in meta-analysis detected by a simple, graphical test. BMJ. 1997;315:629–34.

Searching for Diagnostic Test Accuracy Studies

7

Su Golder and Julie Glanville

7.1 Introduction

This chapter describes methods used to search for studies to inform systematic reviews of diagnostic test accuracy (DTA). Literature searching is a key component of any review [1–3], and an information professional should be involved from the proposal stage, to check that the review has not already been carried out, estimate the volume of literature through scoping searches and help to develop the review question. To be useful to decision makers and to minimise some of the effects of publication bias [4, 5], reviews should aim to be as comprehensive as possible under the constraints of time, other resources and the difficulties of identifying some data (such as unpublished studies, manufacturers' data, documents in languages other than English or older studies). In addition, the methods used to conduct the systematic review, including the methods used to conduct the searches, should be robust, reproducible and transparent, to enable readers to assess the quality of the review and to update it if required.

Searching for DTA studies is particularly challenging. Although a number of research projects [6–9] have attempted to develop a search filter with an appropriate level of sensitivity to consistently identify DTA studies, none have as yet been successful because studies tend to be inadequately reported, authors do not use consistent terminology to describe DTA studies, suitable indexing terms may be absent in some databases and sometimes, where indexing terms are available, indexers may not have not assigned them appropriately [10]. These challenges reinforce the need for researchers to involve a healthcare librarian or information specialist from the

S. Golder (✉)
Department of Health Sciences, University of York, York, UK
e-mail: su.golder@york.ac.uk

J. Glanville
York Health Economics Consortium, University of York, York, UK
e-mail: julie.glanville@york.ac.uk

G. Biondi-Zoccai (ed.), *Diagnostic Meta-Analysis*,
https://doi.org/10.1007/978-3-319-78966-8_7

outset when planning a systematic review, to inform the selection of relevant and appropriate resources to search and to achieve effective search strategies.

7.2 Searching for Diagnostic Test Accuracy Systematic Reviews

One of the first steps in a systematic review should be a thorough search for published reviews and ongoing protocols addressing the researcher's question to ensure that a new review is required. This search is undertaken to avoid unplanned duplication of existing research and to identify information to inform the new review, such as relevant studies (see section on reference checking below). There may even be cases where a review is identified which is suitable for updating. There are a number of resources which may help with identifying published systematic reviews:

The Cochrane Database of Systematic Reviews (CDSR) can be searched via the Cochrane Library at http://www.cochranelibrary.com. This database contains the protocols and full text of all Cochrane reviews and protocols including all Cochrane Systematic Reviews of Diagnostic Test Accuracy. At the time of going to press, there were 70 full reviews (including 6 updates) and 97 protocols of DTA reviews published in the Cochrane Library (Issue 11, 2016).

Epistemonikos is a wider collection of systematic reviews, and it also lists the primary studies included in the reviews. It is available at http://www.epistemonikos.org/en/ and is searchable via the Cochrane Library at http://www.cochranelibrary.com.

The Health Technology Assessment (HTA) database is available via the Centre for Reviews and Dissemination (CRD) website (https://www.crd.york.ac.uk/CRDWeb/). This database contains over 1000 systematic reviews of diagnostic evaluations. The records in this database are quite brief and few have abstracts, so searches need to be sensitive and use synonyms, ideally focusing on the target condition only. In addition individual Health Technology Assessment (HTA) agency websites may be explored for diagnostic test guidance, for example, National Institute for Health and Care Excellence (NICE) guidance is available at https://www.nice.org.uk/guidance/published?type=dg.

The Centre for Reviews and Dissemination (CRD) also used to produce DARE (Database of Abstracts of Reviews of Effects) and its archive (covering DTA reviews published 1994 to March 2015) is still searchable via the CRD website at https://www.crd.york.ac.uk/CRDWeb/.

The Aggressive Research Intelligence Facility (ARIF) database is produced by the Department of Public Health, Epidemiology and Biostatistics at the University of Birmingham, UK, and is available at http://www.birmingham.ac.uk/research/activity/mds/projects/HaPS/PHEB/ARIF/databases/index.aspx. About 2000 DTA reviews and reviews of screening studies are included in this database. The records in this database are quite brief and few have abstracts, so searches need to be sensitive and use synonyms, ideally focusing on the target condition only. If the volume of records retrieved is too large, then the results could be combined with 'diagnosis OR diagnostic' in the Keywords field.

TRIP is a search engine at https://www.tripdatabase.com/ which contains research evidence from numerous sources including PubMed and Cochrane and includes some coverage of diagnostics.

PDQ Evidence is a collection of systematic reviews specifically about health systems and also includes the primary studies from these reviews. Despite its focus on health systems, it does contain DTA reviews (see http://www.pdq-evidence.org/).

In addition to databases focusing on systematic reviews, major biomedical bibliographic databases, such as MEDLINE or Embase, can be searched to identify DTA systematic reviews. There are a number of search strategies or search filters to identify systematic reviews that may assist with this process. Filters to identify systematic reviews can be found on the UK InterTASC Information Specialists Subgroup (ISSG) Search Filter Resource (https://sites.google.com/a/york.ac.uk/issg-search-filters-resource/filters-to-identify-systematic-reviews). Each filter will have been designed for a specific database and search interface, and with specific objectives in mind, so filters should be chosen and used with care. Critical appraisal tools are available to help assess the quality of search filters and are listed on the Filter Resource website (https://sites.google.com/a/york.ac.uk/issg-search-filters-resource/critical-appraisal-of-search-filters).

In addition to searching for published systematic reviews, a search of the international prospective register of systematic reviews in health and social care (PROSPERO) will help to establish whether there are any ongoing or unpublished systematic reviews that address the research question. PROSPERO is freely available to search on the CRD website http://www.crd.york.ac.uk/PROSPERO/.

Once it has been established that the research question does require a new or updated review, the systematic review protocol can be developed. A search strategy specifying the databases and additional resources to be searched and the likely search terms to be used to search those resources is an essential part of the protocol. PRISMA-P can facilitate the development and reporting of the systematic review protocol [11].

7.3 Searching for DTA Studies to Populate a Diagnostic Test Accuracy Review

7.3.1 Resources

It is generally recommended that searches for diagnostic test accuracy studies should search resources beyond MEDLINE to ensure coverage of journals not indexed by this database. As MEDLINE only indexes journals, other publication types such as conference abstracts, reports and dissertations need to be identified using other databases. Even where journals are indexed MEDLINE, records can be missed by specific strategies because of the reasons noted in the introduction to this chapter. Cochrane and other health technology assessment organisations currently recommend that in addition to MEDLINE and searches for other systematic reviews, searches should be conducted in Embase [10, 12–15].

Case studies have shown that searching bibliographic databases other than MEDLINE can retrieve additional relevant studies to those identified in MEDLINE including Science Citation Index (SCI) (available as part of Web of Science), BIOSIS Previews and LILACS (Literatura Latino Americana em Ciências da Saúde) [15]. Whilst three recent analyses have suggested that fewer databases might be adequate, an analysis of ten meta-analyses found that only using studies indexed in MEDLINE did not impact significantly on the sensitivity and specificity estimates of the meta-analyses in those reviews [16]. However, this research was based on known-item searches of MEDLINE: review searches may not detect all the records in MEDLINE that might be relevant to a review, so searching other databases provides opportunities to retrieve (MEDLINE indexed) studies by other routes. Another recent study of nine reviews performed by a single research group found that the reviewers' original searches would have found 85% of their included studies from MEDLINE and Embase (range: 60–100%) [17]. And another study of 16 meta-analyses found that MEDLINE searches alone may capture 91% of all eligible studies [18]. The research, however, has been inconclusive as to the actual value of sources other than MEDLINE. The variability in these results suggests that decisions should be based per individual review depending on the subject area and ease of searching and accepted levels of sensitivity. When developing the literature search for a DTA review, generic databases (such as MEDLINE and Embase) should be considered along with subject-specific databases such as CINAHL and PsycINFO, dependent on the test being reviewed.

Searchers usually choose a large bibliographic database, such as MEDLINE or Embase, as a starting point for searching. However, Embase may be the best database within which to develop a search for DTA studies, particularly for more recent tests. Embase introduced the check tag/publication type 'diagnostic test accuracy study' on 1 December 2010 and was therefore the first of the major electronic medical literature databases to introduce a specific indexing term for DTA studies. As of 18 January 2017, 69,600 records in Embase have the check tag 'diagnostic test accuracy study'. The performance of this check tag, in terms of sensitivity and precision, is unknown, but it can be recommended for scoping searches and as part of a multistranded search approach (see below).

Literature searching to identify DTA studies for inclusion in a systematic review may involve a range of activities in addition to searching bibliographic databases. These activities can include checking reference lists, citation searching, searching for conference abstracts and grey literature, contacting experts and manufacturers, and handsearching [1, 3, 10, 19].

Checking the reference lists of primary studies (particularly those identified for inclusion in the review) and the reference lists of published existing reviews has been shown to be useful in finding DTA studies [15, 20, 21].

Citation searching, which begins with a set of known journal articles, or key authors, and identifies further journal articles that have cited those known articles, has been found to be a useful technique to supplement database searching for DTA studies [15]. Citation searching is available through a number of subscription-only resources, such as Science Citation Index (SCI), Social Science Citation Index (SSCI) and Scopus, as well as freely available resources such as Google Scholar http://scholar.google.co.uk/.

Usually reviewers will try to identify unpublished (or 'grey') materials, such as theses and conference presentations or information that might only be available via the Internet such as reports and presentations. Such publications can be identified by searching databases that focus on specific kinds of publication, such as dissertations (e.g. ProQuest Dissertations and Theses Databases) or conferences (e.g. ISI Proceedings). For some topics it may be beneficial to identify the conference proceedings of specific organisations and browse programmes or conference abstracts online. Unpublished documents can also be identified by scanning the websites of relevant organisations such as those of the test manufacturer, national regulatory and reimbursement bodies and research centres [22, 23].

Sometimes researchers may carry out general Internet searches using a search engine such as Google or Google Scholar. This approach has the potential for retrieving an unmanageable number of records, and searches may also be challenging to reproduce. To cope with these issues, the review team may choose to scan a predefined number of the records resulting from Internet searches [24, 25]. This method should be used as a supplement to other forms of searching.

The proportion of ongoing trials investigating diagnostic test accuracy is relatively low [26]. However, trial registries are an increasingly useful resource of information as many records incorporate the results of trials or references to the results and can provide detailed information on the conduct of the DTA study. Trial registries include ClinicalTrials.gov. The key gateway to clinical trial registry databases is the WHO International Clinical Trials Registry Platform (ICTRP) (www.who.int/ictrp/). Useful links to registries can be found at https://sites.google.com/a/york.ac.uk/yhectrialsregisters/. New initiatives to improve access to trial data include OpenTrials (http://opentrials.net/) and AllTrials (http://www.alltrials.net/). The importance of registries and other resources for unpublished data is found on the AllTrials site (http://www.alltrials.net/).

7.4 Searching Bibliographic Databases Such as MEDLINE and Embase

7.4.1 Search Strategies

The search strategies used with bibliographic databases such as MEDLINE and Embase need to reflect the research question being asked and may sometimes be complex. Search strategies should, where databases permit, contain both thesaurus/indexing terms and 'free text' terms for maximum sensitivity. For example, MEDLINE records are assigned subject index terms from the Medical Subject Headings (MeSH) thesaurus (a controlled hierarchical set of keywords) so that records about a topic theoretically receive the same MeSH no matter how the authors have chosen to describe their work. Embase has its own thesaurus called Emtree. Some databases (such as Science Citation Index (SCI)) do not have a thesaurus (or controlled vocabulary), but do provide the keywords that the authors have added to the records. Other databases have no controlled vocabulary at all.

Free text terms are usually the words in the title and abstract fields, but may also include author, keywords and other information from other fields, which may vary by database. When developing a search strategy, searchers should usually include synonyms, spelling variants and abbreviations of the free text terms of interest. Within Embase there are additional specific fields, such as .dm. (device manufacturer) and .dv. (device trade name) which can be useful additional access points when searching, particularly for very new diagnostic technologies.

The searcher's objective is to create a search strategy with a high degree of sensitivity to ensure that as many potentially relevant records as possible are identified from the searches, with as few irrelevant records as possible. Unfortunately, achieving this objective is often difficult due to inconsistent terminology in the title and abstracts of records, the absence of appropriate indexing terms in some databases and inconsistently applied indexing terms. The search strategy will also need to be adapted to suit the requirements of the search interface for each database or resource selected.

As well as the search terms, a search strategy needs a structure. This is developed from the review question. A DTA review question needs to be broken down into its component parts (or concepts) which are usually expressed in the review eligibility criteria for the included studies. In DTA reviews the component parts or key concepts are usually:

- The study participants (P)
- The index test (I)
- The comparator tests/reference standard
- The target condition (T) being diagnosed
- The types of studies [10]

A good example of a search strategy can be found in the Cochrane Handbook for Systematic Reviews of Diagnostic Test Accuracy chapter on searching for studies [10] shown in Table 7.1. This strategy has three concepts: the index test, the target condition and the patient population.

The search should reflect or contain at least some of the key concepts, but it is unlikely, and usually undesirable, to reflect all of these concepts. It is usually best to start off with identifying the smallest yielding concept, which is also likely to be the most specific concept. Often this will be the index test. Only if the search results for the index test are too large to process should additional concepts be added to the strategy. The most likely additional concept to be included in the strategy, if needed, is the target condition (clinical disorder or disease stage being diagnosed). If the results of a strategy structured as index test AND target condition are too numerous to process, then a further concept may be added. Additional concepts might include sets of terms for the patient population (such as children or women) or the reference standard (usually the best available test or test strategy).

Search terms that capture the diagnostic test are likely to include both general terms (such as dipstick) and specific terms (such as named dipsticks, e.g. Multistix). MeSH or Emtree subheadings (sometimes called qualifiers) may also be useful. The MeSH subheading 'diagnosis' can be used either as a floating subheading (not attached to any indexing term) or as an attached subheading, for example, attached to the indexing term for the index test or the target condition. For example, in Ovid MEDLINE 'Exp urinary tract infections/di' identifies records where the 'diagnosis' subheading has been attached to the condition

Table 7.1 Demonstration search strategy for PubMed (MEDLINE), for the topic 'Clinical assessment for diagnosing congenital heart disease in newborn infants with Down syndrome'

Search terms	Notes
('Physical Examination'[MeSH Terms] OR 'Electrocardiography'[MeSH Terms:noexp] OR 'Oximetry'[MeSH Terms:noexp] OR auscultat*[tw] OR palpat*[tw] OR electrocardiogra*[tw] OR ECG[tw] OR pulse[tw] OR oximet*[tw] OR (chest[tw] AND (radiogra*[tw] OR roentgenogra*[tw] OR x-ray*[tw] OR xray*[tw])) OR (thora*[tw] AND (radiogra*[tw] OR roentgenogra*[tw] OR x-ray*[tw] OR xray*[tw])) OR (physical*[tw] AND (examin*[tw] OR assess*[tw] OR sign[tw] OR signs[tw])) OR (clinical*[tw] AND (examin*[tw] OR assess*[tw] OR sign[tw] OR signs[tw])))	Index test(s) set
AND	
('Heart Defects, Congenital'[MeSH Terms] OR (congenital*[tw] **AND** (cardia*[tw] OR cardiol*[tw] OR cardiovasc*[tw])) OR (congenital*[tw] AND (cardia*[tw] OR cardiol*[tw] OR cardiovasc*[tw])) OR (congenital*[tw] AND heart[tw]) OR (septal[tw] AND defect*[tw]) OR (septum[tw] AND defect*[tw]) OR AVSD[tw] OR VSD[tw] OR 'patent ductus arteriosus'[tw] OR 'Eisenmenger syndrome'[tw] OR 'Eisenmengers syndrome'[tw] OR 'Eisenmenger's syndrome'[tw] OR (tetralogy[tw] AND fallot[tw]))	Target condition set
AND	
('Infant, Newborn'[MeSH Terms] OR neonate*[tw] OR newborn*[tw] OR baby[tw] OR babies[tw]) AND ('Down Syndrome'[MeSH Terms] OR 'Down syndrome'[tw] OR 'Downs syndrome'[tw] OR 'Down's syndrome'[tw] OR 'trisomy 21'[tw])	Patient description set

[MeSH Terms] restricts the search to Medical Subject Headings and automatically 'explodes' the term to include all the more specific terms associated with it
[MeSH Terms:noexp] restricts the search to Medical Subject Headings but does not 'explode' the term
[tw] searches text words across the record included in the title, abstract
MeSH, Publication Types or Substance Names
* is the truncation symbol used to retrieve variant endings

indexing term 'urinary tract infections', whereas 'di.fs' identifies any records where the subheading 'diagnosis' appears, no matter to which indexing term it has been attached. Other MeSH subheadings are available. In December 2016, NLM introduced the new MeSH subheading '/diagnostic imaging', which replaced deleted subheadings: /radiography, /radionuclide imaging and /ultrasonography. However, subheadings tend to be inconsistently applied so they should be used with caution.

The challenges of constructing search strategies for some DTA reviews has led to the use of multistranded strategies when trying to find records for challenging or complex topics. Instead of a single concept combination, a series of concept combinations might be developed to capture the various ways that records express the topic of interest. For example, multiple different approaches could be run sequentially and then combined using the OR operator. Using the concepts (rather than actual search terms), an example might be as follows:

1. Index test AND condition
2. Condition AND reference standard
3. Index test AND diagnostic test accuracy terms (search filters)
4. 1 OR 2 OR 3

This approach allows for the cautious use of DTA search filters in approach 3. Despite the availability of search filters designed to capture DTA studies, review evidence suggests that the performance of these filters is inconsistent and that using such filters is likely to result in an unacceptable proportion of relevant studies being missed without significantly reducing the number of studies that have to be assessed [6]. Using DTA filters (https://sites.google.com/a/york.ac.uk/issg-search-filters-resource/filters-for-diagnostic-test-accuracy-studies) in multistranded approaches is seen as a useful extra option, since they are not the only approach being used. Table 7.2 shows an example of a multistranded search strategy used in practice to identify diagnostic test accuracy studies for diagnosing urinary tract infections in children.

Overall, the effort and time involved in developing and carrying out an extensive and robust search to identify studies for inclusion in a DTA systematic review can be considerable. Developing the strategy may involve several iterations. Random samples of results from search strategy drafts should be assessed for relevance to provide estimations of sensitivity, and the retrieval performance of a strategy can be tested by checking whether strategies find known relevant records. Any limits that are applied to

Table 7.2 Example of a multistranded search strategy in Ovid MEDLINE [27]

Search terms	Notes
1 exp urinary tract infections/ 2 bacterial infections/ or exp pseudomonas infections/ or exp klebsiella infections/ or gram negative infections/ or exp escherichia coli/ or exp proteus/ or exp enterococcus/ 3 exp Staphylococcus/ 4 exp leukocytes/ 5 (microbial infection? or bacterial infection?).ti,ab. 6 (urinary or urine or urethra or bladder or ureter? or kidney or kidneys or renal).ti,ab. 7 exp urinary tract/ 8 or/2–5 9 or/6–7 10 8 and 9 11 1 or 10	Target condition terms: urinary tract infections Line 1 is the very specific MeSH for the topic Lines 2–5 are MeSH and title and abstract words that capture the concept of infections as well as bacteria involved in the infections Lines 6–7 are search terms related to the urinary tract The infections and urinary tract terms are combined in set 10 The results of set 1 and set 10 are gathered together in set 11
12 exp child, preschool/ or exp infant/ 13 (infant? or baby or babies or toddler? or preschooler?).ti,ab. 14 or/12–13	Patient description set: children These search lines use MeSH and title and abstract words to capture records which report research in children
15 11 and 14	Target condition set AND Patient description set This seeks to identify records that report urinary tract infections in children

Table 7.2 (continued)

Search terms	Notes
16 (risk assessment? or exam or examination or feeding or slow weight gain or fever or vomiting or diarrh?).ti,ab. 17 (((sepsis or failure) adj2 thrive) or malaise or frequent urination or abdominal discomfort or abdominal pain).ti,ab. 18 (delayed bladder control or dysuria or (pain adj3 urination) or painful urination or difficult urination). ti,ab. 19 (urinalysis or urine analysis or urine sample? or urine specimen? or (urine adj3 collect?)).ti,ab. 20 (urine bags or dipstick? or dip stick? or urine microscopy).ti,ab. 21 (reagent strip? or colorimetric test? or gas analysis or impedance or luminescence).ti,ab. 22 (immunological test? or elisa or enzyme test? or bacterial oxygen consumption or turbidimetry or urine culture).ti,ab. 23 (bacterial culture or dipslide? or renal ultrasonography or planar imaging or radiography or urography or pyelography or kub or bladder imaging).ti,ab. 24 (cystography or cystourethrography or nuclear medicine or scintigraphy or cystogram?).ti,ab. 25 exp physical examination/ or exp fever/ or exp body weight changes/ or exp abdominal pain/ or exp urological manifestations/ or failure to thrive/ 26 exp vomiting/ or diarrhea/ or exp sepsis/ or urinalysis/ 27 exp microscopy/ or exp "indicators and reagents"/ 28 colorimetry/ or electric impedance/ or exp immunoassay/ or exp fluorescent antibody technique/ 29 exp diagnostic imaging/ 30 exp nuclear medicine/ or exp cystoscopy/ or exp diagnostic techniques, urological/ 31 or/16–30	Index test(s) set: symptoms and signs of infection as well as diagnostic processes and tools These search lines (all gathered together in line 31) look for general and specific search terms suggesting or reporting that diagnosis may have been undertaken
32 15 and 31	Target condition set AND Patient description set AND Index test(s) set. These records contain terms from all three concepts. Diagnosis of urinary tract infections in children
33 vesico-ureteral reflux/ or pyelonephritis/ or bacteriuria/ or cystitis/	These terms are further MeSH terms indicative of urinary tract infection

(continued)

Table 7.2 (continued)

Search terms	Notes
34 (failure adj2 thrive).ti,ab. 35 sepsis.tw. 36 ultrasonography.ti,ab. 37 exp succimer/ or exp organometallic compounds/ or technetium/ or exp sulfhydryl compounds/ or exp culture media/ 38 urinary catheterization/ or ammonium chloride/ or c-reactive protein/ or urodynamics/ or urine/mi 39 (dmsa or urogram? or ultrasound? or (renal adj scan?)).ti,ab. 40 (spect or (planar adj image?) or (dip adj slide?) or cystoscopy).ti,ab. 41 ((bladder adj aspiration) or (acidification adj test?) or (cortical adj echogenicity)).ti,ab. 42 workup.ti,ab. 43 (radiographic or cystomanometry).ti,ab. 44 (bladder adj3 (investigat? or detect?)).ti,ab. 45 (kidney adj3 (investigat? or detect?)).ti,ab. 46 (urethra adj3 (investigat? or detect?)).ti,ab. 47 (renal adj3 (investigat? or detect?)).ti,ab. 48 (kidneys adj3 (investigat? or detect?)).ti,ab. 49 (urinary adj3 (investigat? or detect?)).ti,ab.	These terms and words in close proximity form another set of search terms indicative of the presence of infection or causes of infection or diagnosing urinary tract infection These records are all gathered into a set in line 54
50 (infection? adj3 (urinary or urine or urethra or bladder or ureter? or kidney or kidneys or renal)).ti,ab.	This search looks for words in close proximity that suggest urinary tract infections
51 (2 or 3 or 4 or 33) and 7	This gathers records which report bacterial infections in the urinary tract (set 7)
52 1 or 50 or 51	This set gathers together the records which are most explicit about urinary tract infections
53 52 and 14	This combines the urinary tract infection records with children
54 or/34–49	These terms and words in close proximity to search terms indicative of the presence of infection or causes of infection or diagnosing urinary tract infection
55 53 and 54	This line combines urinary tract infections in children with other terms indicative of the presence of infection or causes of infection or diagnosing urinary tract infection
56 55 OR 32	This line selects records from two strands together: (a) Urinary tract infections in children with other terms indicative of the presence of infection or causes of infection or diagnosing urinary tract infection (b) Diagnosis of urinary tract infections in children

searches need to be applied with caution, and the trade-offs of applying them should be described in the search methods. Even in cases where limits have to be made for resource issues, it is still possible to provide information on the impact of the limit. For example, even when translation services are unavailable, it can be preferable to not limit the search strategies by language, so that an indication to the size of the literature that has been missed can be presented along with a list of potentially relevant studies. Evidence suggests that all search strategies should be peer reviewed before use [28]. The PRESS (Peer Review of Electronic Search Strategies) tool can assist with structured peer review of search strategies [29], and we note that the search strategies of all Cochrane DTA reviews are peer reviewed. This process has potential for enormous benefit when errors are detected and corrected and additional key terms are identified.

In time, improvements in reporting and indexing and in search interfaces should enable more effective searching. This is likely to be one of the results of the increased advocacy for and uptake of reporting guidance such as STARD which encourages more informative reporting of study methods (http://www.stard-statement.org/) [30].

7.5 Managing References/Libraries

It is usual practice to search several databases to take account of differences in publication and topic coverage and also to compensate for poor or inconsistent indexing that can result in a search strategy failing to identify relevant records [1–3, 19]. Inevitably this approach leads to some records being identified multiple times from several databases, but duplicates can usually be identified and removed using bibliographic software. Bibliographic management software such as EndNote, Reference Manager, ProCite, RefWorks and Mendeley can be used to load, store, deduplicate and record references from searches of individual databases and non-database resources. These software can also be used to record screening decisions on the inclusion and exclusion of records and details of papers ordered and received. Using one of these software packages makes it quicker and easier to locate references, produce data required for publication (such as the numbers of records retrieved and screened) and create a list of included and excluded studies. These records may also enable production of a flow diagram as recommended by reporting guidance such as the Preferred Reporting Items for Systematic Reviews and Meta-Analysis (PRISMA) statement [31].

Another advantage of bibliographic management software packages is that they usually interface with word processing packages so that bibliographies/reference lists for reports can be created easily in a choice of citation styles. In addition, the export options from bibliographic management software means that records can be exported and loaded into other software packages such as Covidence or Access, where screening and further record management can be undertaken.

7.6 Updating Literature Searches

Depending on the timescale and scope of the review, it may be appropriate to include an update of the literature searches towards the end of the project to check for recent relevant papers. The value of this is not just to find studies which have been added to the databases since the search but also to find records which have been indexed or reindexed since the original search.

We recommend for systematic review purposes that, since database interfaces may not offer easy or consistent update search options and since records that are reindexed in databases might be missed if date limits are applied, an update search should involve a full rerun of the original search (for the complete time period). Results can then be loaded into the original reference library and duplicates removed, enabling new records to be identified and processed.

7.7 Current Awareness

Setting up current awareness alerts can help reviewers to identify research published after the initial searches. Automated email alerts from specified journal titles and RSS feeds from databases or websites can be set up easily. Researchers should be aware that there is likely to be a high level of duplication in the records received so it is good practice to check whether records have been identified by previous searches before adding to the project's reference library.

7.8 Documenting the Search

The search process should be reported in such a way that it is reproducible and transparent to the reader and so that searchers are able to re-run or update the searches [1–3, 10, 19]. To ensure the search is reproducible, key items of information need to be recorded:

- names of the resources searched and the platform/interface used (some databases are available from multiple providers)
- dates when searches were executed
- full search strategies used
- database date ranges searched
- numbers of records retrieved [1–3, 19]

Guidelines on reporting standards of systematic reviews are available. Examples include MECIR (Methodological standards for the conduct of Cochrane Intervention Reviews) and PRISMA (Preferred Reporting Items for Systematic Reviews and Meta-Analysis) (and at the time of going to press there is a PRISMA-DTA and the PRISMA-S (PRISMA-Search) extension in development http://www.prisma-statement.org/Extensions/InDevelopment.aspx and http://www.equator-network.org/wp-content/uploads/2009/02/Protocol-PRISMA-S-Delphi.pdf). Literature search reporting in these guidelines focuses on reporting the full search strategy and providing a full listing of the information resources (database and non-database) searched.

Since many journals now offer authors the facility to submit online appendices and supplementary material, it is usually possible to provide full search strategies for all of the searches to enhance transparency and replicability. Journal editors encourage adherence to systematic review reporting guidelines.

Examples of search reports are provided in guides such as the *Cochrane Handbook* [2], the *DTA Handbook* [10] and *Systematic Reviews: CRD's Guidance for Undertaking Systematic Reviews in Health Care* [19].

7.9 Quality Assessment of the Search

Before submitting a review for publication it should be checked to ensure that it meets reporting requirements (PRISMA), and these include aspects that relate to the searches. A useful check may also be to assess the review using a tool to assess the methodological quality of systematic reviews, including the search process, such as AMSTAR (Assessment of Multiple Systematic Reviews) [32] and ROBIS tool to assess risk of bias in systematic reviews [33].

7.10 Keeping Up to Date

The methods of searching for DTA studies are constantly being evaluated and improved. To keep up to date with the current recommendations, we recommend visiting the diagnostic test accuracy chapter within SuRe Info (Summarized Research in Information Retrieval for HTA) web resource [14] which is updated every 6 months and the Cochrane Handbook for DTA Reviews (http://methods.cochrane.org/sdt/handbook-dta-reviews) (which is updated less frequently).

The National Institute for Health and Care Excellence (NICE) (https://www.nice.org.uk/about/what-we-do/our-programmes/nice-guidance/nice-diagnostics-guidance) and other health technology assessment agencies review diagnostic tests and their methods guidance and websites are also useful to check regularly for new advice and methods.

7.11 Summary

Identifying diagnostic studies suitable for inclusion in a systematic review is a fundamental step to ensure the validity of the review findings in terms of minimising publication bias or similar threats to accuracy. Since there are no dedicated databases of diagnostic test accuracy studies, a range of databases should be searched.

The search should contain concepts for the index test and possibly the target condition. Search filters to identify diagnostic test accuracy studies are not recommended, except when used in multistranded searches.

Searching for studies is challenging and often complex and early collaboration with an information specialist is recommended to achieve searches that best reflect the review requirements.

Acknowledgements We would like to thank Kath Wright, CRD, and Kate Misso, Kleijnen Systematic Reviews Ltd for comments on an earlier draft.

Funding None.

References

1. EUnetHTA—European network for Health Technology Assessment. Process of information retrieval for systematic reviews and health technology assessments on clinical effectiveness. Belgium: European network for Health Technology Assessment; 2015.
2. Higgins J, Green S, editors. Cochrane Handbook for Systematic Reviews of Interventions Version 5.1.0 [updated March 2011]: The Cochrane Collaboration, 2011. www.cochrane-handbook.org. Accessed 28 June 2018.
3. Institute of Medicine. Finding what works in health care: standards for systematic reviews. Washington, DC: The National Academies Press; 2011.
4. Cohen JF, Korevaar DA, Wang J, Leeflang MM, Bossuyt PM. Meta-epidemiologic study showed frequent time trends in summary estimates from meta-analyses of diagnostic accuracy studies. J Clin Epidemiol. 2016;77:60–7.
5. Korevaar DA, van Es N, Zwinderman AH, Cohen JF, Bossuyt PM. Time to publication among completed diagnostic accuracy studies: associated with reported accuracy estimates. BMC Med Res Methodol. 2016;16:68.
6. Beynon R, Leeflang MM, McDonald S, Eisinga A, Mitchell RL, Whiting P, Glanville JM. Search strategies to identify diagnostic accuracy studies in MEDLINE and EMBASE. Cochrane Database of Syst Rev. 2013;MR000022.
7. Leeflang MMG, Scholten RJ, Rutjes AWS, Reitsma JB, Bossuyt PM. Use of methodological search filters to identify diagnostic accuracy studies can lead to the omission of relevant studies. J Clin Epidemiol. 2006;59:234–40.
8. Ritchie G, Glanville J, Lefebvre C. Do published search filters to identify diagnostic test accuracy studies perform adequately? Health Inf Libr J. 2007;24:188–92.
9. Whiting P, Westwood M, Beynon R, Burke M, Sterne JA, Glanville J. Inclusion of methodological filters in searches for diagnostic test accuracy studies misses relevant studies. J Clin Epidemiol. 2011;64:602–7.
10. de Vet HCW, Eisinga A, Riphagen II, Aertgeerts B, Pewsner D. Chapter 7: searching for studies. In: Cochrane handbook for systematic reviews of diagnostic test accuracy version 0.4 [updated September 2008]: The Cochrane Collaboration; 2008.
11. Moher D, Shamseer L, Clarke M, Ghersi D, Liberati A, Petticrew M, Shekelle P, Stewart LA. Preferred reporting items for systematic review and meta-analysis protocols (PRISMA-P) 2015 statement. Syst Rev. 2015;4:1.
12. Fraser C, Mowatt G, Siddiqui R, Burr J. Searching for diagnostic test accuracy studies: an application to screening for open angle glaucoma (OAG) [abstract]. XIV Cochrane Colloquium, 23–26 Oct 2006; Dublin, Ireland. p. 88.
13. Glanville J. Searching for diagnostic tests: which databases, which filters? Fourth Annual Meeting of Health Technology Assessment International (HTAi): Pushing the frontiers of information management; 2007; Barcelona, Spain.
14. Glanville J, Spijker R, Ormstad SS, Higgins C, Fitzgerald A. SuRe Info: diagnostic accuracy. HTAi Vortal. 2016. http://vortal.htai.org/?q=node/339. Accessed 28 June 2018.
15. Whiting P, Westwood M, Burke M, Sterne J, Glanville J. Systematic reviews of test accuracy should search a range of databases to identify primary studies. J Clin Epidemiol. 2008;61:357–64.
16. van Enst WA, Scholten RJ, Whiting P, Zwinderman AH, Hooft L. Meta-epidemiologic analysis indicates that MEDLINE searches are sufficient for diagnostic test accuracy systematic reviews. J Clin Epidemiol. 2014;67:1192–9.

17. Preston L, Carroll C, Gardois P, Paisley S, Kaltenthaler E. Improving search efficiency for systematic reviews of diagnostic test accuracy: an exploratory study to assess the viability of limiting to MEDLINE, EMBASE and reference checking. Syst Rev. 2015;4:82.
18. Rice DB, Kloda LA, Levis B, Qi B, Kingsland E, Thombs BD. Are MEDLINE searches sufficient for systematic reviews and meta-analyses of the diagnostic accuracy of depression screening tools? A review of meta-analyses. J Psychosom Res. 2016;87:7–13.
19. Centre for Reviews and Dissemination. Systematic Reviews: CRD's guidance for undertaking systematic reviews in health care. In. York: University of York, Centre for Reviews and Dissemination; 2009. http://www.york.ac.uk/inst/crd/SysRev/!SSL!/WebHelp/SysRev3.htm. Accessed 28 June 2018.
20. Devillé WL, Buntinx F. Guidelines for conducting systematic reviews of studies evaluating the accuracy of diagnostic tests. In: Knottnerus JA, editor. The evidence base of clinical diagnosis. London: BMJ Books; 2002. p. 145–65.
21. Devillé WL, Buntinx F, Bouter LM, Montori VM, de Vet HC, van der Windt DA, Bezemer PD. Conducting systematic reviews of diagnostic studies: didactic guidelines. BMC Med Res Methodol. 2002;2:9.
22. CADTH. Grey Matters: a practical tool for searching health-related grey literature. 2015. Canadian Agency for Drugs and Technologies in Health (CADTH): Toronto. Available from: https://www.cadth.ca/resources/finding-evidence/grey-matters. Accessed 28 June 2018.
23. Giustini D. Finding the hard to finds: searching for grey literature (2012 update). 2012. http://www.slideshare.net/giustinid/finding-the-hard-to-finds-searching-for-grey-gray-literature-2010. Accessed 28 June 2018.
24. Haddaway NR, Collins AM, Coughlin D, Kirk S. The role of Google scholar in evidence reviews and its applicability to grey literature searching. PLoS One. 2015;10:e0138237.
25. Haddaway NR, Collins AM, Coughlin D, Kohl C. Including non-public data and studies in systematic reviews and systematic maps. Environ Int. 2016;99:351–65.
26. Korevaar DA, Bossuyt PMM, Hooft L. Infrequent and incomplete registration of test accuracy studies: analysis of recent study reports. BMJ Open. 2014;4:e004596.
27. Whiting P, Westwood M, Bojke L, Palmer S, Richardson G, Cooper J, et al. Clinical effectiveness and cost-effectiveness of tests for the diagnosis and investigation of urinary tract infection in children: a systematic review and economic model. Health Technol Assess. 2006;10:iii–v, xi–xiii, 1–154.
28. Sampson M, McGowan J, Lefebvre C, Moher D, Grimshaw J. PRESS: peer review of electronic search strategies. Ottawa: Canadian Agency for Drugs and Technologies in Health; 2008.
29. PRESS—Peer Review of Electronic Search Strategies: 2015 Guideline Explanation and Elaboration (PRESS E&E). Ottawa: CADTH; 2016.
30. Noel-Storr AH, et al. Reporting standards for studies of diagnostic test accuracy in dementia: the STARDdem initiative. Neurology. 2014;83:364–73.
31. Moher D, Liberati A, Tetzlaff J, Altman DG, PRISMA Group. Preferred reporting items for systematic reviews and meta-analyses: the PRISMA statement. J Clin Epidemiol. 2009;62:1006–12.
32. Shea BJ, Grimshaw JM, Wells GA, Boers M, Andersson N, Hamel C, Porter AC, Tugwell P, Moher D, Bouter LM. Development of AMSTAR: a measurement tool to assess the methodological quality of systematic reviews. BMC Med Res Methodol. 2007;7:10.
33. Whiting P, Savović J, Higgins JP, Caldwell DM, Reeves BC, Shea B, Davies P, Kleijnen J, Churchill R, ROBIS Group. ROBIS: a new tool to assess risk of bias in systematic reviews was developed. J Clin Epidemiol. 2016;69:225–34.

8 Abstracting Evidence

Luca Testa and Mario Bollati

Nothing has such power to broaden the mind as the ability to investigate systematically and truly [1].

Marcus Aurelius, 121–180 AD, Rome

8.1 Introduction

Data are the backbone of any reviewing effort, and their careful yet efficient abstraction is crucial to enable the production of valid and similarly efficient umbrella reviews, overview of reviews, or meta-epidemiologic studies. Despite their obvious role, data and their collection means have often been overlooked or treated superficially. This is unfortunate as no statistical technique, even if highly sophisticated, can remedy bias due to suboptimal data abstraction (e.g., information bias). Indeed, the key aims which should inform data abstraction for tertiary research should be transparency, error minimization, and efficiency [2, 3].

Despite such importance and the self-evident relevance of the above goals, the evidence informing on best practices in data collection for systematic reviews is quite limited and practically absent for umbrella reviews, overview of reviews, or meta-epidemiologic studies [4–6]. We thus need to borrow from sources of evidence focused more on systematic reviews and meta-analyses and concomitantly rely largely on expert opinion (combining experience and expertise). Nonetheless, there is still room for credible recommendations on effective and efficient data collection methods. Careful application of such methods will typically yield high-quality data and maximize the validity of any reviewing exercise.

In general and apparently tautological terms, the minimum set of data requiring abstraction are those that are essential for the review of interest (e.g., details on populations, interventions/comparisons/exposures of interest, and outcomes), supplemented by those ancillary data which are required to let the reader and decision-maker put the findings into context and check their plausibility and applicability. In addition, a thorough data collection process will ensure that the data already abstracted may be useful to other researchers in the future, a practice which will become more and more common in the era of open dataset access and online data

L. Testa (✉) · M. Bollati
Department of Cardiology, IRCCS Pol. S. Donato, S. Donato Milanese, Milan, Italy

G. Biondi-Zoccai (ed.), *Diagnostic Meta-Analysis*,
https://doi.org/10.1007/978-3-319-78966-8_8

repositories, such as the Systematic Review Data Repository (SRDR) [7, 8]. On top of the following recommendations, the reader is referred to other important documents and in particular the *Cochrane Handbook for Systematic Reviews of Interventions* and the *Joanna Briggs Institute Reviewers' Manual* sections devoted to overviews of reviews and umbrella reviews, respectively, for other important insights [4, 5].

8.2 Collection of Review Data

In keeping with our default definitions of umbrella reviews, overviews of reviews, and meta-epidemiologic studies, the key unit for data collection in such reviewing efforts is a systematic review, a meta-analysis, or any other type of secondary research. First, research source has to be carefully chosen: not only the "classic" MEDLINE but also other sources as CENTRAL, Embase, or the Cochrane review database have to be explored.

Having said this, great attention should be given to the peculiarities of this study design, notwithstanding the ultimate focus on the goal of summarizing, in most cases, the available evidence in terms of populations, interventions/comparisons/exposures of interest, and outcomes (Table 8.1) [4, 9–14]. In other words, while apparently the unit of study is a review, ultimately the focus of the reader and user will likely be on patients. In addition, details on the persons undertaking the umbrella review, bibliographic and bibliometric features of the review under analysis, and any ancillary information which may be considered relevant for confounding and/or effect modification (e.g., funding and conflicts of interest) can be abstracted [15]. Finally, the data abstraction process should be planned in keeping with the preferred approach for validity assessment, as a one-stop collection process is usually preferable to minimize time loss and inconsistency. Accordingly, the specific items of the different tools to appraise the validity of reviews should be borne in mind in this phase of planning and reviewing [9–13].

Table 8.1 Critical appraisal tools (CATs) for study validity

Topic
– Is the trial/registry specific in scope and application?
Methods
– Is the authorship transparent? – Are the research methods transparent and comprehensive? – Is the evidence grading system transparent and translatable?
Conclusions/discussion
– Are the conclusions consequent from the trials' findings? – Are the other sources correctly cited? – Are the conclusions unbiased? – Is the trial/registry updated?
Application
– Can the trial/registry be applied to our patients?

8.3 Collection of Study Data

In many cases, reviewers aiming for an umbrella review, overview of review, or meta-epidemiologic study may rely on the data presented in the shortlisted reviews to gather details on primary sources of evidence (e.g., randomized controlled trials, observational studies). In such instances, it is important though to make sure that the original data collection process had been valid and that no systematic error had been entered in the processes taken to complete and report the review (e.g., typographical errors in publishing the review). Thus, it may be useful to double-check at least some of the shortlisted trials, either from the original source document or through another review including the same study.

In other cases, it may be needed to collect additional details from the primary studies, either because they had not been collected or because some primary studies had not been included at all. In such settings then an umbrella review, overview of review, or meta-epidemiologic study entails the same methodological aspects and skills required for a traditional systematic review. This specific topic is largely beyond our present scope, and high-quality recommendations are available elsewhere [3–5, 16–18]. As previously clarified, it is paramount to collect details informing on populations, interventions/comparisons/exposures of interest, and outcomes, as well as reviewer, bibliographic, and validity data, to enable comprehensive and detailed reporting and analysis. In addition, validity appraisal of such primary studies may be of interest, and in such cases details sufficient to enable the application of established appraisal, such as the Cochrane Risk of Bias Tool or the Newcastle-Ottawa Scale, are also required [4, 14].

8.4 Troubleshooting

Besides the minimal and optimal set of data to be collected, it is important to define and plan how to best abstract data [8]. In most cases, data retrieval should be performed by two or more reviewers, independently, with divergences traced and solved after consensus or involvement of another reviewer [19]. It may occasionally be accepted that one reviewer extracts data, while a different one checks all of them for accuracy. In any case, divergences should be solved constructively, tracking explicitly the consensus development. In addition, agreement between different reviewers may be explicitly appraised with specific tests, such as the Cohen's kappa coefficient, to ensure consistency.

Data collection forms, being them on paper or electronic, should be piloted in order to ensure validity and agreement among different reviewers, especially if the reviewing effort is substantial (e.g., >10 reviews included). Reviewers should be trained, though, notwithstanding the apparently limited impact of reviewer experience on data quality [20]. The transition from paper forms to spreadsheets, all-purpose databases, web surveys, and, eventually, specialized software is already occurring, and the benefits of the latter type of tools are clear especially when the number of included reviews and trials is substantial [9, 21–24]. The use of standardized forms and definitions is also going to be particularly welcome in the, hopefully near, future, when authors will most likely upload their data on public repositories, such as the SRDR, to enable other researchers check and use them at their will [7, 8].

While blinding reviewers to the identification details of the authors of the shortlisted reviews is conceivable, it may be logistically challenging, and to date there is no irrefutable evidence to support it [25, 26]. In addition, it is recommended to quote verbatim in the abstraction forms those sections of the shortlisted reviews which guide a specific labeling. Moreover, quantitative data as originally reported should be preferred to back-computed values, which may lead to biased results if mathematical transformations are used inconsistently [27]. Accordingly, denominators, counts, and samples at risk should always be explicitly stated, especially when different outcomes at varying risk of attrition are considered. Whenever data are missing, are inconsistent, or need confirmation, authors of the shortlisted reviews or even authors of the original primary studies can be contacted. Such efforts should be based on an explicit plan, recorded and transparently reported to avoid duplicate efforts. Whereas there is an ongoing push to perfect automated data abstraction and validity appraisal in systematic reviewing efforts, to date there is no room for their prime-time use [28, 29]. Summarizing, every review has to be conducted as per the critical appraisal tools (CATs), evaluating studies' methodological validity (see Table 8.1).

Another very important issue is the potential clustering of multiple systematic reviews including different reports all stemming from the same initial trial [30].

This phenomenon, which can be considered similar to a snowball effect, should be taken into account when describing the umbrella review results and even more importantly by means of hierarchical models in case of formal inferential analysis [31]. Indeed, meta-epidemiologic studies may aptly exploit duplicate reviewing efforts to highlight important mediators of review results [32–34], but such duplicate entries may instead significantly bias effect estimates in umbrella reviews if not recognized and managed correctly.

Finally, and more pragmatically, it is best to limit the amount of collected data to a reasonably small to moderate set, at least when the number of included systematic reviews is large, to avoid creating an exceedingly extensive dataset which only dilutes the core inferential message and can also raise the temptation of multiplicity and cherry picking. Doing the research, the sensitivity vs. precision balance has to be considered, where sensitivity is defined as the number of relevant reports identified divided by the total number of relevant reports in existence. Precision is defined as the number of relevant reports identified divided by the total number of reports identified. The combination between these two elements represents a review key point [4].

Conclusion

Data collection represents a very important aspect of any reviewing effort. Given the lack of a large evidence base on best practices in this step of an umbrella review, overview of review, or meta-epidemiologic study, it is necessary to apply sound judgment and balance the desire for detailed datasets with pragmatism, without however risking being superficial. It is clear that bias forced into a reviewing effort at this stage is very difficult to recognize later on, and thus, robust methods must be employed. In the future, it is likely that the duplication of data collection efforts will be minimized by uploading standardized data abstraction forms for clinical studies and systematic reviews into dedicated online data repositories.

References

1. https://www.brainyquote.com/quotes/quotes/m/marcusaure118558.html. Accessed 28 June 2018.
2. Guyatt G, Rennie D, Meade MO, Cook DJ. Users' guide to the medical literature. A manual for evidence-based clinical practice. 2nd ed. New York: McGraw-Hill Professional; 2008.
3. Biondi-Zoccai G, editor. Network meta-analysis: evidence synthesis with mixed treatment comparison. Hauppauge: Nova; 2014.
4. Higgins JPT, Green S, editors. Cochrane handbook for systematic reviews of interventions. Version 5.1.0 [updated March 2011]. The Cochrane Collaboration. 2011. Available from: www.cochrane-handbook.org. Last accessed 28 June 2018.
5. The Joanna Briggs Institute. The Joanna Briggs Institute Reviewers' manual. Methodology for JBI umbrella reviews. Adelaide: The University of Adelaide; 2014.
6. Li L, Tian J, Tian H, Sun R, Liu Y, Yang K. Quality and transparency of overviews of systematic reviews. J Evid Based Med. 2012;5:166–73.
7. Systematic Review Data Repository (SRDR). Available at: srdr.ahrq.gov. Last accessed 28 June 2018.
8. Li T, Vedula SS, Hadar N, Parkin C, Lau J, Dickersin K. Innovations in data collection, management, and archiving for systematic reviews. Ann Intern Med. 2015;162:287–94.
9. Oxman AD, Guyatt GH. Validation of an index of the quality of review articles. J Clin Epidemiol. 1991;44:1271–8.
10. Shea BJ, Grimshaw JM, Wells GA, Boers M, Andersson N, Hamel C, Porter AC, Tugwell P, Moher D, Bouter LM. Development of AMSTAR: a measurement tool to assess the methodological quality of systematic reviews. BMC Med Res Methodol. 2007;7:10.
11. Diekemper RL, Ireland BK, Merz LR. Development of the documentation and appraisal review tool for systematic reviews. World J Meta Anal. 2015;3:142–50.
12. Pieper D, Buechter RB, Li L, Prediger B, Eikermann M. Systematic review found AMSTAR, but not r(evised)-AMSTAR, to have good measurement properties. J Clin Epidemiol. 2015;68:574–83.
13. La Torre G, Backhaus I, Mannocci A. Rating for narrative reviews: concept and development of the International Narrative Systematic Assessment tool. Senses Sci. 2015;2:31–5.
14. Stang A. Critical evaluation of the Newcastle-Ottawa scale for the assessment of the quality of nonrandomized studies in meta-analyses. Eur J Epidemiol. 2010;25:603–5.
15. Jørgensen AW, Maric KL, Tendal B, Faurschou A, Gøtzsche PC. Industry-supported meta-analyses compared with meta-analyses with non-profit or no support: differences in methodological quality and conclusions. BMC Med Res Methodol. 2008;8:60.
16. Centre for Reviews and Dissemination. Systematic reviews: CRD's guidance for undertaking reviews in healthcare. York: University of York; 2009.
17. Eden J, Levit L, Berg A, Morton S. Finding what works in health care. Standards for systematic reviews. Washington, DC: The National Academies Press; 2011.
18. Agency for Healthcare Research and Quality. Methods guide for effectiveness and comparative effectiveness reviews. Rockville: Agency for Healthcare Research and Quality (US); 2008.
19. Buscemi N, Hartling L, Vandermeer B, Tjosvold L, Klassen TP. Single data extraction generated more errors than double data extraction in systematic reviews. J Clin Epidemiol. 2006;59:697–703.

20. Horton J, Vandermeer B, Hartling L, Tjosvold L, Klassen TP, Buscemi N. Systematic review data extraction: cross-sectional study showed that experience did not increase accuracy. J Clin Epidemiol. 2010;63:289–98.
21. Bachmann LM, Coray R, Estermann P, Ter Riet G. Identifying diagnostic studies in MEDLINE: reducing the number needed to read. J Am Med Inform Assoc. 2002;9:653–8.
22. Elamin MB, Flynn DN, Bassler D, Briel M, Alonso-Coello P, Karanicolas PJ, Guyatt GH, Malaga G, Furukawa TA, Kunz R, Schünemann H, Murad MH, Barbui C, Cipriani A, Montori VM. Choice of data extraction tools for systematic reviews depends on resources and review complexity. J Clin Epidemiol. 2009;62:506–10.
23. Ip S, Hadar N, Keefe S, Parkin C, Iovin R, Balk EM, Lau J. A web-based archive of systematic review data. Syst Rev. 2012;1:15.
24. Doctor evidence. Available at: drevidence.com. Last accessed 28 June 2018.
25. Berlin JA. Does blinding of readers affect the results of meta-analyses? University of Pennsylvania Meta-analysis Blinding Study Group. Lancet. 1997;350:185–6.
26. Jadad AR, Moore RA, Carroll D, Jenkinson C, Reynolds DJ, Gavaghan DJ, McQuay HJ. Assessing the quality of reports of randomized clinical trials: is blinding necessary? Control Clin Trials. 1996;17:1–12.
27. Gøtzsche PC, Hróbjartsson A, Maric K, Tendal B. Data extraction errors in meta-analyses that use standardized mean differences. JAMA. 2007;298:430–7.
28. Jonnalagadda SR, Goyal P, Huffman MD. Automating data extraction in systematic reviews: a systematic review. Syst Rev. 2015;4:78.
29. Marshall IJ, Kuiper J, Wallace BC. Automating risk of bias assessment for clinical trials. IEEE J Biomed Health Inform. 2015;19:1406–12.
30. Tramèr MR, Reynolds DJ, Moore RA, McQuay HJ. Impact of covert duplicate publication on meta-analysis: a case study. BMJ. 1997;315:635–40.
31. Caldwell DM, Welton NJ, Ades AE. Mixed treatment comparison analysis provides internally coherent treatment effect estimates based on overviews of reviews and can reveal inconsistency. J Clin Epidemiol. 2010;63:875–82.
32. Biondi-Zoccai GG, Lotrionte M, Abbate A, Testa L, Remigi E, Burzotta F, Valgimigli M, Romagnoli E, Crea F, Agostoni P. Compliance with QUOROM and quality of reporting of overlapping meta-analyses on the role of acetylcysteine in the prevention of contrast associated nephropathy: case study. BMJ. 2006;332:202–9.
33. Nowbar AN, Mielewczik M, Karavassilis M, Dehbi HM, Shun-Shin MJ, Jones S, Howard JP, Cole GD, Francis DP, DAMASCENE Writing Group. Discrepancies in autologous bone marrow stem cell trials and enhancement of ejection fraction (DAMASCENE): weighted regression and meta-analysis. BMJ. 2014;348:g2688.
34. Peruzzi M, De Falco E, Abbate A, Biondi-Zoccai G, Chimenti I, Lotrionte M, Benedetto U, Delewi R, Marullo AG, Frati G. State of the art on the evidence base in cardiac regenerative therapy: overview of 41 systematic reviews. Biomed Res Int. 2015;2015:613782.

Appraising Evidence

9

Valentina Pecoraro

9.1 Introduction

Diagnostic accuracy studies compare results of index test and reference standard in the same patients with the objective to evaluate the accuracy of a new test. Incorrect assessment of the accuracy can lead to inappropriate diagnostic testing, unnecessary costs and inaccurate clinical decision [1].

In the systematic review development, the question leading the research is the most critical step. The approach to build the clear and explicit question is based on the acronym PICO. For a diagnostic accuracy study, the PICO parameters are relevant population (P), diagnostic intervention or index test (I) (including its role, such as triage, replacement, or an add-on test), comparator or reference test (gold standard) (C), and patient important outcomes (O) [2, 3].

Another critical step is the appraisal of the methodological quality of diagnostic accuracy studies included in the review. The assessment of methodological quality is a critical evaluation of the study methodology that allows for appropriate interpretation of results and conclusions. It is essential to assess the reliability of a study and to identify elements leading the correct interpretation of results. The lack of methodological rigor may introduce bias or variations in results between studies, limiting their applicability. A large number of tools and checklist have been proposed to assess the methodological quality of diagnostic accuracy studies [4].

The quality of studies can be evaluated in terms of internal and external validity.

Internal validity refers to how well a study is conducted, whereby the diagnostic accuracy estimate was not bias due to shortcomings in study design, conduction, analysis, or reporting [5, 6].

V. Pecoraro
Laboratory of Toxicology, Department of Laboratory Medicine and Pathological Anatomy, Azienda USL of Modena, Modena, Italy

G. Biondi-Zoccai (ed.), *Diagnostic Meta-Analysis*,
https://doi.org/10.1007/978-3-319-78966-8_9

External validity refers to how the results of a study can be applied to patients in clinical practice. Diagnostic accuracy studies could enroll patients who are not similar to those in whom the test is used, or the test may be used in a different way than in practice [6]. External validity depends on the spectrum of disease, patients' characteristics, conduction of diagnostic test, and cut-off used [5].

The relevance of the quality assessment is highlighted by some authors. Lijemer et al. showed that studies enrolling nonrepresentative patients, using different reference standard or interpreting the test result knowing the reference test result, overestimate the diagnostic performance of a test examined [7]. Likewise, Rutjes and colleagues demonstrated that studies with nonconsecutive patients' inclusion or retrospective data collection tend to overestimate the test accuracy, whereas studies selecting patients relying on the index test result or on clinical symptoms produce lower estimates of diagnostic accuracy [8].

In this chapter, available tools to critically appraise the evidence for a systematic review of diagnostic test accuracy studies will be discussed. In particular, possible type of bias (Sect. 9.2), criteria to perform a critical appraisal of a diagnostic test (Sect. 9.3), and tools for the appropriate reporting of a diagnostic test study (Sect. 9.4), for the evaluation of the methodological quality of individual studies (Sect. 9.5), and for assessment of quality of evidence (Sect. 9.6) will be described.

9.2 Source of Bias in Diagnostic Test Accuracy Studies

To avoid inappropriate use of diagnostic test, researchers and clinicians should be able to critically review the diagnostic accuracy studies and identify those studies containing reliable information. However, they should recognize different source of bias and how these could lead erroneous test results [9]. The term "bias" indicates any systematic deviation from the true value. Methodological quality relates to the risk of bias. Bias could be introduced following the loss of details in study design or conduction, loss of blindness in the process of test interpretations, or loss of study reporting completeness [10].

Diagnostic test studies are susceptible to bias that will overestimate or underestimate the sensitivity and specificity of the test. Furthermore, a source of variation could determine possible difference in the diagnostic accuracy across studies, in terms of population, disease, setting, or definition of target condition, limiting the applicability of results [11].

In the evaluation of diagnostic accuracy studies, it is important to consider possible source of bias and variation (Table 9.1).

Methodological deficiency may influence the results' interpretation and the clinicians' decision. Common methodological shortcomings are [12]:

- Use of inappropriate gold standard
- Spectrum bias
- Lack of blinding
- Use of inappropriate cutoffs
- Presence of inconclusive results

Table 9.1 Source of bias and source of variation (adapted from [10] with permission from Elsevier)

	Source of bias	Source of variation
Patients	Study design	Demographic characteristics
	Patients' recruitment	Disease prevalence
	Prospective data collection	Disease severity
	Consecutive patient enrollment	Prior testing
		Participant selection
Index test	Test review bias	Observer variation
	Threshold selection	Availability of clinical information
		Test technology
		Test execution
Reference standard	Use of inappropriate reference standard	Definition of target condition
	Diagnostic review bias	
	Incorporation bias	
	Partial verification	
	Differential verification	
Flow and timing	Disease progression	Observer
	Treatment paradox	
	Partial verification bias	
	Differential verification bias	
	Incorporation bias	
	Withdrawals	

The main type of bias that can occur in diagnostic test accuracy studies are the following [13, 14] (Table 9.2):

Spectrum bias: it occurs when patients with or without a disease were wrongly selected. Patients enrolled in a diagnostic study should have assorted features, such as different sex, age, and severity disease, in order to represent the general population and produce valid and generalizable results [15, 16]. However, spectrum bias exists when the population under investigation does not reflect the review target population or the general population [3] and determine an overestimation of both sensitivity and specificity [17].

Information bias: it occurs when assessors were not blinded to previous results and could be influenced in the interpretation of results and conclusion. This type of bias can lead to overestimation of the test accuracy.

Misclassification bias: it occurs when the reference test does not correctly classify patients with target condition [3].

Verification (or work-up) bias: it occurs when patients with a positive or negative test result are preferentially selected to be tested by the gold standard for verification of the disease [9]. Verification bias included:

(a) **Partial verification bias**: it occurs when patients with positive index test result were tested by the gold standard more likely than patients negative to index test [1, 17]. Usually, all patients tested for index test should be verified by reference

Table 9.2 Types of bias in diagnostic accuracy studies (adapted from Roever 2016 [14])

	Type of bias	When does it occur?	Impact on accuracy
Patients	Spectrum bias	When a study included patients who do not represent the broad spectrum of those that the test is intended to use and spectrum of target or alternative conditions	Depends on which end of the disease spectrum the included patients represent
	Selection bias	When eligible patients are not enrolled consecutively or randomly	Usually leads to overestimation of accuracy
Index test	Information bias	When the index test results are interpreted with knowledge of the reference test results	Usually leads to overestimation of accuracy
Reference test	Misclassification bias	When the reference test does not correctly classify patients with target condition	Depends on whether both the reference and index test make the same mistakes
	Partial verification bias	When not all patients undergo the reference test	Usually leads to overestimation of sensitivity
	Differential verification bias	When not all patients are verified with a second or third reference test, especially when this selection depends on index test results	Usually leads to overestimation of accuracy
	Information bias	When the reference test data is interpreted with the knowledge of the index test results	Usually leads to overestimation of accuracy
	Incorporation bias	When the index test is incorporated in a (composite) reference test	Usually leads to overestimation of accuracy
	Disease/condition progression bias	When the patients' condition changes between administering the index and reference test	Under- on overestimation of accuracy
Data analysis	Excluded data	When uninterruptable or intermediate test results and withdrawals are not included in the analysis	Usually leads to overestimation of accuracy

standard. This bias is common when reference test is invasive or more expensive and could determine the overestimation of sensitivity and the underestimation of specificity.

Withdrawals: when the rate of withdrawals depends on the results of the index test, they can have the similar impact of partial verification bias.

(b) **Differential verification bias**: it occurs when an alternative reference standard was used in those patients, usually in patients positive to index test, for whom the preferred reference test cannot be used (e.g., invasive procedure) [1], or when two different reference standards (such as clinical follow-up) were used to verify the result [3]. Sensitivity and specificity were overestimated respect to a study in which all patients receive the same reference standard, independently of the index test result [17].

Incorporation bias: it occurs when the result of the index test is explicitly used as criteria for the reference standard. If the index test is included in the reference standard, it can lead to an overestimation of test accuracy. Index test should have no role in determining whether the reference standard classifies patients as disease positive or negative [17]. Sensitivity and specificity were raised.

9.3 Critical Appraisal of a Diagnostic Test

The aim of a diagnostic test is to determine whether it is able to accurately identify patients with and without the disease of interest as defined by a gold standard test. To evaluate a diagnostic test, it is essential to appraise critically the validity of the study and the applicability of the results [18]. The process of critical appraisal examines the methodology of a study following pre-defined criteria, considering individual sources of bias [19].

To evaluate if a study is likely to provide a reliable estimate of the diagnostic parameters, you should apply three essential queries [18, 20, 21]:

1. Are the results of the study valid?
2. What are the results of the study?
3. Will the results help me look after my patient?

1. *Are the results of the study valid?*
   (a) Did the patients sample include an appropriate spectrum of patients?
   The patients enrolled in a diagnostic study should be representative of the population whom the test will apply in the clinical practice, and the test should be applied to the full **spectrum of patients** (*spectrum bias*).
   (b) Does everyone get the gold standard?
   Both the **index test** and the **reference standard** should be **carried out on all patients** enrolled in a study, or alternative reference standard could be applied in case of invasiveness or expensive test. The validity of the index test should be compromised if its result influences the decision to submit or not patients to gold standard for confirmation (*verification bias* or *work-up bias*) [18, 20].
   (c) Is there an independent, blind, or objective comparison with the gold standard?
   The ideal reference standard should be safe, easy to administer, and able to differentiate patients with and without disease [18, 20]. Patients enrolled in a study should have undergone **appropriate gold standard** or combination of tests. However, the person interpreting the index test result should be **blind** in respect to the result of reference standard. Likewise, the person interpreting gold standard should be blind in respect to the index test result.

Table 9.3 Statistical measures used to express diagnostic test utility (adapted from [12] with permission from Taylor and Francis Ltd.)

Statistical measures	Definition	Calculation
Sensitivity	The proportion of patients with disease who have tested positive	TP/(TP + FN)
Specificity	The proportion of patients without disease who have tested negative	TN/(FP + TN)
Positive predictive value (PPV)	The proportion of patients with a positive test who have the diseases	TP/(TP + FP)
Negative predictive value (NPV)	The proportion of patients with a negative test who do not have the diseases	TN/(FN + TN)
Positive likelihood ratio (LR+)	The ratio of the probability that a positive test result will occur in subjects with the disease; in respect to that, the same result will occur in subjects without the disease	Sensitivity/(1 − specificity)
Negative likelihood ratio (LR−)	The ratio of the probability that a negative result will occur in subjects with the disease; in respect to that, the same result will occur in subjects without the disease	(1 − sensitivity)/specificity

Lack of blindness will lead to overestimation of sensitivity and specificity (*observed bias*) [18, 20].

2. *What are the results of the study?*
   The properties of diagnostic test are usually described in terms of accuracy and expressed as sensitivity, specificity, positive and negative likelihood ratio, and in terms of positive and negative predictive value (Table 9.3) [12].
3. *Will the results help me look after my patient?*
   (a) Were methods for performing the test described with sufficient details to permit its replication?
   The study should be described with sufficient details to permit its replication. The accuracy of the diagnostic test depends also on its reproducibility, in other words, its ability to reproduce the same results when reapplied to patients.
   (b) Are the results applicable to my patients?
   The study results can be applied to real clinical scenario, and the study population can be comparable with the patients in own clinical practice.
   (c) Will the results change my management?
   Study results may influence the clinicians' decision about a diagnosis or therapeutic strategy to adopt.

9.4 Tool for the Reporting of Diagnostic Accuracy Studies: The STARD Statement

Diagnostic test accuracy studies should be transparently reported to permit both the critical appraisal of methodology and the studies' replication [22]. Sometimes essential elements of study's methods are poorly reported, patients' recruitment is insufficiently described, study results are selectively reported, clinical context is omitted, and the accuracy estimate does not correspond to real value, making studies at high risk of bias [23].

When the study reporting is inadequate, the information originating from the quality assessment limits the understanding of the design and conduction of the test accuracy study. Furthermore, there are some evidence that papers of diagnostic studies often omit important methodological details [8, 22, 23], making it difficult for readers to judge if a study uses a good methodology but inadequate reporting, or if a study applies inadequate methods introducing bias [19].

To improve the quality and promote the completeness and transparency in reporting of diagnostic accuracy studies, the STARD (Standard for Reporting of Diagnostic Accuracy Studies) was developed [24]. This guideline (published for the first time in 2003 and updated in 2015) contains a checklist of 30 essential items, included in seven sections (title, abstract, introduction, methods, results, discussion, and other information), that should be reported in any diagnostic accuracy study (Table 9.4). Moreover, a diagram to report the flow of participants through the study (Fig. 9.1) and the key terms (Table 9.5) are proposed [25].

The mean journals suggest to adopt the STARD checklist to improve the quality of reporting of diagnostic test accuracy studies [26, 27], but the compliance of laboratory studies is suboptimal [28]. In these types of studies, some items are

Table 9.4 Standard for Reporting of Diagnostic Accuracy Studies (STARD) checklist 2015 [24]

Section and topic	No	Item
Title or abstract	1	Identification as a study of diagnostic accuracy using at least one measure of accuracy (such as sensitivity, specificity, predictive values, or AUC)
Abstract		
	2	Structured summary of study design, methods, results, and conclusions (for specific guidance, see STARD for abstracts)
Introduction		
	3	Scientific and clinical background, including the intended use and clinical role of the index test
	4	Study objectives and hypotheses
Methods		
Study design	5	Whether data collection was planned before the index test and reference standard were performed (prospective study) or after (retrospective study)
Participants	6	Eligibility criteria
	7	On what basis potentially eligible participants were identified (such as symptoms, results from previous tests, inclusion in registry)
	8	Where and when potentially eligible participants were identified (setting, location, and dates)
	9	Whether participants formed a consecutive, random, or convenience series

(continued)

Table 9.4 (continued)

Section and topic	No	Item
Test methods	10a	Index test, in sufficient detail to allow replication
	10b	Reference standard, in sufficient detail to allow replication
	11	Rationale for choosing the reference standard (if alternatives exist)
	12a	Definition of and rationale for test positivity cutoffs or result categories of the index test, distinguishing pre-specified from exploratory
	12b	Definition of and rationale for test positivity cutoffs or result categories of the reference standard, distinguishing pre-specified from exploratory
	13a	Whether clinical information and reference standard results were available to the performers/readers of the index test
	13b	Whether clinical information and index test results were available to the assessors of the reference standard
Analysis	14	Methods for estimating or comparing measures of diagnostic accuracy
	15	How indeterminate index test or reference standard results were handled
	16	How missing data on the index test and reference standard were handled
	17	Any analyses of variability in diagnostic accuracy, distinguishing pre-specified from exploratory
	18	Intended sample size and how it was determined
Results		
Participants	19	Flow of participants, using a diagram
	20	Baseline demographic and clinical characteristics of participants
	21a	Distribution of severity of disease in those with the target condition
	21b	Distribution of alternative diagnoses in those without the target condition
	22	Time interval and any clinical interventions between index test and reference standard
Test results	23	Cross tabulation of the index test results (or their distribution) by the results of the reference standard
	24	Estimates of diagnostic accuracy and their precision (such as 95% confidence intervals)
	25	Any adverse events from performing the index test or the reference standard
Discussion		
	26	Study limitations, including sources of potential bias, statistical uncertainty, and generalizability
	27	Implications for practice, including the intended use and clinical role of the index test
Other information		
	28	Registration number and name of registry
	29	Where the full study protocol can be accessed
	30	Sources of funding and other support; role of funders

frequently reported, but others, such as methods for calculating reproducibility, are omitted, making this type of studies more sensitive to reporting bias [28].

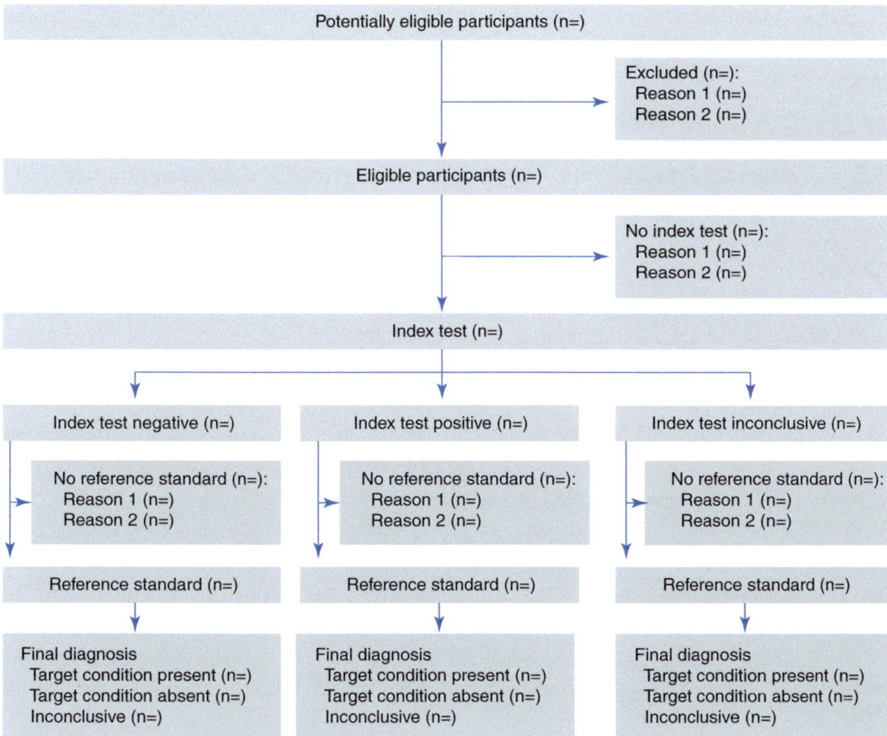

Fig. 9.1 Flow diagram, from Cohen 2016 [24]

Table 9.5 Key STARD terminology [24]

Term	Explanation
Medical test	Any method for collecting additional information about the current or future health status of a patient
Index test	The test under evaluation
Target condition	The disease or condition that the index test is expected to detect
Clinical reference standard	The best available method for establishing the presence or absence of the target condition; a gold standard would be an error-free reference standard
Sensitivity	Proportion of those with the target condition who test positive with the index test
Specificity	Proportion of those without the target condition who test negative with the index test
Intended use of the test	Whether the index test is used for diagnosis, screening, staging, monitoring, surveillance, prediction, prognosis, or other reasons
Role of the test	The position of the index test relative to other tests for the same condition (e.g., triage, replacement, add-on, new test)

STARD statement was proposed to apply for several diagnostic accuracy studies evaluating the performance of all types of medical tests, and many methodology experts stress its adoption by authors, peer reviewers, and journal editors.

9.5 Tool to Assess the Quality of Diagnostic Accuracy Studies: QUADAS-2

Quality assessment of individual studies included in a systematic review is necessary to identify potential source of bias and to limit the effect that these distortions could have on estimations and interpretation of results [29].

A large number of tools, such as scales or checklists, are available for the quality assessment of diagnostic accuracy studies, and they are different from the items considered [4]. The tool recommended for the quality assessment of diagnostic test accuracy studies is the QUADAS-2 (Quality Assessment of Diagnostic Accuracy Studies) [30]. This checklist was developed in 2003 [31, 32] and later updated.

QUADAS-2 consists of four phases: (1) to report the review question in terms of patients, index test, reference standard, and target condition; (2) to develop review-specific guidance choosing to consider all signaling questions or just some of these and use the information recovered in the paper to judge the risk of bias; (3) to review the flow diagram of primary study or build it to understand the flow of recruited participants; (4) and to assess bias and applicability through the signaling questions [30].

QUADAS-2 is composed of four domains: patients' selection, index test, reference standard, and flow and timing (Table 9.6).

Patients' selection should be realized consecutively or randomly and may be distorted by a case-control design or inappropriate exclusion of patients, resulting in an overestimation of diagnostic accuracy. The index test and the reference standard should be evaluated in blind, without knowing the other test result or diagnosis. Knowledge of the first test result may influence the interpretation of the second test. The result of the meta-analysis could also be distorted if the cutoff value reported was selected specifically, or if the reference standard does not correctly classify the target condition. Likewise, different test technologies, methods, or interpretations may affect estimates of the diagnostic accuracy. In the end, the domain "flow and timing" refers to the time interval elapsing between executions of the two tests. Results of index test and reference standard should be collected in the same patients at the same time to avoid misclassification of disease [30].

Each domain is evaluated in terms of risk of bias and the first three domains also in terms of concerns about applicability. Signaling questions are included to judge the risk of bias, and the possible answers are "yes," "no," or "unclear." Risk of bias and concerns about applicability are judged as "low," "high," or "unclear" according to information reported in each study.

At least two review authors, with knowledge of diagnostic accuracy study's methodology, should independently perform the quality assessment and resolve disagreement.

Table 9.6 Quality Assessment of Diagnostic Accuracy Studies (QUADAS-2) checklist (From [30]. Reprinted with the permission of American College of Physicians, Inc.)

Domain	Patient selection	Index test	Reference standard	Flow and timing
Description	Describe methods of patient selection. Describe included patients (prior testing, presentation, intended use of index test, and setting)	Describe the index test and how it was conducted and interpreted	Describe the reference standard and how it was conducted and interpreted	Describe any patients who did not receive the index test(s) and/or reference standard or who were excluded from the 2 × 2 table (refer to flow diagram). Describe the time interval and any interventions between index test(s) and reference standard
Signaling questions (yes/no/unclear)	Was a consecutive or random sample of patients enrolled?	Were the index test results interpreted without knowledge of the results of the reference standard?	Is the reference standard likely to correctly classify the target condition?	Was there an appropriate interval between index test(s) and reference standard?
	Was a case-control design avoided?	If a threshold was used, was it pre-specified?	Were the reference standard results interpreted without knowledge of the results of the index test?	Did all patients receive a reference standard?
	Did the study avoid inappropriate exclusions?			Did all patients receive the same reference standard?
				Were all patients included in the analysis?
Risk of bias (low/unclear/high)	Could the selection of patients have introduced bias?	Could the conduct or interpretation of the index test have introduced bias?	Could the reference standard, its conduct, or its interpretation have introduced bias?	Could the patient flow have introduced bias
Concerns regarding applicability (low/unclear/high)	Are there concerns that the included patients do not match the review question?	Are there concerns that the index test, its conduct, or interpretation differ from the review question?	Are there concerns that the target condition as defined by the reference standard does not match the review question?	

There are several ways to incorporate results of quality assessment into a systematic review: (1) excluding studies at lower quality from analysis or from review, (2) exploring the effect of methodological quality on diagnostic accuracy in a sensitivity or meta-regression analysis, and (3) highlighting the domains of poor quality and using these as recommendations for future research.

Moreover, QUADAS Group members recommend to no generate an overall quality score combining the individual items but to report risk of bias for each domain. Whiting and colleagues [33] report that different methods used to weigh individual items from the same quality assessment tool produce different quality scores that led to different conclusions.

9.6 Assessing the Quality of Evidence: The GRADE Approach

Clinicians, usually, refer to diagnostic test in terms of sensitivity and specificity, in other words, how better a test classifies patients with or without a specific disease. This assumption does not imply that patients inevitably benefit from the correct diagnosis. A possible benefit should be measured in terms of patient important outcomes [34]. The use of a test is not recommended if it does not improve patient outcomes.

The patient important outcomes are defined as "the desirable and undesirable consequence related to patients as consequence of a correct or incorrect diagnosis," generating four accuracy categories: true positives and negatives and false positives and negatives. Therefore, diagnostic accuracy is considered a surrogate outcome to patient important outcomes [35].

In the GRADE system, valid studies can provide high-quality evidence concerning the diagnostic accuracy [36]. A diagnostic test could be evaluated comparing the impact of the new test with the previous test or reference standard in randomized or crossover studies [34].

To develop a recommendation about the use of a diagnostic test, the GRADE approach for diagnostic test provides a transparent framework and comprehensive methodology to rate the quality of evidence related to each patient important outcome of interest and to grade the recommendation [34, 37]. According to the GRADE approach, outcomes of diagnostic accuracy studies are the true positives and negatives and false positives and negatives. This system permits to evaluate the quality of evidence in four domains reflecting the grade of confidence in estimates of the diagnostic test related to patient outcome [36].

Factors that decrease the quality of evidence of diagnostic accuracy studies are classified in five categories (Table 9.7) [34].

1. **Study design and risk of bias**: the best evidence of test performance comes from large randomized trials of different diagnostic strategies that directly measure patient important outcomes. But other valid study designs for diagnostic tests are crossover and observational studies. In diagnostic accuracy studies,

Table 9.7 Factors that decrease the quality of evidence in the GRADE approach for studies of diagnostic accuracy

Factors that decrease the quality of evidence	Explanations and differences from quality of evidence for other interventions
Study design	Different criteria for accuracy studies—Cross-sectional or cohort studies in patients with diagnostic uncertainty and direct comparison of test results with an appropriate reference standard are considered high quality and can move to moderate, low, or very low depending on other factors
Limitations (risk of bias)	Different criteria for accuracy studies—Consecutive patients should be recruited as a single cohort and not classified by disease state, and selection as well as referral process should be clearly described. Seven tests should be done in all patients in the same patient population for new test and well-described reference standard; evaluators should be blind to results of alternative test and reference standard
Indirectness	
Outcomes	Similar criteria—Panels assessing diagnostic tests often face an absence of direct evidence about impact on patient important outcomes. They must make deductions from studies of diagnostic tests about the balance between the presumed influences on patient important outcomes of any differences in true and false positives and true and false negatives in relation to complications and costs of the test. Therefore, accuracy studies typically provide low-quality evidence for making recommendations owing to indirectness of the outcomes, similar to surrogate outcomes for treatments
Patient populations, diagnostic test, comparison test, and indirect comparisons	Similar criteria—Quality of evidence can be reduced if important differences exist between populations studied and those for whom recommendation is intended (in previous testing, spectrum of disease, or comorbidity), if important differences exist in tests studied and diagnostic expertise of people applying them in studies compared with settings for which recommendations are intended, or if tests being compared are each compared with a reference (gold) standard in different studies and not directly compared in same studies
Important inconsistency in study results	Similar criteria—For accuracy studies, unexplained inconsistency in sensitivity, specificity, or likelihood ratios (rather than relative risk or mean differences) can reduce the quality of evidence
Imprecise evidence	Similar criteria—For accuracy studies, wide confidence intervals for estimates of test accuracy or true and false positive and negative rates can reduce the quality of evidence
High probability of publication bias	Similar criteria—High risk of publication bias (e.g., evidence from small studies for new intervention or test, or asymmetry in funnel plot) can lower the quality of evidence

Reproduced from [34] with permission from BMJ Publishing Group Ltd.

usually, representative patients were enrolled consecutively, index test was compared with an appropriate reference (or gold) standard, and results were interpreted in blind.

2. **Directness**: new test could produce false positives and negatives reducing the test accuracy and the quality of evidence. Minimizing these results, the test may improve the patient outcomes. Likewise, the test accuracy may be different across

patients, so authors should consider if the patients enrolled in the study correspond to patients receiving the final recommendations. This domain refers also to indirect comparison of two tests and to differences in terms of population, test, and outcome of interest between evaluated study and objective of the systematic review.

3. **Inconsistency**: unexplained heterogeneity in the results across studies could reduce the quality of evidence for all outcomes. For diagnostic accuracy review, the heterogeneity among studies was expected, not only because the studies usually have small sample size but also for differences in patients' characteristics, study methods, and consequently accuracy results [29].
4. **Imprecision**: high confidence interval for the test accuracy estimates can reduce the quality of evidence.
5. **Publication bias**: this bias may be suspected in the presence of small study effect or asymmetry in the funnel plot and could reduce the quality of evidence.

The overall quality of the evidence for each outcome could be stated as "high," "moderate," "low," or "very low" according to the number of domains satisfied. The overall quality of evidence is, usually, determined by the lowest grade of quality for any outcomes indicated as critical.

The quality of evidence assessed through GRADE approach could be represented in a "Summary of findings" table produced using GRADEpro software summarizing the results of critical outcomes.

Conclusions

The appraising evidence of diagnostic accuracy studies is an essential part in the systematic review development. The quality of any study can be considered in terms of internal and external validity, other than the quality of data analysis and reporting.

Diagnostic accuracy studies are characterized by some methodological elements not in common with clinical trials, such as features in study design and test assessment, leading to different types of bias (e.g., spectrum or verification bias). Authors should be able to identify various sources of bias to avoid misinterpretation of results.

Structured and suitable tools for diagnostic accuracy studies exist for the quality assessment, while formalized tools to assess the systematic review quality are not currently available. STARD and QUADAS-2 are recommended for reporting studies and evaluating the methodological quality, respectively. GRADE approach is also suggested for rating the quality of evidence.

References

1. de Groot JA, Bossuyt PM, Reitsma JB, Rutjes AW, Dendukuri N, Janssen KJ, Moons KG. Verification problems in diagnostic accuracy studies: consequences and solutions. BMJ. 2011;343:d4770.
2. Schünemann HJ, Oxman AD, Brozek J, Glasziou P, Bossuyt P, Chang S, Muti P, Jaeschke R, Guyatt GH. GRADE: assessing the quality of evidence for diagnostic recommendations. Evid Based Med. 2008;13:162–3.

3. Schmidt RL, Factor RE. Understanding sources of bias in diagnostic accuracy studies. Arch Pathol Lab Med. 2013;137:558–65.
4. Whiting P, Rutjes AW, Dinnes J, Reitsma JB, Bossuyt PM, Kleijnen J. A systematic review finds that diagnostic reviews fail to incorporate quality despite available tools. J Clin Epidemiol. 2005;58:1–12.
5. Manchikanti L, Derby R, Wolfer L, Singh V, Datta S, Hirsch JA. Evidence-based medicine, systematic reviews, and guidelines in interventional pain management: part 5. Diagnostic accuracy studies. Pain Physician. 2009;12:517–40.
6. Reitsma JB, Moons KG, Bossuyt PM, Linnet K. Systematic reviews of studies quantifying the accuracy of diagnostic tests and markers. Clin Chem. 2012;58:1534–45.
7. Lijmer JG, Mol BW, Heisterkamp S, Bonsel GJ, Prins MH, van der Meulen JH, Bossuyt PM. Empirical evidence of design-related bias in studies of diagnostic tests. JAMA. 1999;282:1061–6.
8. Rutjes AW, Reitsma JB, Di Nisio M, Smidt N, van Rijn JC, Bossuyt PM. Evidence of bias and variation in diagnostic accuracy studies. CMAJ. 2006;174:469–76.
9. Mower WR. Evaluating bias and variability in diagnostic test reports. Ann Emerg Med. 1999;33:85–91.
10. Whiting PF, Rutjes AW, Westwood ME, Mallett S, QUADAS-2 Steering Group. A systematic review classifies sources of bias and variation in diagnostic test accuracy studies. J Clin Epidemiol. 2013;66:1093–104.
11. Whiting P, Rutjes AW, Reitsma JB, Glas AS, Bossuyt PM, Kleijnen J. Sources of variation and bias in studies of diagnostic accuracy: a systematic review. Ann Intern Med. 2004;140:189–202.
12. Cook C, Cleland J, Huijbregts P. Creation and critique of studies of diagnostic accuracy: use of the STARD and QUADAS methodological quality assessment tools. J Man Manip Ther. 2007;15:93–102.
13. http://www.joannabriggs.org/assets/docs/sumari/Reviewers-Manual_The-systematic-review-of-studies-of-diagnostic-test-accuracy.pdf. Accessed 28 June 2018.
14. Roever L. Types of bias in studies of diagnostic test accuracy. Evid Based Med Pract. 2016;1:e113.
15. Mulherin SA, Miller WC. Spectrum bias or spectrum effect? Subgroup variation in diagnostic test evaluation. Ann Intern Med. 2002;137:598–602.
16. Willis BH. Spectrum bias—why clinicians need to be cautious when applying diagnostic test studies. Fam Pract. 2008;25:390–6.
17. Kohn MA, Carpenter CR, Newman TB. Understanding the direction of bias in studies of diagnostic test accuracy. Acad Emerg Med. 2013;20:1194–206.
18. Chien T, Malhotra R, Bhandari M. The 3-min appraisal of a diagnostic test. Indian J Orthop. 2011 Sep;45:389–91.
19. Reitsma JB, Rutjes AWS, Whiting P, Vlassov VV, Leeflang MMG, Deeks JJ. Chapter 9: assessing methodological quality. In: Deeks JJ, Bossuyt PM, Gatsonis C, editors. Cochrane handbook for systematic reviews of diagnostic test accuracy version 1.0.0: The Cochrane Collaboration; 2009. Available from: http://srdta.cochrane.org/. Accessed 28 June 2018.
20. Manikandan R, Dorairajan LN. How to appraise a diagnostic test. Indian J Urol. 2011;27: 513–9.
21. http://www.cebm.net/wp-content/uploads/2014/04/diagnostic-study-appraisal-worksheet.pdf. Accessed 28 June 2018.
22. Glasziou P, Altman DG, Bossuyt P, Boutron I, Clarke M, Julious S, Michie S, Moher D, Wager E. Reducing waste from incomplete or unusable reports of biomedical research. Lancet. 2014;383:267–76.
23. Bossuyt PM. The quality of reporting in diagnostic test research: getting better, still not optimal. Clin Chem. 2004;50:465–6.
24. Cohen JF, Korevaar DA, Altman DG, Bruns DE, Gatsonis CA, Hooft L, Irwig L, Levine D, Reitsma JB, de Vet HC, Bossuyt PM. STARD 2015 guidelines for reporting diagnostic accuracy studies: explanation and elaboration. BMJ Open. 2016;6:e012799.
25. Bossuyt PM, Reitsma JB, Bruns DE, Gatsonis CA, Glasziou PP, Irwig L, Lijmer JG, Moher D, Rennie D, de Vet HC, Kressel HY, Rifai N, Golub RM, Altman DG, Hooft L, Korevaar

DA, Cohen JF, STARD Group. STARD 2015: an updated list of essential items for reporting diagnostic accuracy studies. BMJ. 2015;351:h5527.
26. Ochodo EA, Bossuyt PM. Reporting the accuracy of diagnostic tests: the STARD initiative 10 years on. Clin Chem. 2013;59:917–9.
27. Korevaar DA, Wang J, van Enst WA, Leeflang MM, Hooft L, Smidt N, Bossuyt PM. Reporting diagnostic accuracy studies: some improvements after 10 years of STARD. Radiology. 2015;274:781–9.
28. Pecoraro V, Banzi R, Trenti T. Quality of reporting of diagnostic test accuracy studies in medical laboratory journals. Clin Chem Lab Med. 2016;54:e319–21.
29. Leeflang MM, Deeks JJ, Gatsonis C, Bossuyt PM, Cochrane Diagnostic Test Accuracy Working Group. Systematic reviews of diagnostic test accuracy. Ann Intern Med. 2008;149(12):889–97.
30. Whiting PF, Rutjes AW, Westwood ME, Mallett S, Deeks JJ, Reitsma JB, Leeflang MM, Sterne JA, Bossuyt PM, QUADAS-2 Group. QUADAS-2: a revised tool for the quality assessment of diagnostic accuracy studies. Ann Intern Med. 2011;155:529–36.
31. Whiting P, Rutjes AW, Reitsma JB, Bossuyt PM, Kleijnen J. The development of QUADAS: a tool for the quality assessment of studies of diagnostic accuracy included in systematic reviews. BMC Med Res Methodol. 2003;3:25.
32. Whiting PF, Weswood ME, Rutjes AW, Reitsma JB, Bossuyt PN, Kleijnen J. Evaluation of QUADAS, a tool for the quality assessment of diagnostic accuracy studies. BMC Med Res Methodol. 2006;6:9.
33. Whiting P, Harbord R, Kleijnen J. No role for quality scores in systematic reviews of diagnostic accuracy studies. BMC Med Res Methodol. 2005;5:19.
34. Schünemann HJ, Oxman AD, Brozek J, Glasziou P, Jaeschke R, Vist GE, Williams JW Jr, Kunz R, Craig J, Montori VM, Bossuyt P, Guyatt GH, GRADE Working Group. Grading quality of evidence and strength of recommendations for diagnostic tests and strategies. BMJ. 2008;336:1106–10.
35. Gopalakrishna G, Mustafa RA, Davenport C, Scholten RJ, Hyde C, Brozek J, Schünemann HJ, Bossuyt PM, Leeflang MM, Langendam MW. Applying Grading of Recommendations Assessment, Development and Evaluation (GRADE) to diagnostic tests was challenging but doable. J Clin Epidemiol. 2014;67:760–8.
36. Brozek JL, Akl EA, Jaeschke R, Lang DM, Bossuyt P, Glasziou P, Helfand M, Ueffing E, Alonso-Coello P, Meerpohl J, Phillips B, Horvath AR, Bousquet J, Guyatt GH, Schünemann HJ, GRADE Working Group. Grading quality of evidence and strength of recommendations in clinical practice guidelines: Part 2 of 3. The GRADE approach to grading quality of evidence about diagnostic tests and strategies. Allergy. 2009;64:1109–16.
37. Balshem H, Helfand M, Schünemann HJ, Oxman AD, Kunz R, Brozek J, Vist GE, Falck-Ytter Y, Meerpohl J, Norris S, Guyatt GH. GRADE guidelines: 3. Rating the quality of evidence. J Clin Epidemiol. 2011;64:401–6.

Synthesizing Evidence 10

Paul-Christian Bürkner

10.1 Introduction

Results of diagnostic studies are typically reported in terms of 2 × 2 tables that capture the relation of the true state of participants with the state that is diagnosed by the test under evaluation (see Table 10.1). The approaches presented in this chapter all assume that the true state is known and measured without error. In practice, the true state may not always be known exactly, but we can assume that a sufficiently accurate *gold standard* test exists that can serve as a benchmark for other tests.

Synthesizing evidence in diagnostic meta-analyses comes with more challenges than typical meta-analyses such as those evaluating clinical trials [1]. This is due to the fact that diagnostic studies always have two relevant outcomes: (1) the accuracy of the diagnostic test for participants who have the target condition and (2) the accuracy for participants who do not have the target condition. The former is measured by the *sensitivity* that is the proportion of participants with the target condition who are correctly identified as such:

$$\text{Sen} = \frac{y_{11}}{n_1} \tag{10.1}$$

The latter is measured by the *specificity* that is the proportion of participants without the target condition who are correctly identified as such:

$$\text{Spe} = \frac{y_{00}}{n_0} \tag{10.2}$$

It is critical to incorporate both outcomes in the evaluation of the test's performance. For instance, one could easily achieve 100% sensitivity through diagnosing everyone as positive, but this would not lead to a meaningful test since the

P.-C. Bürkner
Institute of Psychology, University of Münster, Münster, Germany

G. Biondi-Zoccai (ed.), *Diagnostic Meta-Analysis*,
https://doi.org/10.1007/978-3-319-78966-8_10

Table 10.1 Data from a diagnostic study in a 2 × 2 table

		True state		
		With target condition	Without target condition	Total
Diagnostic Test	Positive	y_{11}	y_{01}	m_1
	Negative	y_{10}	y_{00}	m_0
	Total	n_1	n_2	N

specificity would be 0% in this case. Generally, there is a trade-off between sensitivity and specificity: Depending on where we set the threshold at which participants are diagnosed as positive, we will favor sensitivity over specificity or vice versa. The fact that studies often use different thresholds further complicates meta-analyses of diagnostic studies. Even in the same study, multiple thresholds with corresponding sensitivities and specificities might be reported, but in the present chapter, we assume that only one pair of sensitivity and specificity is selected for each diagnostic study.

In addition to sensitivity and specificity, there are other bivariate statistics used in diagnostic studies. The *positive predictive value* (PPV) measures the probability that, given a positive test result, the diagnosed participant indeed has the target condition, while the *negative predictive value* (NPV) measures the probability that, given a negative test result, the diagnosed participant does not have the target condition. With the above introduced notation, PPV and NPV can be written as follows:

$$\mathrm{PPV} = \frac{y_{11}}{m_1} \tag{10.3}$$

$$\mathrm{NPV} = \frac{y_{00}}{m_0} \tag{10.4}$$

An important property of these two measures is that they depend on the prevalence of the target condition, that is, the proportion of participants in the population having the target condition at a certain point in time. Thus, we always have to keep the prevalence in mind when interpreting PPV and NPV. Also, since the prevalence might vary across studies, using these quantities for meta-analyses is somewhat more complicated.

A pair of diagnostic quantities derived directly from sensitivity and specificity are the *positive likelihood ratio* (PLR) and the *negative likelihood ratio* (NLR). They are defined as the odds that a positive and negative test result, respectively, is obtained for participants having the target condition versus those not having the target condition. More formally:

$$\mathrm{PLR} = \frac{\mathrm{Sen}}{1 - \mathrm{Spe}} \tag{10.5}$$

$$\mathrm{NLR} = \frac{1 - \mathrm{Sen}}{\mathrm{Spe}} \tag{10.6}$$

While intuitively appealing, [2] have argued against the use of likelihood ratios in meta-analyses, as summarizing them across studies may lead to impossible summary estimates for sensitivity and specificity.

Quite a few statistical methods have been proposed to tackle the problem of synthesizing evidence in diagnostic meta-analysis. In the present chapter, we will focus on the currently most common and important ones and briefly mention less common approaches at the end of the chapter.

10.2 The SROC Curve

One of the oldest methods developed to summarize diagnostic studies is the *summary receiver operating characteristic curve* (SROC curve; [3]). While the basic SROC approach is rarely applied in practice to date, because of the development of more advanced methods, understanding it is vital to the understanding of most other methods, and so we introduce the SROC approach first. The basic SROC curve can be obtained as follows. First, compute the quantities

$$D_i = \text{logit}(\text{Sen}_i) - \text{logit}(1 - \text{Spe}_i) \tag{10.7}$$

$$S_i = \text{logit}(\text{Sen}_i) + \text{logit}(1 - \text{Spe}_i) \tag{10.8}$$

for each study i. The logit transform $\text{logit}(p) = \log(p/(1 - p))$ is used to transform probabilities or rates in the unit interval [0, 1] to values on the complete real line. The quantity D_i is the log of the diagnostic odds ratio that may also be used as a one-dimensional measure of diagnostic accuracy (see Sect. 10.5). Second, fit a linear regression with D as response variable and S as predictor variable:

$$D_i = a + bS_i + e_i \tag{10.9}$$

The regression may also be weighted to account for differences in the measurement uncertainty between studies typically originating from varying sample sizes. Studies with less measurement uncertainty/higher sample sizes will receive higher weights. In Eq. (10.9), a and b are the model intercept and slope, respectively, and e_i is the error term, which is assumed to be normally distributed. Third, having estimated a and b, we can back-transform values to the original scales to obtain the SROC curve capturing the relation between the sensitivity and the false-positive rate (FPR), which is just one minus specificity.

$$\text{Sen}(\text{FPR}) = \left(1 + \exp\left(-\hat{a} / \left(1 - \hat{b}\right)\right)\left(\frac{1 - \text{FPR}}{\text{FPR}}\right)^{\left(1+\hat{b}\right)/\left(1-\hat{b}\right)}\right)^{-1}. \tag{10.10}$$

In the above equation, $\hat{a}$ and $\hat{b}$ denote the estimates of a and b computed from the data. Consider the following example of four hypothetical diagnostic studies with sensitivities and specificities given in Table 10.2. Using linear regression, the estimates of a and b can be computed as $\hat{a} = 3.06$ and $\hat{b} = 0.05$. Applying formula

Table 10.2 Hypothetical data from four diagnostic studies

Study	Sensitivity	Specificity	Logit(Sen)	Logit(Spe)	*D*	*S*
1	0.74	0.88	1.05	1.99	3.04	−0.95
2	0.84	0.83	1.66	1.59	3.24	0.07
3	0.95	0.57	2.94	0.28	3.23	2.66
4	0.82	0.79	1.52	1.32	2.84	0.19

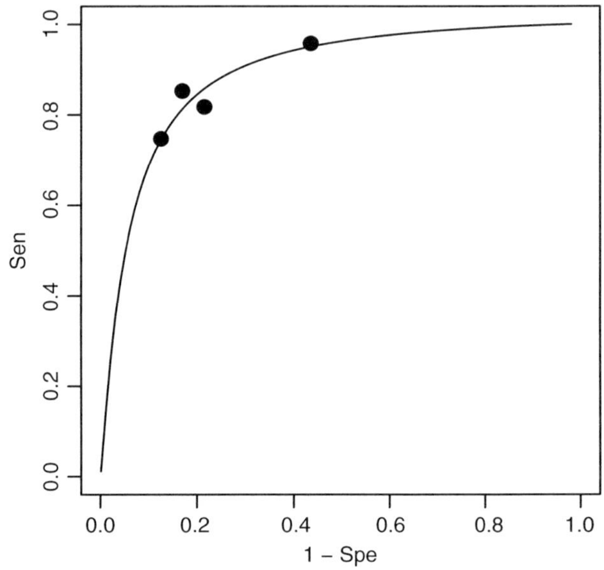

Fig. 10.1 SROC curve based on four hypothetical diagnostic studies. Dots indicate pairs of sensitivity and false-positive rate obtained from the studies

(10.10) yields the SROC curve for the four diagnostic studies (see Fig. 10.1). We see that studies differ to a non-negligible amount with respect to sensitivity and specificity, but apparently, the SROC curve provides a good fit to the data. Hence, it is plausible that differences between studies originate simply from different thresholds.

A common method to summarize (S)ROC curves is the *area under the curve* (AUC). It can be interpreted as the average sensitivity of the diagnostic test taken over all possible values of the specificity [4]. The higher the AUC, the higher the accuracy of the diagnostic test, with AUC = 0.5 describing a useless test, classifying participants at random, and AUC = 1 describing a perfect test, classifying all participants correctly. The AUC might also be interpreted as follows: If pairs of participants—one with and one without the target condition—are randomly drawn and tested, the AUC is equal to the probability that the participant getting the higher test result is the one with the target condition. When only a certain range of specificity values is of interest, one may compute the partial AUC, which is simply the average sensitivity over the desired range of specificity values.

The basic SROC approach is easy to apply and provides a nice visualization of the relationship of sensitivity and specificity across studies. The main problem with this method is, however, that it assumes all variation between studies to originate from differences in the applied thresholds. Hence, we call the basic SROC approach a *fixed effects* model to indicate that we do not allow for systematic variation between studies apart from the applied threshold. This assumption is quite unrealistic since studies often differ considerably in other aspects such as the investigated population or the exact testing procedure. Thus, more advanced methods have been developed over the years, and we will explain the two most important ones in the two upcoming sections.

10.3 The Hierarchical Model

To overcome the main problem of the basic SROC approach and incorporate systematic variation between studies, Rutter and Gatsonis [5] introduced their hierarchical model, which we will call the HSROC (hierarchical SROC) model in the following. It formally originates from a binomial regression model for the number of positively diagnosed participants in both study arms. We assume that y_{ij1}—where $j \in \{0, 1\}$ indexes study arms (i.e., participants with and without the target condition)—are binomially distributed with probabilities π_{ij} and sample sizes n_{ij}:

$$y_{ij1} \sim \text{Binomial}\left(\pi_{ij}, n_{ij}\right) \tag{10.11}$$

The probabilities π_{i1} and π_{i0} are to be predicted in a regression model. The former probability refers the sensitivity of study i, whereas π_{i0} refers to the false-positive rate of study i. The logit of π_{ij} should be regressed as:

$$\text{logit}\left(\pi_{ij}\right) = \left(\theta_i + \alpha_i X_{ij}\right)\exp\left(-\beta X_{ij}\right). \tag{10.12}$$

The dummy variable X_{ij} indicates the true state of the participants being coded as $X_{i0} = -1/2$ and $X_{i1} = 1/2$. The parameters of the model, which are to be estimated, are θ_i, α_i, as well as β. The model intercepts θ_i are called accuracy parameters since they model the difference between sensitivity and false-positive rate. The slopes α_i are called accuracy parameters since they model the difference between sensitivity and false-positive rate. Both θ_i and α_i are allowed to vary between studies (as indicated by the index i) and are assumed to come from independent normal distributions:

$$\theta_i \sim N\left(\theta, \sigma_\theta\right) \tag{10.13}$$

$$\alpha_i \sim N\left(\alpha, \sigma_\alpha\right) \tag{10.14}$$

This is a so called *random effects* assumption contrasting with the fixed effects assumption of the basic SROC approach. The parameters θ, α, σ_θ, and σ_α are hyperparameters, which are also estimated from the data. Finally, the parameter β in Eq. (10.12) is a scale parameter, which allows for differences in the variance of diagnostic outcomes in the populations having/not having the target condition. It requires information from multiple studies and hence cannot be assumed to vary across studies.

The authors of the HSROC model proposed to fit it using fully Bayesian techniques, but it may also be fitted using classical statistical methods [6]. Having estimated the model parameters, the HSROC curve can be computed as

$$\mathrm{Sen}(\mathrm{FPR}) = \mathrm{logit}^{-1}\left(\left(\mathrm{logit}(\mathrm{FPR})\exp\left(\hat{\beta}/2\right)+\hat{\alpha}\right)\exp\left(\hat{\beta}/2\right)\right), \tag{10.15}$$

where $\mathrm{logit}^{-1}(x) = \dfrac{\exp(x)}{1+\exp(x)}$ is the inverse of the logit-transform.

Adding covariates—sometimes also called (effect) moderators—to the HSROC model is straightforward: One may simply replace θ and / or α with linear predictor terms that is:

$$\theta = \theta_0 + \sum_{k=1}^{K_\theta} \theta_k Z_k \tag{10.16}$$

$$\alpha = \alpha_0 + \sum_{k=1}^{K_\alpha} \alpha_k Z_k, \tag{10.17}$$

where Z_k are the covariates and θ_k and α_k are the corresponding regression parameters. For instance, if the aim of the test is to diagnose lung cancer, one may add the type of lung cancer investigated in each study as a dummy-coded covariate. Of course, one may choose to use different covariates for θ and α or only predict one of them.

The HSROC model is a flexible and powerful approach for performing diagnostic meta-analysis. However, another (under certain conditions equivalent) random effect model is more frequently applied and is introduced in the upcoming section.

10.4 The Bivariate Model

Similar to the hierarchical model, the bivariate model proposed by [7], extended in [8], brought to greater attention by [9], and refined by [10] preserves the bivariate nature of diagnostic outcomes and allows for systematic variation (i.e., random effects) between studies. As noted earlier, diagnosticians have to make a trade-off between sensitivity and specificity since lowering the threshold increases sensitivity but at the same time decreases specificity. Thus, there is an inherent negative correlation between sensitivity and specificity, which is explicitly considered in the bivariate model. Formally, the logit-transformed sensitivities of each study are assumed to come from a bivariate normal distribution with mean vector (θ_{Sen}, θ_{Spe}) and covariance matrix Σ estimated from the data. We write:

$$\begin{pmatrix} \mathrm{logit}(\mathrm{Sen}_i) \\ \mathrm{logit}(\mathrm{Spe}_i) \end{pmatrix} \sim N\left(\begin{pmatrix} \theta_{\mathrm{Sen}} \\ \theta_{\mathrm{Spe}} \end{pmatrix}, \Sigma\right) \tag{10.18}$$

and

$$\Sigma = \begin{pmatrix} \sigma_{\text{Sen}}^2 & \rho\sigma_{\text{Sen}}\sigma_{\text{Spe}} \\ \rho\sigma_{\text{Sen}}\sigma_{\text{Spe}} & \sigma_{\text{Spe}}^2 \end{pmatrix}, \tag{10.19}$$

where σ_{Sen} and σ_{Spe} denote the standard deviation across studies of logit sensitivity and specificity, respectively, and ρ denotes their correlation. Sensitivities and specificities are measured with different precision due to varying sample sizes both within and between studies. Studies including more participants achieve higher precision/lower variance and should thus receive higher weights in the meta-analysis. The within study variances $s_{\text{Sen}_i}^2$ and $s_{\text{Spe}_i}^2$ of logit sensitivity and specificity of study i can be approximated as follows:

$$s_{\text{Sen}_i}^2 = \frac{1}{n_{i1}\,\text{Sen}_i\left(1-\text{Sen}_i\right)} \tag{10.20}$$

$$s_{\text{Spe}_i}^2 = \frac{1}{n_{i0}\,\text{Spe}_i\left(1-\text{Spe}_i\right)} \tag{10.21}$$

For smaller sample sizes or in case of zero sensitivity or specificity, these approximations may not be accurate [11]. Therefore, one should rather use the binomial parameterization of the bivariate model as noted by [10]. Denoting with S_i the within study variance matrix that is:

$$S_i = \begin{pmatrix} s_{\text{Sen}_i}^2 & 0 \\ 0 & s_{\text{Spe}_i}^2 \end{pmatrix}, \tag{10.22}$$

the complete bivariate model for diagnostic meta-analysis is given by:

$$\begin{pmatrix} \text{logit}\left(\text{Sen}_i\right) \\ \text{logit}\left(\text{Spe}_i\right) \end{pmatrix} \sim N\left(\begin{pmatrix} \theta_{\text{Sen}} \\ \theta_{\text{Spe}} \end{pmatrix}, \Sigma + S_i\right). \tag{10.23}$$

The parameters θ_{Sen} and θ_{Spe} denote the meta-analytic logit sensitivity and specificity, respectively. Together with their estimated confidence intervals, they may be transformed back to the original metric by applying the inverse of the logit-transform. The standard deviations σ_{Sen} and σ_{Spe} provide information on the variation of sensitivity and specificity across studies, for instance, due to different thresholds or other systematic differences between studies. Finally, ρ captures the (usually negative) correlation between sensitivity and specificity. Similar to the HSROC model, moderators may easily be introduced by replacing θ_{Sen} and θ_{Spe} with linear predictors, that is:

$$\theta_{\text{Sen}} = \theta_{\text{Sen}0} + \sum_{k=1}^{K_{\text{Sen}}} \theta_{\text{Sen}k} Z_k \tag{10.24}$$

$$\theta_{\text{Spe}} = \theta_{\text{Sen}0} + \sum_{k=1}^{K_{\text{Spe}}} \theta_{\text{Spe}k} Z_k. \tag{10.25}$$

The bivariate model can easily be fit using standard statistical software (cf. Chap. 12). Although the HSROC and the bivariate model may look rather different at first glance, it has been shown by [12] and likewise and independently by [13] that they are very closely related and even equivalent in the absence of covariates. Since the bivariate model is easier to fit and perhaps also easier to understand, it has become the standard approach for meta-analysis of diagnostic studies, and we highly recommend its application when only one diagnostic test is being evaluated [1]. The bivariate model can also be applied if quantities other than sensitivity and specificity—such as the positive and negative likelihood ratio—are of primary interest, as one can generate samples for observed sensitivities and specifities based on the fitted model parameters and then use these samples to obtain estimates for other quantities [2]. In fact, models that directly target alternative quantities may be so complicated that using the bivariate model, instead, is advised even in these cases [2].

10.4.1 Other Bivariate Models

Several other methods have been proposed that provide either extentions or alternatives to the standard bivariate model. More advanced methods of fitting the bivariate model include composite likelihood [14] or simulation-based methods [15]. Alternative models include the method of [16] using the Lehmann family, the method of [17] based on the Youden index, nonparametric approaches [18, 19], semi-parametric mixtures [20], or copulas [21]. Due to the large number of alternative models, we will not discuss them in more detail in the present chapter. Generalizations of the bivariate model for the comparison of multiple diagnostic tests are introduced in Chap. 13.

10.5 Univariate Approaches

Although it is highly recommended to keep the bivariate nature of diagnostic data in order not to lose information, we want to briefly note the possibility of univariate diagnostic meta-analysis. In order to apply standard meta-analytic techniques such as those used for clinical trials, one has to find a univariate measure of diagnostic accuracy that is approximately normally distributed. Glas et al. [22] proposed to use the log diagnostic odds ratio D for this purpose, which we have already introduced in Eq. (10.7). The log diagnostic odds ratio has some favorable properties as compared to other univariate measures such that it is relatively robust to varying threshold across studies [22]. The variance of its estimator can be computed as

$$\mathrm{Var}\left(\hat{D}_i\right) = \frac{1}{y_{i11}} + \frac{1}{y_{i10}} + \frac{1}{y_{i01}} + \frac{1}{y_{i00}}. \tag{10.26}$$

Meta-analysis may be performed using the standard univariate model for normally distributed outcomes:

$$\hat{D}_i \sim N\left(\theta, \sigma_\theta^2 + \mathrm{Var}\left(\hat{D}_i\right)\right), \tag{10.27}$$

where θ is the meta-analytic estimate across studies and σ_θ^2 is the between study variance. We do not recommend using a univariate approach to diagnostic meta-analysis, but if one still wants to apply it for some reason, the log diagnostic odds ratio should be the measure of choice.

Conclusion

In the present chapter, we introduced several methods to synthesize evidence of diagnostic studies. Emphasis was put on the bivariate nature of diagnostic outcomes, as performance of diagnostic tests is evaluated for participants who have the target condition and participants who do not have the target condition. Thus, appropriate methods analyze pairs of sensitivity and specificity. Despite other reasonable methods, we recommend applying the bivariate model—or one of its extensions—as it allows for systematic variation between studies in addition to differences in the applied thresholds while still being relatively easy to fit using standard statistical software.

Acknowledgments I want to thank Prof. Philipp Doebler and Prof. Gerta Rücker for their very helpful comments on this chapter.

References

1. Macaskill P, Gatsonis C, Deeks J, Harbord R, Takwoingi Y. Cochrane handbook for systematic reviews of diagnostic test accuracy. London: The Cochrane Collaboration; 2010.
2. Zwinderman AH, Bossuyt PM. We should not pool diagnostic likelihood ratios in systematic reviews. Stat Med. 2008;27:687–97.
3. Moses LE, Shapiro D, Littenberg B. Combining independent studies of a diagnostic test into a summary roc curve: data-analytic approaches and some additional considerations. Stat Med. 1993;12:1293–316.
4. Gatsonis C, Paliwal P. Meta-analysis of diagnostic and screening test accuracy evaluations: methodologic primer. Am J Roentgenol. 2006;187:271–81.
5. Rutter CM, Gatsonis CA. A hierarchical regression approach to meta-analysis of diagnostic test accuracy evaluations. Stat Med. 2001;20:2865–84.
6. Macaskill P. Empirical Bayes estimates generated in a hierarchical summary roc analysis agreed closely with those of a full Bayesian analysis. J Clin Epidemiol. 2004;57:925–32.
7. Van Houwelingen HC, Zwinderman KH, Stijnen T. A bivariate approach to meta-analysis. Stat Med. 1993;12:2273–84.
8. Van Houwelingen HC, Arends LR, Stijnen T. Advanced methods in meta-analysis: multivariate approach and meta-regression. Stat Med. 2002;21:589–624.
9. Reitsma JB, Glas AS, Rutjes AWS, Scholten RJPM, Bossuyt PM, Zwinderman AH. Bivariate analysis of sensitivity and specificity produces informative summary measures in diagnostic reviews. J Clin Epidemiol. 2005;58:982–90.
10. Chu H, Cole SR. Bivariate meta-analysis of sensitivity and specificity with sparse data: a generalized linear mixed model approach. J Clin Epidemiol. 2006;59:1331–2.
11. Sweeting MJ, Sutton AJ, Lambert PC. What to add to nothing? Use and avoidance of continuity corrections in meta-analysis of sparse data. Stat Med. 2004;23:1351–75.

12. Harbord RM, Deeks JJ, Egger M, Whiting P, Sterne JAC. A unification of models for meta-analysis of diagnostic accuracy studies. Biostatistics. 2007;8:239–51.
13. Arends LR, Hamza H, Van Houwelingen HC, Heijenbrok-Kal MH, Hunink MGM, Stijnen T. Bivariate random effects meta-analysis of roc curves. Med Decis Mak. 2008;28:621–38.
14. Chen Y, Liu Y, Ning J, Nie L, Zhu H, Chu H. A composite likelihood method for bivariate meta-analysis in diagnostic systematic reviews. Stat Methods Med Res. 2017;26:914–30.
15. Annamaria Guolo. A double simex approach for bivariate random-effects meta-analysis of diagnostic accuracy studies. BMC Med Res Methodol. 2017;17:6.
16. Holling H, Böhning W, Böhning D. Meta-analysis of diagnostic studies based upon sroc-curves: a mixed model approach using the Lehmann family. Stat Model. 2012;12:347–75.
17. Rücker G, Schumacher M. Summary roc curve based on a weighted Youden index for selecting an optimal cutpoint in meta-analysis of diagnostic accuracy. Stat Med. 2010;29:3069–78.
18. Martínez-Camblor P. Fully non-parametric receiver operating characteristic curve estimation for random-effects meta-analysis. Stat Methods Med Res. 2017;26:5–20.
19. Zapf A, Hoyer A, Kramer K, Kuss O. Nonparametric meta-analysis for diagnostic accuracy studies. Stat Med. 2015;34:3831–41.
20. Doebler P, Holling H. Meta-analysis of diagnostic accuracy and roc curves with covariate adjusted semiparametric mixtures. Psychometrika. 2015;80:1084–104.
21. Kuss O, Hoyer A, Solms A. Meta-analysis for diagnostic accuracy studies: a new statistical model using beta-binomial distributions and bivariate copulas. Stat Med. 2014;33:17–30.
22. Glas AS, Lijmer JG, Prins MH, Bonsel GJ, Bossuyt PMM. The diagnostic odds ratio: a single indicator of test performance. J Clin Epidemiol. 2003;56:1129–35.

Appraising Heterogeneity 11

Antonia Zapf

11.1 Introduction

In the *Cochrane Handbook for Systematic Reviews of Diagnostic Test Accuracy* ([1], Section 10.1.3), the authors name as one difference between interventional and diagnostic meta-analyses that heterogeneity is to be expected in the diagnostic context. This means that heterogeneity is not an exception but the rule in diagnostic meta-analyses. This variability can be caused by chance alone or by true heterogeneity. To consider this heterogeneity in an appropriate way is a crucial point in diagnostic meta-analysis.

11.1.1 Structure of the Chapter

Naaktgeboren et al. [2] evaluated in a systematic overview how authors explored potential sources of heterogeneity in diagnostic meta-analysis and how they handle it in analysis and reporting. The result was that heterogeneity was explored in the majority of the meta-analyses, but that the methods used for exploration varied widely. For this reason, Naaktgeboren et al. [2] made suggestions what should be considered and reported when heterogeneity is explored. The general recommendation of the Cochrane Collaboration is to group the studies in categories for graphical illustration and to investigate the relationship between diagnostic accuracy and covariates by meta-regression models ([1], Section 10.1.4.2). To put a finer point of it, Naaktgeboren et al. [3] recommend a five-step approach for the assessment of the variability: (1) Visualize total

A. Zapf
Department of Medical Statistics, University Medical Center Göttingen, Göttingen, Germany

Department of Medical Biometry and Epidemiology, University Medical Center Hamburg-Eppendorf, Hamburg, Germany
e-mail: a.zapf@uke.de

G. Biondi-Zoccai (ed.), *Diagnostic Meta-Analysis*,
https://doi.org/10.1007/978-3-319-78966-8_11

variability, (2) judge, whether there is more variability in sensitivity and specificity than can be expected by chance, (3) measure the total between-study variability, (4) attribute some of the between-study variability to the threshold effect, and (5) explore what study features might explain some of the variability' (see Fig. 11.1). As a memento, sensitivity is the true positive (TP) rate, and specificity is the true negative (TN) rate, meaning

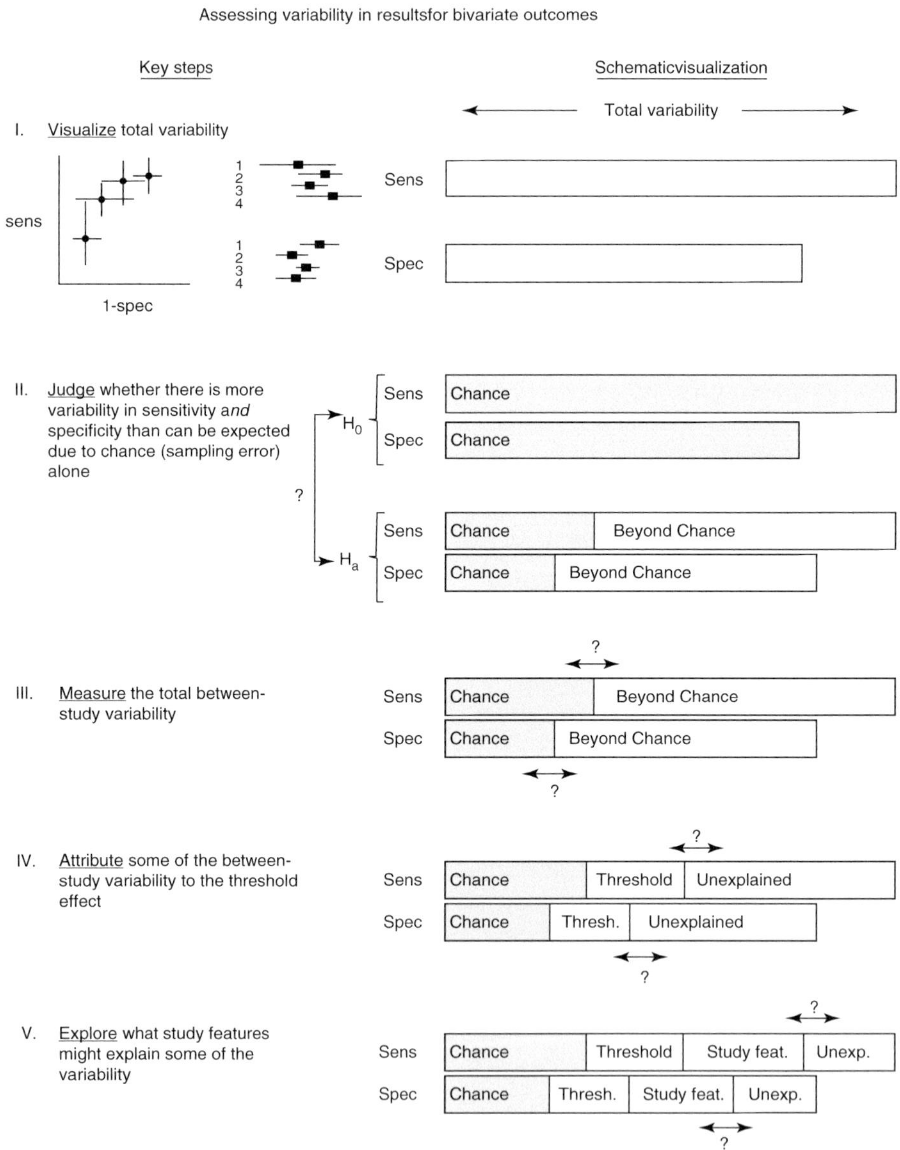

Fig. 11.1 Process of the assessment of variability suggested from Naaktgeboren et al. [3]

Table 11.1 Diagnostic fourfold table with the used notation

		Reference standard		
		Diseased	Non-diseased	Total
Index test	Positive	TP	FP	n_p
	Negative	FN	TN	n_n
	Total	n_1	n_2	N

$$\mathrm{se} = \frac{\mathrm{TP}}{n_1} \quad \text{and} \quad \mathrm{sp} = \frac{\mathrm{TN}}{n_2}$$

with TP, TN, n_1, and n_2 from the diagnostic fourfold table (Table 11.1).

Accordingly, the structure of this chapter is as it follows: First, the different sources of variation and bias and the consequences for diagnostic meta-analysis will be described. Afterwards, in Sect. 11.3 graphical approaches for illustration of variability will be presented (*visualize*). Statistical tests (*judge*) and measures for quantification of variability (*measure*) will be discussed in Sects. 11.4 and 11.5. In Sect. 11.6 modelling approaches for multiple thresholds are introduced (*attribute*), and in Sect. 11.7 the different approaches for 'standard' meta-analysis of heterogeneous diagnostic accuracy studies will be presented (*explore*). The focus will be set on sensitivity and specificity as co-primary endpoints and on the comparison of an index test with the reference standard. The comparison of two or more index tests will be addressed in Chap. 9 about network meta-analysis. In Sect. 11.8 approaches for diagnostic meta-analysis with 'special features' as, for example, multiple thresholds, individual patient data, or other accuracy measures will be presented. In the last section of this chapter, in Sect. 11.9, the results will be summarized.

11.1.2 Illustrating Example Meta-analysis

For the illustration of the different approaches, data of the meta-analysis from Roberts et al. [4] about the diagnostic accuracy of the natriuretic peptides in heart failure in the acute care setting are used. In the original meta-analysis, the diagnostic accuracy of serum natriuretic peptide levels (BNP and NTproBNP) and of mid-regional proatrial natriuretic peptide (MRproANP) was investigated. However, in the following, the focus will be set on the data of BNP. This meta-analysis was selected because quite many primary studies are included, several covariates are reported, and different and multiple thresholds were investigated in the individual studies. Roberts et al. [4] distinguished three groups regarding the used threshold: below 110 ng/L, between 110 and 500 ng/L, and above 500 ng/L. Each study occurred in one group only once but can occur in more than one group (the maximum number of considered thresholds per study is three). In the first group, all thresholds were very similar (between 100 and 110 ng/L); therefore, this group will be used for approaches, which cannot handle different thresholds. In the other two groups, the threshold varied strongly (between 110 and 400 ng/L in the second group and between 500 and

1000 ng/L in the third group). The second group was used for approaches, which can handle different but not multiple thresholds, and all three groups were used for approaches which can handle different and multiple thresholds. Roberts et al. analysed the BNP data in the low- and in the medium-threshold group. For the visualization of the heterogeneity, they used ROC plots including the SROC curves, funnel plots, and forest plots. To test for publication bias, the authors performed the Deeks' funnel plot asymmetry test. They measured the heterogeneity with the I^2 index and investigated in the case of large heterogeneity the variation in sensitivity and specificity by adding covariates in the bivariate meta-analysis model. Furthermore, they compared models with and without covariates with the likelihood ratio test. All these methods will be described and discussed in this chapter.

In some studies zero false-positive or false-negative results were reported. If an approach cannot handle such zero cells, a continuity correction of 0.5 was added to all entries (TP, FP, TN, FN) of all studies. The characteristics of the included primary studies (obtained from [4]) are summarized in Table 11.2. For the analysis of the data, the packages 'mada' [5, 6] and 'meta' [7, 8] for the statistical computing environment R [9] were used.

11.2 Sources of Bias and Variation

In the meta-analysis of diagnostic accuracy studies, the reason for heterogeneity can be variation and bias. Variation can be caused by different research questions in the individual studies, leading, for example, to study populations with differences in disease prevalence. Another important source of variation is the chosen threshold to define a positive test result. In contrast, bias relates to the individual studies and is caused by inappropriate study design, study conduct, or data analysis. Therefore, the challenge for the meta-analysis is to address the variation and to correct for the bias to obtain interpretable and reliable results. Lijmer et al. [35] explored the sources of heterogeneity using the diagnostic odds ratio as summary measure and pointed out that there are artefactual, methodological, and clinical causes of heterogeneity.

11.2.1 Sources in Different Dimensions of Diagnostic Studies

Whiting et al. [36] investigated and summarized the different sources of variation and bias in diagnostic accuracy studies in five dimensions: study population, index test, reference standard, reading process, and data analysis.

- Differences in the study populations regarding demographic features, disease severity, disease prevalence, and distorted selection of participants may lead to a variation of the diagnostic accuracy estimates.
- Regarding the index test, variation can result from differences in test execution and test technology, while a delay between the reference standard and the index

Table 11.2 Characteristics of the included primary studies, obtained from Roberts et al. [4]

Study number	Study identifier	Design	BNP index test	Overall study quality (QUADAS II)	Number of participants	Prevalence in %	Threshold
1	Alibay 2005 [10]	Cross-sectional	Triage	High	160	38	100, 150
2	Arques 2005 [11]	Prospective	Triage	High	70	46	100, 146
3	Arques 2007 [12]	Prospective	Triage	Low	41	54	253
4	Barcase 2004 [13]	Prospective	Triage	High	98	58	100, 300
5	Blonde-Cynober 2011 [14]	Prospective	Triage	Low	64	41	100, 129, 635
6	Chenevier-Gobeaux 2010 [15]	Prospective	Triage	High	378	30	100
7	Chung 2006 [16]	Prospective	Triage	High	143	50	100, 400
8	Dao 2001 [17]	Cross-sectional	Triage	High	250	39	100, 150
9	Davis 1994 [18]	Prospective	In-house	Low	52	62	100, 195
10	Dokainish 2004 [19]	Cross-sectional	Triage	High	122	57	250
11	Fleischer 1997 [20]	Prospective	In-house	High	123	35	173
12	Gorissen 2007 [21]	Retrospective	Triage	High	80	50	225
13	Karmpaliotis 2007 [22]	Prospective	Triage	High	74	31	1000
14	Lainchbury 2003 [23]	Prospective	Triage	High	205	34	104, 347
15	Logeart 2002 [24]	Cross-sectional	Triage	High	163	71	100, 250

(continued)

Table 11.2 (continued)

Study number	Study identifier	Design	BNP index test	Overall study quality (QUADAS II)	Number of participants	Prevalence in %	Threshold
16	Lokuge 2010 [25]	Retrospective	Abbott	High	612	45	101, 265
17	Maisel 2002 [26]	Prospective	Triage	Low	1586	47	100, 150
18	Maisel 2010 [27]	Prospective	Triage	Low	1641	35	100
19	Mueller 2005 [28]	Prospective	Abbott	Low	251	55	100, 295
20	Parab 2005 [29]	Retrospective	Triage	High	70	67	100, 300, 500
21	Ray 2004 [30]	Cross-sectional	Triage	Low	308	46	100, 250
22	Kevin Rogers 2009 [31]	Prospective	Triage	High	740	50	100
23	Sanz 2006 [32]	Prospective	Access	High	75	60	100, 116
24	Villacorta 2002 [33]	Cross-sectional	Triage	Low	70	51	200
25	Wang 2010 [34]	Prospective	Abbott	Low	84	58	100, 500

test may lead to biased results, if the disease is progressive or/and a treatment is started in the meantime.

- Regarding the reference standard, the authors describe three sources of bias, namely, if the reference standard is inappropriate, if not all index test results are verified by the same reference standard (differential verification bias), or if only a selected sample of the index test results is verified by the reference standard (partial verification bias).
- The reading process, i.e. the interpretation of the test results, can lead to bias if the reference standard and the index test are not interpreted without knowledge of the other test (review bias), if the index test is part of the reference standard (incorporation bias), or if information on clinical data is available (clinical review bias). Variation results from inter- and intra-observer variability.
- In data analysis inappropriate handling of indeterminate test results can lead to bias, while the different selection of the threshold value leads to variation between the studies.

To assess the potential variation and bias of the individual diagnostic accuracy studies, the QUADAS-2 tool [37] shall be used. Using this tool, which is an improved version of the original QUADAS tool [38], the domains patient selection, index test, reference standard, and flow and timing are assessed in terms of risk and bias and in terms of concerns regarding applicability. For details, the signalling questions and a suggested tabular presentation of the results are provided in [37].

11.2.2 Effect of Variation and Bias on the Results

Several authors addressed the effect of variation and bias on the results of a diagnostic meta-analysis. Rutjes et al. [39] evaluated the effect of design deficiencies on bias and variation in diagnostic accuracy studies (only one meta-analysis had no deficiencies). Comparing seriously diseased patients with healthy controls (case-control study design) leads to the largest overestimation of the diagnostic accuracy. Other factors leading to an overestimation were non-consecutive inclusion of patients, retrospective data collection, random inclusion of eligible patients, and verification bias. Furthermore, the accuracy was lower when patients were not selected based on clinical symptoms but if they had been referred to the index test. Song et al. [40] investigated the effect of study design bias on the diagnostic accuracy in the field of magnetic resonance imaging (MRI) to detect silicone breast implant ruptures. The result was again that patient selection (symptomatic versus asymptomatic) has a large effect on sensitivity and specificity and that in ultrasound studies with partial verification bias the specificity was lower than in studies without. Regarding different study designs, Parker et al. [41] stated that including studies with different designs within the same meta-analysis may lead to a higher estimated diagnostic accuracy than including studies with a comparable study design. The reason could be that case-control studies lead in general to a larger accuracy. Furthermore, there is a clear association between disease prevalence and diagnostic accuracy in the sense that higher prevalence leads to a lower specificity and by tendency to a higher sensitivity [42]. Noteworthy here is that the prevalence explained the variation better than other study characteristics. Ochodo et al. [43] found out that most authors of diagnostic meta-analysis are aware of the association between study quality and diagnostic accuracy and assess the study quality in their review. However, they often do not consider the assessed quality in the conclusions [43] .

Because some reviews cover a long lapse of time, Cohen et al. [44] investigated a possible time trend in summary estimates from diagnostic meta-analyses. Their conclusion is that such time trends are relatively frequent and that the validity of early diagnostic meta-analyses with few studies is limited [44].

11.3 Visualization of the Variability

In meta-analysis of interventional studies, heterogeneity is in general illustrated with the forest and the funnel plot. These two graphics are also often used in diagnostic meta-analyses. However, more often the ROC plot is used (in the review of Naaktgeboren et al. [3], the ROC plot was used in 75% of the diagnostic meta-analyses and the forest plot in 64% of the meta-analyses). Another graphic for the visualization of the variability in diagnostic meta-analyses is the cross-hairs plot.

11.3.1 The ROC Plot

In the ROC plot, the pairs (1 − specificity, sensitivity) of all individual studies are displayed. With this graphic one can get a good impression of the variability, and in addition the heterogeneity of sensitivity and specificity can be compared. Furthermore, by grouping the studies by potential sources of heterogeneity (e.g. test technique or study type) and corresponding illustration by different colours or symbols, the heterogeneity between the subgroups can be assessed. In addition to the pairs (1 − specificity, sensitivity) also the SROC curves and the prediction ellipses are plotted. The SROC curve (proposed by Moses et al. [45]) was already explained in Chap. 6 and will be discussed again later on in this chapter. Comparing the SROC curves of different groups, one gets an idea of the heterogeneity between the groups. The prediction ellipse results from the bivariate model and represents the prediction region around sensitivity and specificity considering the correlation between them (for details see Leeflang et al. [46]).

In Fig. 11.2 the ROC plot for the BNP meta-analysis (threshold <110 ng/L) is displayed, grouped for prospective and non-prospective (cross-sectional and retrospective) study design.

However, with SROC plots it is difficult to differentiate between random variability and heterogeneity ([1], Section 10.3.1). A further disadvantage is that the allocation from the points in the SROC curve to the individual studies is difficult.

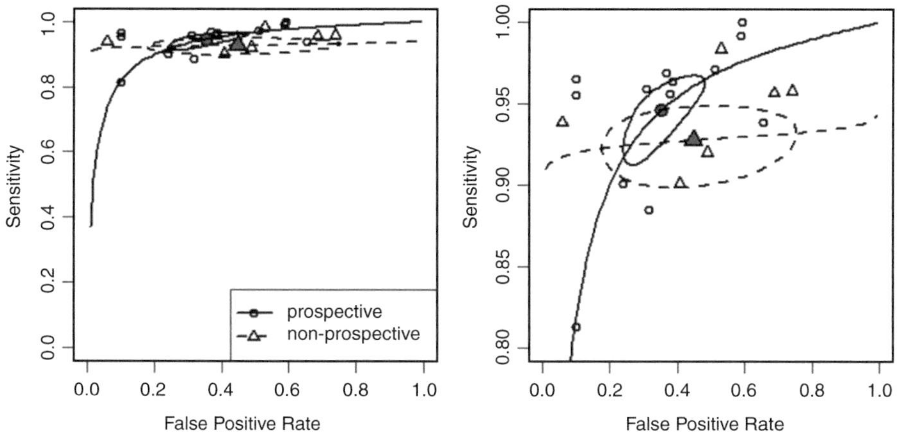

Fig. 11.2 The ROC plot grouped for prospective and non-prospective studies from the BNP meta-analysis data from Roberts et al. [4] created with the R package 'mada' [5, 6]: on the left side the whole ROC space [0;1] × [0;1], on the right side the upper part enlarged [0;1] × [0.8;1]. The grey symbols are the meta-analysis estimators

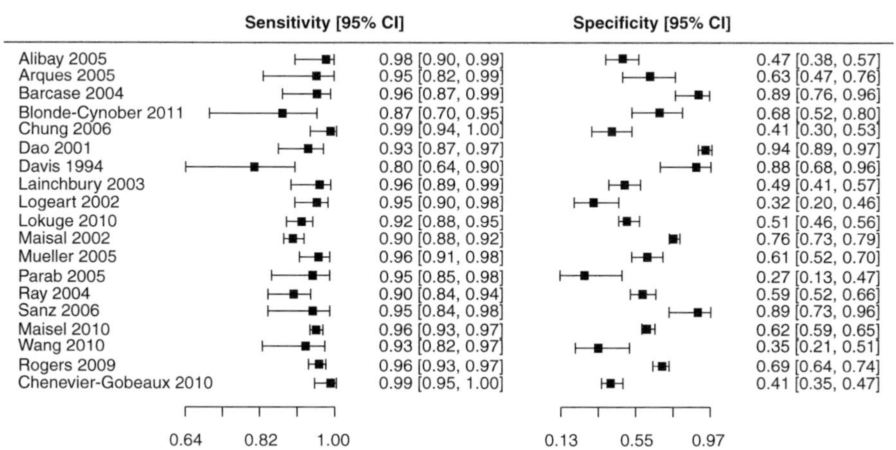

Fig. 11.3 Coupled forest plot from the BNP meta-analysis from [4], created with the R package mada [5, 6]

11.3.2 The Coupled Forest Plot

Another graphical approach for the assessment of heterogeneity is the coupled forest plot. The advantage here is that sensitivity and specificity and the corresponding confidence intervals are displayed in connection with the label of the individual study. Also the raw numbers of the diagnostic fourfold table (true positives, false positives, true negatives, false negatives) can be provided. In Fig. 11.3 the coupled forest plot from the BNP meta-analysis is presented.

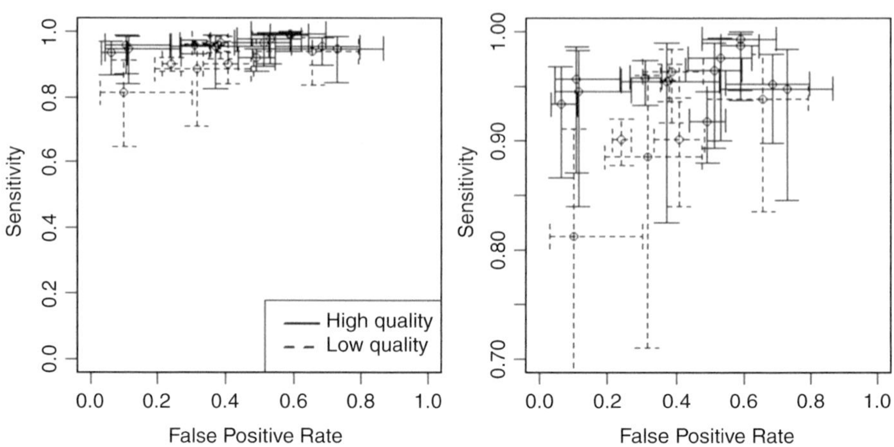

Fig. 11.4 Cross-hairs plot for the BNP meta-analysis, grouped for studies with high (solid lines) and low (dashed lines) study quality, according to QUADAS II (created with the R package 'mada' [5, 6]). On the left side the whole ROC space [0;1] × [0;1], on the right side the upper part enlarged [0;1] × [0.7;1]

11.3.3 Cross-Hairs Plot

A sort of mixture between coupled forest plot and SROC curve is the so-called 'cross-hairs' plot, proposed by Phillips et al. [47]. This graphic is a SROC curve where also the confidence intervals of sensitivity and specificity of the individual studies are plotted. The advantage is that the key information of both graphics is combined in one. Though, the disadvantage of missing study allocation remains and a further problem is that, especially in the case of many studies, the plot can be very confusing. As example a cross-hairs plot for the BNP meta-analysis is given in Fig. 11.4, again for the studies with a threshold <110 ng/L.

11.3.4 The Funnel Plot

The funnel plot [48] is a standard graphic in interventional meta-analyses to check whether publication bias exists. To this aim, the treatment effect is plotted against the study size or the study variation. The idea is that in general smaller studies have a larger variation, and that by tendency large studies and positive small studies are published. If small studies with unfavourable results are not published, one expects a gap on one side of the funnel plot. Accordingly an asymmetric funnel plot indicates publication bias. However, this is not necessarily true for diagnostic meta-analyses. Song et al. [49] investigated the association between asymmetric funnel plots and publication bias and came to the following conclusions: First, the smaller the number of primary studies is, the greater is the asymmetry in the funnel plot. Second, the asymmetry becomes smaller with an increasing number of searched

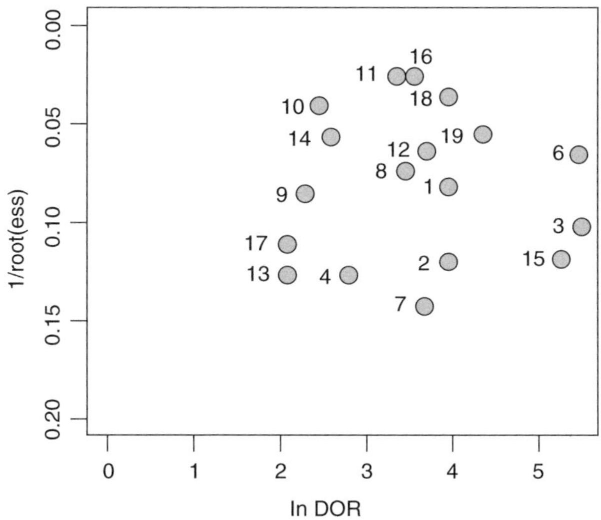

Fig. 11.5 Funnel plot which displays the ln DOR versus reciprocal of the square root of the effective sample size ESS for the BNP meta-analysis (suggested by [50], created with the R package 'meta' [7, 8])

databases. Third, smaller studies tend to report higher accuracy. Accordingly, if funnel plots are used in diagnostic meta-analyses, they have to be interpreted very carefully. Deeks et al. [50] suggested in their article about tests of publication bias a funnel plot for the logarithm of the diagnostic odds ratio (DOR) from Glas et al. [51] as summary measure. The DOR is defined as it follows:

$$\mathrm{DOR} = \frac{\mathrm{TP}/\mathrm{FP}}{\mathrm{FN}/\mathrm{TN}}$$

with TP as true positives, FP as false positives, FN as false negatives, and TN as true negatives as in Table 11.1. By the logarithm transformation of the DOR, one obtains an effect measure in analogy to the log odds ratio in meta-analyses of interventional studies. In the article from Deeks et al. [50], the ln DOR was plotted against the reciprocal of the square root of the effective sample size ESS = $(4n_1n_2)/(n_1 + n_2)$ with n_1 and n_2 as the number of the diseased and the non-diseased, respectively. For the BNP meta-analysis, the corresponding funnel plot is presented in Fig. 11.5.

Two other graphics, proposed by Lijmer et al. [35], are the Galbraith plot, where the log of the diagnostic odds ratio (ln DOR) divided by its standard error is plotted against the reciprocal of the standard error, and a plot of the log odds ratio versus the sum of the logits of sensitivity and 1 − specificity. However, these graphics are rarely applied, probably mainly because the DOR cannot be interpreted directly.

11.4 Judging the Variability

11.4.1 The Cochran' Q Test

The standard statistical test for heterogeneity in interventional meta-analysis is the Cochran Q test. In the review of Naaktgeboren et al. [3], the Cochran' Q test was used in 53% of the diagnostic reviews to judge whether the variability was larger than expected due to chance alone. In each review the univariate Cochran's Q test was used, evaluating sensitivity and specificity separately. But in the univariate analyses, the correlation between sensitivity and specificity is not considered, which may introduce bias. Therefore, Jackson et al. [52] proposed as a multivariate extension of the Q statistic the matrix

$$\boldsymbol{Q} = \begin{bmatrix} \sum\limits_{i \in \boldsymbol{R}_{\mathrm{se}}} \dfrac{\left(\mathrm{se}_i - \overline{\mathrm{se}_1}\right)^2}{\sigma^2_{\mathrm{se}_i}} & \sum\limits_{i \in \boldsymbol{R}_{\mathrm{se,sp}}} \dfrac{\left(\mathrm{se}_i - \overline{\mathrm{se}_2}\right)\left(\mathrm{sp}_i - \overline{\mathrm{sp}_2}\right)}{\sigma_{\mathrm{se}_i}\sigma_{\mathrm{sp}_i}} \\ \sum\limits_{i \in \boldsymbol{R}_{\mathrm{se,sp}}} \dfrac{\left(\mathrm{se}_i - \overline{\mathrm{se}_2}\right)\left(\mathrm{sp}_i - \overline{\mathrm{sp}_2}\right)}{\sigma_{\mathrm{se}_i}\sigma_{\mathrm{sp}_i}} & \sum\limits_{i \in \boldsymbol{R}_{\mathrm{sp}}} \dfrac{\left(\mathrm{sp}_i - \overline{\mathrm{sp}_1}\right)^2}{\sigma^2_{\mathrm{sp}_i}} \end{bmatrix}$$

where R_{se}, R_{sp}, and $R_{\mathrm{se,\,sp}}$ denote the sets of studies where sensitivity, specificity, and both are reported, respectively. The weighted average sensitivity and specificity of all studies of R_{se} and R_{sp} are denoted by $\overline{\mathrm{se}_1}$ and $\overline{\mathrm{sp}_1}$, whereas the weighted average sensitivity and specificity of all studies of $R_{\mathrm{se,\,sp}}$ are denoted by $\overline{\mathrm{se}_2}$ and $\overline{\mathrm{sp}_2}$. Details are provided in [52].

For the BNP meta-analysis with a threshold below 110 ng/L, the Q test statistic was 90.94 leading to a p-value <0.01 (with the 'trimfill' function of the 'meta' package [7, 8] with the fixed random model—fixed effect for the number of missing studies, random effects for summary estimates—and the restricted maximum likelihood (REML) for the estimation of the between-study variance). A disadvantage of the Cochran Q statistic is that, at least for the univariate case, it has been shown that the statistic has low power in the case of few and small studies [53, 54].

11.4.2 Tests for Funnel Plot Asymmetry

While the meta-analysis itself should be performed with bivariate models for sensitivity and specificity (because these are in general the co-primary endpoints), for the assessment of a possible publication bias univariate measures like the diagnostic odds ratio are reasonable. For tests for asymmetry of the above-mentioned funnel plot to assess publication bias (originally proposed by Egger et al. [55]), it is known that they are only appropriate for an odds ratio close to one. However, the DOR is in general much larger. Because of this and because of the above-mentioned characteristics of the funnel plot, these tests are inappropriate and should not be used for diagnostic meta-analyses ([1], Section 10.6.3). Deeks et al. [50] demonstrated that these tests reject the hypothesis of publication bias too often incorrectly in the case of large DOR's, imbalanced sample size in the status groups, and when sensitivity and specificity are not weighted equally. Therefore, the authors proposed for illustration the above depicted funnel plot, where the ln DOR is plotted against $1/\sqrt{\text{ESS}}$. Furthermore, Deeks et al. [50] proposed two tests: (1) the regression approach from Macaskill et al. [56], where the total sample size is replaced by the effective sample size, leading to

$$\ln\ \text{DOR} = b_0 + b_1\text{ESS} + \varepsilon,$$

with ε as prediction error, and (2) an adaptation of Begg's rank correlation test [57]

$$\ln\ \text{DOR}_i^* = \frac{\ln \text{DOR}_i - \overline{\ln \text{DOR}}}{\sqrt{v_i^*}}$$

with $v_i^* = \text{ESS}_i - \left(\sum_j \text{ESS}_j^{-1}\right)^{-1}$, and then correlating $\ln \text{DOR}_i^*$ with ESS_i. The authors demonstrated that both tests are robust to study characteristics but recommend the regression because it has greater statistical power than the correlation test. However, when the ln DOR varies more than expected by chance alone, independent from the sample size, all tests for funnel plot asymmetry have low power [50].

Bürkner and Doebler [58] compared in their article the properties of four approaches for four univariate diagnostic accuracy measures. Beside the already mentioned DOR and ln DOR, the authors investigated the Youden index [59]

$$Y = \text{se} + \text{sp} - 1,$$

and a summary measure from Le [60]. Le proposed to model the ROC function by the proportional hazards model

$$\text{se} = (1 - \text{sp})^{\theta}.$$

Then the summary measure is the natural logarithm of θ

$$\ln \theta = \ln\left(\frac{\ln(\text{se})}{\ln(1 - \text{sp})}\right)$$

[58, 60], whereas Bürkner used $-\ln\theta$ to obtain the same order as for the other measures (because $\ln\theta$ is lower for higher accuracy). As approaches Bürkner and Doebler [58] investigated the above-mentioned Macaskill regression, Begg's correlation test, and in addition the Egger regression and the trim and fill approach. In the Egger regression equation sensitivity or specificity divided by their standard errors is the dependent variable, and the corresponding precision (one divided by the standard error) is the independent variable [55, 58].

The trim and fill approach was proposed by Duval and Tweedie [61] and is a nonparametric method. The underlying assumption is that originally $k + k_0$ studies were

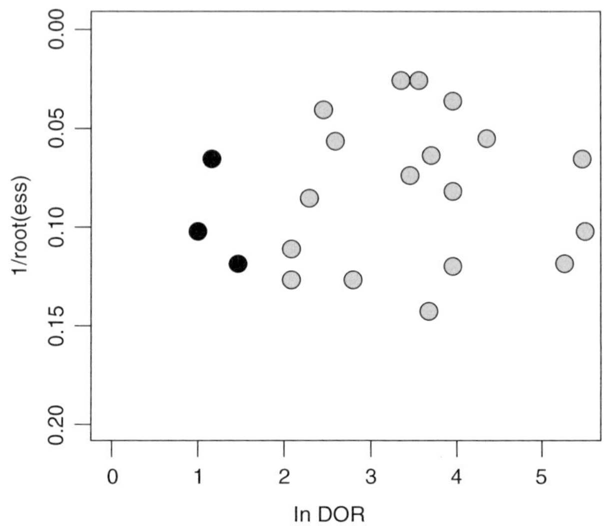

Fig. 11.6 Funnel plot illustrating the trim and fill method (using the estimator R_0) for the BNP meta-analysis with the results of the included studies (grey dots) and three assumed not published studies (black dots). The graphic was created with the R package 'meta' [7, 8]

performed but that the k_0 studies with the 'most extreme negative ranks' were not published [61]. This might lead to an asymmetric funnel plot. So, in a first step the studies in the asymmetric outlying part of the funnel plot are trimmed off. Then the true centre of the funnel plot Θ is estimated based on the remaining studies. Afterwards, the trimmed studies and their assumed counterparts are replaced symmetric to the centre. The final estimates are then based on the resulting filled funnel plot. For illustration of the approach regarding the BNP meta-analysis, the 'trimfill' function of the 'meta' package [7, 8] with the same settings as for the Q test statistic above was used to create Fig. 11.6. The key point is the estimation of the number of missing studies, k_0, for which Duval and Tweedie defined three estimators (for details see [61]). As a result of their simulation study, Bürkner and Doebler [58] recommend the trim and fill methods for the ln DOR because for this combination the type one error was not or only slightly inflated and the power was medium to high. If the number of studies was large enough, the approach was also robust to extreme circumstances.

However, the general issue of limited interpretability remains, because asymmetry is not necessarily caused by publication bias. In fact, there are several study characteristics, which are associated with the sample size as well as with the accuracy, like the patient selection (case-control or cohort).

11.5 Measuring the Variability

11.5.1 The I^2 Index

A standard statistical measure of heterogeneity in interventional meta-analyses is the inconsistency index I^2, which is the estimated ratio of the between-study variance to the sum of the between- and the within-study variance [62]. Following

Higgins et al., an I^2 larger than 50% implies moderate and larger than 75% high heterogeneity [62]. However, Deeks et al. ([63], Section 9.5.2) mention that thresholds for the interpretation can be misleading, because the importance of the observed I^2 depends on the magnitude and direction of effects and the strength of evidence for heterogeneity. Furthermore, they say that only an I^2 smaller than 40% might not be important ([63], Section 9.5.2). For diagnostic meta-analyses, the index was originally defined for sensitivity and specificity separately, leading to biased results because the correlation between sensitivity and specificity is not taken into account [64]. Therefore, a multivariate version of the index was proposed by Jackson et al. [65], which is based on the R^2 statistic. Because the derivation of this index is based on the normal assumption of the within-study variability, Zhou and Dendukuri [66] proposed the following improved bivariate I^2 index, which takes the mean-variance relationship across the studies into account:

$$I^2_{E(\text{Biv})} = \frac{\left|\hat{\boldsymbol{T}}\right|^{1/2}}{\left|\widehat{\boldsymbol{E}(\Sigma)}\right|^{1/2} + \left|\hat{\boldsymbol{T}}\right|^{1/2}}.$$

Here $|\boldsymbol{T}|$ is the determinant of the between-study variance-covariance matrix, and $|\boldsymbol{E}(\boldsymbol{\Sigma})|$ is the determinant of the expected within-study variance matrix $\boldsymbol{\Sigma}$. However, there are general concerns regarding I^2, like that the confidence interval of the index is very large in the case of few studies, leading to a low meaningfulness [2]. Despite of this, the confidence interval should always be reported in addition to the index. Another weakness of I^2 is that it depends on the sample size of the individual studies [67] and that it does not reflect the variation of the effect size [68]. In their review Naaktgeboren et al. [3] noted that in 58% of the diagnostic reviews I^2 was reported, and all were univariate. Furthermore, from these reviews only 23% included a corresponding confidence interval. In all reviews the authors assumed heterogeneity, when I^2 was larger than 50%. For the BNP meta-analysis with a threshold below 110 ng/L, the I^2 was 77%.

11.5.2 The τ^2 Parameter

Because of the weaknesses of the I^2 index, Rücker et al. [67] recommended to use an estimate of the variance parameter of the random effects model, τ^2. A multivariate version of τ^2, extending the DerSimonian and Laird's (DSL) methodology, was proposed by Jackson et al. [52]:

$$\hat{\tau}^2 = \max\left(0, \frac{Q-(k-1)}{S_1 - \frac{S_2}{S_1}}\right)$$

where $\boldsymbol{Q}$ is the above-mentioned multivariate heterogeneity statistic, k denotes the number of studies, $S_r = \sum_{i=1}^{k} w_i^r \left(r = 1,2\right)$, and $w_i = \sigma_i^{-2}$. Details are provided in [52]. It should be noted that Böhning et al. [69] ascertained that estimating heterogeneity variance with the DSL estimator and using the study-specific variances instead of population-averaged versions can lead to large bias. There are various other approaches for estimating the between-study covariance matrix (see Chap. 6) in random effects models. In the 'reitsma' function of the R package 'mada' [5, 6] for the bivariate model the following methods are provided: the unrestricted and restricted maximum likelihood (ML, REML), using variance components (VC), and the method of moments (MM). Jackson et al. [70] recommend the multivariate method of moments, because it is also applicable in case of incomplete outcomes and covariates can be considered. Naaktgeboren et al. [2] recommend the combination of the between-study variance τ^2 of the sensitivity, the specificity, and the covariance between them. However, they remark that the τ^2 values are hard to interpret, because they are on the log odds scale. In the review from Naaktgeboren et al. [3], only in 13% of the reviews τ^2 was provided, and only in one review it came from a bivariate random effects model.

For the BNP meta-analysis, the between-study standard deviation for the complete dataset was 0.43 and 0.61 for the logit sensitivity and specificity, and the correlation between them was 0.83 (using the 'reitsma' function with the methods of moments in the 'mada' package [5, 6]). Including the study quality (low versus high) as covariate, the between-study standard deviation was reduced to 0.39 and 0.59 for the logit sensitivity and specificity, and the correlation to 0.76.

11.5.3 The Prediction Ellipse

An alternative heterogeneity measure is the area of the above-mentioned prediction ellipse [46]. However, probably because of its poor interpretability, it is in practice not reported as number but used descriptively as visual impression (see, e.g., [71]).

11.6 Attributing the Variability to Different Thresholds

Most index tests do not lead to a binary result positive/negative, but to a metric value (e.g. laboratory tests), to a count (e.g. questionnaires), or to an ordinal score (e.g. imaging techniques). These values have to be dichotomized artificially by defining a threshold. In some cases there are well established thresholds, but often, the researchers choose their own thresholds leading to explicit differences. Here the problem arises that data-driven selection of the threshold can cause bias; for more details see Leeflang et al. [72]. Furthermore, Macaskill et al. ([1], Section 10.4.1) note that even if the threshold is numerically the same in studies, implicit threshold variation can occur because of different calibrations for the equipment, subjective test interpretation, or differences in the implementation of the tests. If there are

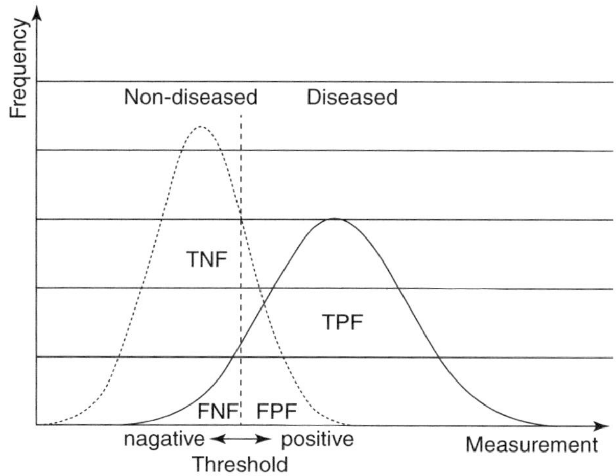

Fig. 11.7 Illustration of the threshold effect. Moving the threshold to the right increases specificity (TNF) and decreases sensitivity (TPF). Moving the threshold to the left has the opposite effect

explicit different thresholds, a threshold effect can be observed in terms of moving the threshold sensitivity increases and specificity decreases or vice versa (for illustration see Fig. 11.7), which implies a negative correlation between the two measures. However, it should be noted that sensitivity and specificity can also be positively correlated. Especially when there are only implicit threshold differences, positive correlation can be caused by different test accuracy in the individual studies ([73], for an example see Janda and Swiston [74]).

Regarding thresholds, three scenarios can be differentiated: (1) In all primary studies, the same explicit threshold is used. Then the aim is to assess the variability due to the implicit threshold differences. (2) In each primary study, sensitivity and specificity are reported for one threshold, whereas the thresholds can differ explicitly between the individual studies. Ignoring the differences between the thresholds would lead to a mean sensitivity and specificity over all present thresholds, which is meaningless and inappropriate. (3) Some or all primary studies report sensitivity and specificity for several thresholds. Selecting only one threshold per study would lead to a relevant loss of information; instead the multiple thresholds should be considered in the analysis [75]. Methods for the appropriate analysis of the last two scenarios will be the topic of the next section (Sect. 11.7) and of Sect. 11.8.2.

Regarding the scenario of primary studies with different thresholds, a pre-analysis step is to assess the amount of variability which is attributable to the different thresholds. Therefore, the criterion for the ROC plot is not how far the pairs of sensitivity and specificity are scattered in the ROC space, but if they lie close to the summary ROC curve ([1], Section 10.4.3). However, in the standard ROC plot, the corresponding threshold cannot be read off. Therefore, a colour coding or an order-representing numbering could be helpful to investigate, whether the order of the points in the ROC plot corresponds to the order of the thresholds (see, e.g., Fig. 11.8).

Naaktgeboren et al. [3] determined in their review that in 38% of the meta-analyses assessed, threshold effects were assessed (from these 75% assessed implicit

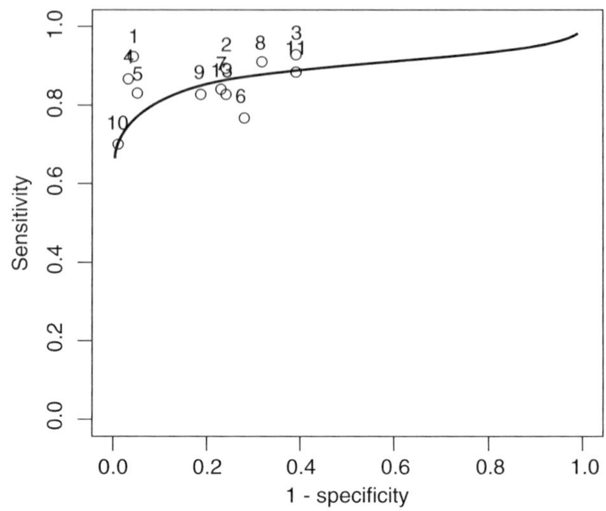

Fig. 11.8 ROC plot for the high-quality studies of the BNP meta-analysis with a threshold between 110 and 400 ng/L, where label numbers represent the threshold (1 means the lowest threshold)

and 35% explicit variations). The authors suggest fitting a bivariate random effects model to obtain the conditional between-study variances (of sensitivity at a fixed specificity and vice versa) and to perform two univariate analyses separately to obtain the unconditional between-study variances. If a threshold effect is present (what implies that sensitivity and specificity are negatively correlated), the conditional between-study variances will be smaller than the unconditional between-study variances [3].

11.7 Exploring the Different Sources of Variability

In the last step, the aim is to explain the heterogeneity by the different sources of variation, like different thresholds or study characteristics. The GRADE (Grades of Recommendation, Assessment, Development and Evaluation) system was developed to grade the quality of evidence [76]. In the part about the quality of evidence and strength of recommendations for diagnostic tests or strategies, one mentioned factor, which can reduce the quality of evidence in diagnostic meta-analyses, is unexplained variability [77]. A prerequisite for the formal investigation of sources of heterogeneity is a sufficient number of studies, a sufficient study quality, and not too similar studies regarding study design and population [2].

11.7.1 Fixed Versus Random Effects Models

As a preliminary point, the difference between fixed and random effects models shall be explained: In a fixed effects model, a common accuracy with variability due to chance is assumed, and the aim is to estimate this common effect. However, in diagnostic meta-analysis in general, the heterogeneity is too large, as it could be explained by chance alone. Therefore, a random effects model is appropriate, where different accuracies are assumed and the aim is to estimate an average accuracy ([1], Section 10.4.3).

11.7.2 Comparison of the Bivariate Model and the HSROC Approach

In general, for meta-analysis of diagnostic accuracy studies, one has to differentiate between approaches where summary measures are point estimators like sensitivity or specificity and approaches where the summary measure is the SROC curve. In general, sensitivity and specificity are co-primary endpoints and approaches with point summary measures are the means of choice. However, if there is large variability between the thresholds, for threshold-specific estimates of sensitivity and specificity, the number of studies is perhaps too small, while the estimation of a mean sensitivity and specificity over all thresholds is (as already noted) meaningless. In such a case, a SROC curve may be preferred ([1], Section 10.4.1). Macaskill et al. [1] recommend reporting both summary measures: clinically informative estimators of sensitivity and specificity at different relevant thresholds and SROC curves for subgroups (e.g. different test types or study designs) to investigate heterogeneity. Approaches with point estimators as summary measures have again to be differentiated in univariate and bivariate models. As mentioned earlier, univariate models cannot be recommended because the threshold effect and the correlation between sensitivity and specificity are not considered.

The bivariate model by Reitsma et al. [78] is a random effects model and accounts for this correlation. Therefore, it is the standard approach for meta-analysis with sensitivity and specificity as co-primary endpoints. When the summary measure is the SROC curve, the main approaches are the Moses-Littenberg model [45, 79] and the hierarchical SROC model (HSROC) [80]. The Moses-Littenberg model is similar to a fixed effects model and cannot be recommended because it does neither account for the correlation between sensitivity and specificity nor for the between-study variability. The HSROC model is a random effects model and accounts for the correlation as well as for the within- and the between-study variability. Therefore, the HSROC model is the standard model for meta-analyses with the SROC curve as endpoint. For a review of these four approaches, which were also explained in detail in Sect. 11.6, see, for example, Lee et al. [81].

For the BNP meta-analysis, the bivariate model (with the method of moments) was used for the studies with a threshold between 100 and 110 ng/L, while the HSROC approach is applied to the studies with the thresholds between 110 and 400 ng/L. Without consideration of covariates, in the low-threshold group the bivariate model estimates the mean sensitivity as 94% and the mean specificity as 40%. With the HSROC approach in the medium-threshold group, the area under the SROC curve is estimated as 0.92.

It should be noted that the bivariate model and the HSROC model are equivalent either when no covariates are included into the model [82, 83] or 'where a covariate (or covariates) is allowed to affect both the sensitivity and the specificity, the Bivariate model is equivalent to an HSROC model in which the covariate or covariates are allowed to affect both the accuracy and the positivity threshold but not the shape parameter' ([1], Section 10.5.3.1).

The bivariate and the HSROC models differ regarding the handling with the included covariates. With the bivariate meta-regression model, it is investigated to what extent the expected values of sensitivity and specificity vary depending on the covariates. In contrast, with the HSROC approach, it is investigated how the position and shape of the estimated SROC curve vary depending on the covariates ([1], Section 10.5.3). With both approaches in principle categorical as well as continuous covariates can be considered. However, in practice usually binary or categorical covariates with few levels are considered, because these comparisons can be well illustrated by grouped SROC curves. If there are too many categories, the problem is often that the number of studies per subgroup becomes too small. If continuous covariates shall be considered, it has to be checked whether the assumption of a linear association (with logit sensitivity and logit specificity or ln DOR) holds true ([1], Section 10.5.3).

11.7.3 The Bivariate Model

In the bivariate model, the logit sensitivity $\mu_{se,\,i}$ and the logit specificity $\mu_{sp,\,i}$ are assumed to be bivariate normal distributed across the studies. Including a linear predictor for a single covariate Z, one obtains

$$\begin{pmatrix} \mu_{se,i} \\ \mu_{sp,i} \end{pmatrix} \sim N\left(\begin{pmatrix} \mu_{se} + v_{se} Z_i \\ \mu_{sp} + v_{sp} Z_i \end{pmatrix}, \Sigma_{se,sp} \right) \quad \text{with} \quad \Sigma_{se,sp} = \begin{pmatrix} \sigma_{se}^2 & \sigma_{se,sp} \\ \sigma_{se,sp} & \sigma_{sp}^2 \end{pmatrix}$$

as covariance matrix for the random effects logit sensitivity and specificity [84]. This model can also be extended for more covariates, if the number of studies in the subgroup is large enough. Furthermore, it is possible that covariates are only modelled for sensitivity or specificity. Assuming a binary covariate ($Z = 0$ or 1) μ_{se} and $\mu_{se} + \nu_{se}$ are the estimators of the logit sensitivity in the both covariate groups. Accordingly are the estimators of the logit specificity in the two covariate groups defined (μ_{sp} and $\mu_{sp} + \nu_{sp}$). The expected sensitivity and specificity in the two covariate groups are obtained using the back-transformation $\text{expit}(\cdot) = \exp(\cdot)/(\exp(\cdot) + 1)$. The effect of the covariate can be assessed by the estimation of $\exp(\nu_{se})$ and $\exp(\nu_{sp})$, which represents the odds ratio for sensitivity and specificity in group $Z = 1$ relative to $Z = 0$. Fitting the model once with and once without ν_{se} and ν_{se}, the effect of the covariate on the accuracy can be investigated. Under the assumption of a normal distributed regression error, the standard error of the resulting estimated sensitivity and specificity can be obtained using the delta method. It should be noted that usually it is assumed that the variance of the random effects and the covariates are not associated ([1], Section 10.5.3.1). In this bivariate model, neither explicit different nor multiple thresholds can be considered [85].

For the BNP meta-analysis for the studies with a threshold below 110 ng/L, the adjustment for the study quality (low vs. high) leads to a lower sensitivity and specificity for low-quality studies (sensitivity 92% vs. 95%, specificity 35% vs. 41%). In contrast, an adjustment for study design (prospective versus non-prospective) leads to an increase in sensitivity and a decrease in specificity (sensitivity 94% vs. 93%, specificity 36% vs. 46%). An adjustment for the type of the index test (Triage versus others) leads to an increase in sensitivity and specificity (sensitivity 95% versus 91%, specificity 40% versus 37%).

11.7.4 The HSROC Model

In the HSROC model by Rutter and Gatsonis [80] covariates can be used to assess heterogeneity regarding the threshold, the position, or the shape of the curve. This means that different thresholds can be considered; however, multiple thresholds cannot. The model is a two-level approach for the within- and the between-study variation. As before, a binary covariate Z (0 or 1) is included in the model; the following notation is based on Macaskill et al. ([1], Section 10.5.3.3). The level I model (within-study variation) for logit sensitivity and specificity in study i, denoted by $\pi_{\text{se},\,i}$ and $\pi_{\text{sp},\,i}$, is given as

$$\operatorname{logit}\left(\pi_{j,i}\right)=\left(\left(\theta_i+\gamma Z_i\right)+\left(\alpha_i+\lambda Z_i\right)\text{dis}_{j,i}\right)\exp\left(-\left(\beta+\delta Z_i\right)\text{dis}_{j,i}\right)\ \text{with} \in \{\text{se,sp}\}.$$

The true disease state j for a patient in study i is denoted by the dummy variable $\text{dis}_{j,i}$ equal to −0.5 for the non-diseased (j = sp) and equal to +0.5 for the diseased (j = se). The parameters θ_i and α_i are the random effects for the threshold and the accuracy (difference of sensitivity and 1 − specificity), and the shape of the SROC curve in the two covariate groups is estimated by β and $\beta + \delta$, respectively. For level II (between-study variation) the distribution of the random effects is given as

$$\theta_i \sim N\left(\Theta+\gamma Z_i,\sigma_\theta^2\right) \quad \text{and} \quad \alpha_i \sim N\left(\Lambda+\lambda Z_i,\sigma_\alpha^2\right).$$

If some heterogeneity regarding the threshold and/or the accuracy is explained by the covariate, the estimated variance of the corresponding random effect should be reduced in the model with the covariate compared to the model without the covariate ([1], Section 10.5.3.3). One aspect of the interpretation of the analysis results is the investigation of the shape of the SROC curve. If the shape of the SROC curves in the two covariate groups is assumed to be the same ($\delta = 0$), but not necessarily symmetric, the relative diagnostic accuracy in the two covariate groups can be summarized with the ratio of the two DOR's (RDOR = exp (λ)). The two SROC curves can be assumed as symmetric, if $\beta = 0$. Assuming the same shape, another aspect regarding the interpretation is the association between the covariate and the accuracy: $\lambda \neq 0$ implies that there is an association, while $\lambda = 0$ means that there is no association and the curves are the same for both covariate groups. In the latter case ($\delta = 0$ and $\lambda = 0$), an association between the covariate and the threshold is assumed if $\gamma \neq 0$. However, such an association is hard to interpret. If the chosen threshold is known for each study, it can be included in the model as a covariate and sensitivity and specificity can be estimated threshold specific. For more details, see ([1], Section 10.5.3.3).

11.7.5 Model Selection

Regarding the model selection, the strategy as well as the selection criterion has to be specified. The strategy means how many covariates are considered together and in which order they are included. Naaktgeboren et al. [2] differentiate here between a motivated and an explorative strategy. Whereas the motivated strategy means the careful selection of few covariates with a strong suspicion of a covariate effect, the exploratory strategy means that many covariates are investigated, independent of a strong suspicion. Using a test statistic, Macaskill et al. ([1], Section 10.5.3.4) recommend the χ^2 test and the likelihood ratio test as selection criterion; as model fit measures the Akaike's or the Bayesian information criterion (AIC or BIC) are appropriate, while the deviance information criterion (DIC) is in general used for Markov chain Monte Carlo (MCMC) simulation.

For the BNP meta-analysis, the χ^2 test for the comparison of the above-presented models (including study quality, study design, or index test type as covariate) demonstrates that study quality is associated with heterogeneity ($p = 0.09$), while the study design and the index test seem not to be ($p = 0.40$ and $p = 0.37$).

11.7.6 Modifications of the Bivariate Model and the HSROC Approach

Since the proposal of the bivariate and the HSROC model, several modifications of the approaches were suggested. Providing details including the notation and the formulas for all methods would go beyond the scope. Therefore, the ideas of the approaches are described, and for details it is referred to the original articles.

For the bivariate model, for example, Chen et al. [86, 87] presented methods based on the composite likelihood approach, which avoid non-convergence problems and model sensitivity and specificity on the original scale. Guolo [88] proposed a double simulation extrapolation (SIMEX) approach for bivariate random effects meta-analysis, which accounts for the presence of measurement errors and can consider covariates.

For the HSROC approach, for example, Rücker and Schumacher [89] proposed a SROC curve based on a weighted Youden index for the selection of an optimal threshold, Doebler et al. [90] recommended the t_α family of transformations (that varies between the logit and the log) instead of the logit transformation, Holling et al. [91] used a mixed model approach using the Lehmann family, and Charoensawat et al. [92] proposed a proportional hazards measure as criterion. A semiparametric approach was proposed by Doebler and Holling [93], which is an extension of the mixed model from Holling et al. [91] using the t_α transformation, which leads to more flexibility regarding the shape of the SROC curve. Using covariate adjusted mixtures, one obtains a meta-regression of the SROC curves, but not sensitivity and specificity, which is a strong limitation. Another extension of the approach from Holling et al. [91], which preserves the bivariate structure of the data, was applied by Schlattmann et al. [94]. They modelled the between-study heterogeneity with a discrete nonparametric distribution of the random effects.

Standard meta-analyses can be performed with these standard approaches (bivariate random effects model or HSROC model). However, the approaches are sometimes reaching their limits. For example, all these approaches have the limitation that multiple thresholds per study cannot be considered. Approaches considering this and other issues will be presented in the next section.

11.8 Further Issues with Heterogeneity

In this section approaches will be presented, which are helpful for non-standard meta-analyses, for example, in the case of multiple thresholds or partial verification bias.

11.8.1 Bayesian Methods

Menke [95] reanalysed 50 meta-analyses with a bivariate Bayesian approach, where the data is taken as fixed and the model parameters as variables. The model fit was evaluated using the deviance information criterion (DIC), and the Bayesian credible interval was used instead of the confidence intervals. However, Dahabreh et al. [96] reanalysed 308 diagnostic meta-analyses with different approaches and concluded among others that 'Fitting the bivariate model using ML and fully Bayesian methods produced almost identical point estimates of summary sensitivity and specificity; however, Bayesian results indicated additional uncertainty around summary estimates'. Novielli et al. [97] investigated Bayesian model selection, also with the DIC, in the field of the Ddimer test for the diagnosis of the deep vein thrombosis. They noticed that the inclusion of covariates in the model improved the model fit.

11.8.2 Multiple Thresholds

Regarding methods for consideration of multiple thresholds, Macaskill et al. ([1], Section 10.6.4) state that they are of particular interest but require further evaluation. Meanwhile several approaches were proposed, which address this issue.

Dukic and Gatsonis [98] extended the HSROC model and presented a fixed effects model and a Bayesian hierarchical approach. However, the fixed effects model is not appropriate because the heterogeneity between the studies is not taken into account. With the hierarchical model, which is fitted with MCMC, the between- as well as the within-study variation can be considered. As a result a SROC curve with sensitivity and specificity for each threshold can be obtained, but it can happen that the resulting sensitivities and specificities are not monotone [99]. Furthermore, Dukic and Gatsonis mention that they did not include covariates in their model but that the Bayesian model could be extended accordingly [98].

Poon [100] proposed a latent normal distribution model for the analysis of ordinal responses, which can be applied for meta-analysis with multiple thresholds. With this approach also covariates can be considered; however, because the approach is a fixed effects model, it cannot be recommended for the meta-analysis of diagnostic accuracy trials.

A multivariate random effects meta-analysis, where multiple thresholds can be included, was suggested by Bipat et al. [101]. The model can be extended for covariates, but the weakness of this approach is that no SROC curves can be derived [102].

Hamza et al. [102] proposed a multivariate random effects meta-analysis where multiple thresholds per study and also covariates can be considered. As for the approach from Dukic and Gatsonis [98], a ROC curve with corresponding (not guaranteed monotone) sensitivities and specificities for the different thresholds can be obtained [99]. Although this approach was intended for an equal number of thresholds in all studies, it is also applicable for different numbers because missing values are allowed. However, if the number of thresholds is too large, the likelihood method may not work [102].

Another approach was used from Putter et al. [99], which applies survival methods to consider multiple thresholds, resulting in a multinomial model with multivariate normal distributed between-study variation. With this model the correlation between sensitivity and specificity is considered, and monotonicity over the different thresholds is guaranteed [99]. Disadvantages of this approach are that the number of thresholds have to be the same for all studies, that the approach is rather inefficient, and that for discrete hazards the overall hazard times frailty are not guaranteed range-preserving, but can become larger than one.

Riley et al. [103] propose a multivariate meta-analysis to consider all thresholds simultaneously and the correlation between them. The idea is that the true logit sensitivity and specificity are modelled as a monotonically decreasing or increasing function of the continuous threshold. As a result one obtains, as with the approach from Putter et al., a SROC curve and the corresponding sensitivity and specificity for each threshold. Covariates can also be included into the model. One problem, the authors mention, is that specific distributions for the test results are assumed and that the results might be biased, if this assumption does not hold true [103]. However, this limitation applies also to other approaches, as, for example, [99] or [102].

Steinhauser et al. [104] estimate with their approach the distribution function of the underlying index test within the non-diseased and the diseased, and the distribution parameters are estimated with linear mixed effects models. The approach also considers between-study variation and correlation between sensitivity and specificity, and the result is again a SROC curve with corresponding sensitivities and specificities. Furthermore, it is possible to choose an optimal threshold according to the Youden index, even if this is only reasonable if the test technique and the interpretation of the result is the same in all studies. However, the approach has also some limitations [104]. For example, the empirical coverage of the estimated distribution parameters and of sensitivity and specificity was very low for some scenarios. Another limitation is that the uncertainty from the first step is ignored in the second step. However, this limitation applies to all two-stage approaches. Regarding the model selection, the standard measures like AIC or BIC are not applicable; thus, the REML criterion was used in the article [104].

Steinhauser et al. [104] used also the meta-analysis from Roberts et al. [4] considering all reported thresholds as example for their approach. The estimated sensitivity and specificity ranged from 94% and 63% for a threshold of 100 ng/L to 41% and 98% for a threshold of 1000 ng/L.

A fully nonparametric approach for the estimation of the SROC curve in the random effects meta-analysis was proposed by Martínez-Camblor [105]. However, this approach makes no use of the threshold information.

A recently published approach was proposed by Hoyer et al. [106], where the ROC curve is interpreted as a bivariate time-to-event model for interval-censored data. The resulting bivariate non-linear mixed effects model, where also covariates can be included, is a single-step approach. This is an advantage of the approach compared to the two-step approaches (see above). The resulting ROC curve is not modelled directly, but sensitivity and specificity are predicted at several thresholds and the AUC can be estimated. One limitation of the approach is that misspecification of the distribution might lead to biased results (see above); another limitation is that the standard measures for model selection are not applicable. In a small simulation study, the approach showed good statistical properties. However, a large simulation study for the comparison with other approaches is yet to be done.

11.8.3 Reference Standard Bias

As already mentioned, when no or only an imperfect reference standard is available or when not all test results were verified by the reference standard or different reference standards were used, this can lead to biased results. Chen et al. [107] used a Bayesian approach for diagnostic meta-analyses with missing data because of partial verification. However, because their approach did not assume between-study heterogeneity, Chu et al. [108] recommended for meta-analyses without a reference standard a non-linear random effects model or a Bayesian hierarchical model. For the approach from Chen et al. [107] as well as from Chu et al. [108], it is assumed that the index and the reference test are conditional independent.

Dendukuri et al. [109] proposed for meta-analysis of studies with imperfect or different reference standards a Bayesian hierarchical model. This model is an extension of the HSROC model, considers between- as well as within-study heterogeneity, and also covariates can be included. A limitation of the approach is that when for all parameters non-informative priors are used, this can lead to meaningless pooled estimators.

Liu et al. [110] compared the approaches from Chu et al. [108] and Dendukuri et al. [109] and noticed that the two approaches are closely related and, as the original bivariate model and HSROC approach, are equivalent when no covariates are considered.

De Groot et al. [111] extended the approach from Begg and Greenes [112] for an individual study to adjust for partial verification bias in the meta-analytic context. Therefore, they use a Bayesian two-level approach. In the first step, the unbiased primary studies are used to estimate the distribution of the index test results. In the second step, based on all studies the positive predictive values are estimated. Combining the results from the two steps, one obtains unbiased sensitivity and specificity estimates [111]. The approach has the further advantage that covariates can be considered, but the limitation that there have to be enough unbiased studies, for the estimation of the distribution in step one.

Menten et al. [113] adjust with their Bayesian approach for the bias resulting from the application of different or imperfect reference standards. With their approach also studies using latent class models can be considered. The informative priors are based on information about the performance of the reference test. The authors determined that the estimation is improved compared to missing adjustment for bias. Furthermore, they mention that the model selection should not be based on the DIC alone. Also the approach of Menten et al. is based on the assumption that the index and the reference test are conditional independent [113].

Recently, Ma et al. [114] proposed a hybrid Bayesian hierarchical model, which combines cohort and case-control studies, accounts for disease prevalence, and can adjust for partial verification bias. The authors come to the conclusion that the novel approach leads to an improved precision of the accuracy estimates. However, the approach cannot adjust for an imperfect gold standard.

11.8.4 Explicit Consideration of the Prevalence

Regarding the consideration of the prevalence, Li and Fine [115] proposed a method especially for the assessment of the association between sensitivity/specificity and the prevalence of the disease in the study population. However, it seems that additional covariates or different/multiple thresholds cannot be considered. Another approach which takes the prevalence information into account is the trivariate generalized linear mixed effects model (TGLMM) [108], which has the limitation that it is only applicable for cohort studies. In the recently published article from Chen et al. [116], a generalized linear mixed effect model is proposed which takes the prevalence into account, is applicable for case-control as well as for cohort studies, and can consider further covariates. As alternative approach, Hoyer and Kuss [117] proposed beta-binomial marginal distributions for sensitivity, specificity, and prevalence linked by trivariate copulas.

11.8.5 Few Studies and Sparse Data

Macaskill et al. ([1], Section 10.5.6) also discuss the topic meta-analysis with small number of studies. They mention the difficulty of model fitting in this case, because in general a high level of uncertainty regarding the estimated variances of the random effects is present. They also bring to mind that in the bivariate regression model as well as in the HSROC model, five parameters have to be estimated. Therefore, the results have to be interpreted very carefully, and it can happen that the models do not converge. The authors give possible reasons for non-convergence: (1) The starting values for the parameter estimates may have been chosen poorly. In this case, a fixeds effect model can be applied and the resulting values then used as starting values. (2) The inclusion or removal of individual studies can be the reason for the non-convergence. (3) When sensitivities are very homogeneous and specificities heterogeneous or vice versa, the model may not converge because the variance of one of the random effects is too small. Then a mixture of random and fixed effects for the two parameters may be helpful. (4) Another reason could be that for the HSROC approach, the standard error for the shape parameter is too large. In this case, a solution could be to assume the shape as symmetric and drop the shape parameter. Anyway, the applied procedure has to be reported and discussed critically ([1], Section 10.5.6).

Takwoingi et al. [118] compared seven approaches for meta-analyses with few studies or sparse data: univariate random effects logistic regression models for sensitivity and specificity separately and six different HSROC models (complete, with symmetric shape, with fixed threshold, with fixed accuracy, with fixed accuracy and threshold, or with symmetric shape and fixed accuracy and threshold). In the simulation study the number of studies varied between 5, 10, and 20, the prevalence between 5, 25, and 50%, and the diagnostic odds ratio went up to 231. The conclusions of the authors were that simpler HSROC models are valid in the case of few studies or sparse data. When a complete bivariate model cannot be fitted, the authors recommend univariate random effects logistic regression models or HSROC models with an assumed symmetric shape of the SROC curve.

11.8.6 Individual Patient Data

In general, for meta-analysis the aggregate data of the primary studies are used. By adjusting for study-specific covariates, one tries to reduce the between-study heterogeneity. However, it is not possible to evaluate the association between the diagnostic accuracy and patient characteristics. Therefore, it would be preferable to perform the meta-analysis based on the individual patient data (IPD). But in general, if any, only some primary studies provide IPD, so approaches are needed, which can consider primary studies with IPD as well as with aggregate data. Riley et al. [119] developed an extension of the bivariate random effects meta-analysis for individual patient data (IPD). This approach allows considering of study-level as well as patient-level covariates, and studies with aggregate data as well as studies with IPD can be included in the meta-analysis. The aim from Riley et al. [119] was to investigate the effect of patient-level covariates on accuracy estimates, between-study heterogeneity, and correlation. Ter Riet et al. [120] discuss in their article the opportunities and challenges of IPD meta-analysis of diagnostic studies. While they list as advantages 'more reliable estimation, particularly in subgroups, and more detailed analysis of thresholds', they mention as main difficulty to obtain the raw data. The recommendation of Ter Riet et al. [120] is to 'establish collaborations ensuring access to the bulk of primary data'.

11.8.7 Non-evaluable Index Test Results

One source of bias is the inappropriate handling of non-evaluable results. Begg et al. [121] differentiate between uninterpretable, intermediate, and indeterminate results. Furthermore, the authors noted that ignoring the non-evaluable may be unbiased (in the case of missing completely at random or missing at random), but as soon as the cause for the non-evaluable results and the disease state are associated (missing not at random), this approach will lead to biased results [121]. This bias in the primary studies will then be transmitted to meta-analyses including such studies. Schütz et al. [122] compared in the context of a meta-analysis regarding coronary computer tomography angiography different approaches handling non-evaluable results: exclusion, which leads to an overestimation of sensitivity and specificity; set to positive, which leads to an overestimation of sensitivity and to an underestimation of specificity; and set to negative, which leads to an underestimation of sensitivity and an overestimation of specificity. Furthermore, they suggested the intention to diagnose principle, where non-evaluable results are set to false positive or negative [122]. This approach is conservative and leads to an underestimation of sensitivity and specificity. Recently, Menke and Kowalski [123] used the mentioned intention to diagnose approach in combination with a multivariate Bayesian random effects meta-analysis. Ma et al. [124] referred to the article from Schütz et al. [122] and mentioned that none of the three approaches can correct biased estimates. Therefore, the authors propose an extension of the trivariate generalized linear mixed model (TGLMM) and compared it to the other three approaches in a simulation study. The authors showed that in the case of missing at random, the TGLMM lead to nearly unbiased estimators of the accuracy and the prevalence.

11.8.8 Further Accuracy Measures

If in the primary studies not individual pairs of sensitivity and specificity are reported, but the whole ROC curve as accuracy measure in general, the area under the ROC curve (AUC) is reported. The AUC is equal to 0.5, if the diagnostic test is completely uninformative, and equal to one, if the test has perfect accuracy. McClish [125] proposed a simple approach for the estimation of a weighted AUC, where only the AUC and the corresponding variance of the primary studies are needed. But covariates can only be considered by stratifying the analysis further. Another approach was used from Kester and Buntinx [126]; they estimated for each primary study the ROC curve by the parameters α (for the position of the curve, denoted by 'central log odds ratio') and β (for the asymmetry of the curve). For the estimation of these two parameters, the authors used weighted linear regression and for the meta-analysis a random effects model with a bivariate normal distribution for the study effect.

Further accuracy measures are the positive predictive value (TP/n_p from Table 11.1) and the negative predictive value (TN/n_n). For the bivariate analysis of the predictive values, Leeflang et al. [46] propose a bivariate random effects logit-normal model. In their article the authors compared two models, one with the predictive values as summary estimates and one with sensitivity and specificity as summary estimates. The conclusion was that 'there were no substantial differences in the goodness of fit or amount of heterogeneity between both models' [46].

In the *Cochrane Handbook*, the authors point out that neither the likelihood ratios (LR, positive LR = sensitivity/(1 − specificity), negative LR = (1 − sensitivity)/specificity) nor the predictive values should be pooled, because the correlation (LR) or the dependence on the prevalence (PV) is ignored, and according impossible or not interpretable results can be obtained ([1], Section 10.4.2, [127]).

Conclusion

In diagnostic meta-analysis heterogeneity is the rule, not the exception. The reason for this heterogeneity can be variation and bias. Variation is particularly caused by different research questions in the individual studies (leading for different study designs) and by different thresholds. In contrast, bias is caused by inappropriate study design, study conduct, or data analysis in the individual studies. Therefore, a proper handling with this heterogeneity is crucial. The aim of this chapter was to give an overview about the different steps in dealing with the heterogeneity (according to Naaktgeboren et al. [3]) and about the latest state of the art to this subject.

1. The variability should be visualized, where the standard graphics are the coupled forest plot, the ROC plot and the funnel plot.
2. The variability should be judged, preferably with the regression test from Deeks et al. [50] or with the trim and fill approach [61] for the ln DOR. In practice often the Cochran Q test is used, but it has relevant limitations ([1], Section 10.4.3].
3. The heterogeneity should be measured with the between-study variance $\hat{\tau}^2$ of a random effects model for sensitivity, specificity, and the covariance between them [2]. When the I^2 index is reported, despite of its weaknesses, then the bivariate version should be used [66].
4. To attribute the variability to different thresholds, a ROC plot can be drawn to check if the sensitivity-specificity pairs follow the SROC curve. Furthermore, a bivariate as well as two univariate random effects models (for sensitivity and specificity) should be fitted, and the conditional and unconditional between-study variances should be compared [3].
5. To explore the different sources of variability in a diagnostic meta-analysis in general, a bivariate random effects model [78] or the HSROC approach [80] with inclusion of covariates is recommended.

However, heterogeneity in diagnostic meta-analysis still is and will remain a current research topic. Therefore, as soon as one moves away from 'standard' diagnostic meta-analysis (e.g. considering multiple thresholds, reference standard bias, or non-evaluable test results), there are no established approaches but many different solutions with advantages and limitations. The claim was to provide a broad overview about the current state of the research. Depending on the specific circumstances of the individual meta-analysis, the researcher has to decide which approach is the most appropriate for his research question.

Reference

1. Macaskill P, Gatsonis C, Deeks JJ, Harbord RM, Takwoingi Y. Chapter 10: analysing and presenting results. In: Deeks JJ, Bossuyt PM, Gatsonis C, editors. Cochrane handbook for systematic reviews of diagnostic test accuracy version 1.0: The Cochrane Collaboration; 2010. http://srdta.cochrane.org/. Accessed 29 June 2018.
2. Naaktgeboren CA, van Enst WA, Ochodo EA, de Groot JA, Hooft L, Leeflang MM, et al. Systematic overview finds variation in approaches to investigating and reporting on sources of heterogeneity in systematic reviews of diagnostic studies. J Clin Epidemiol. 2014;67:1200–9.
3. Naaktgeboren CA, Ochodo EA, Van Enst WA, de Groot JAH, Hooft L, Leeflang MMG, et al. Assessing variability in results in systematic reviews of diagnostic studies. BMC Med Res Methodol. 2016;16:6.
4. Roberts E, Ludman AJ, Dworzynski K, Al-Mohammad A, Cowie MR, McMurray JJ, et al. The diagnostic accuracy of the natriuretic peptides in heart failure: systematic review and diagnostic meta-analysis in the acute care setting. BMJ. 2015;350:h910.
5. Doebler P, Holling H. Meta-analysis of diagnostic accuracy with mada. 2015. 29 June 2018.
6. Doebler P. Mada: meta-analysis of diagnostic accuracy. R package version 0.5.7. 2015. https://CRAN.R-project.org/package=mada. Accessed 29 June 2018.
7. Schwarzer G. Package 'meta'. 2017. https://cran.r-project.org/web/packages/meta/index.html. Accessed 29 June 2018.
8. Schwarzer G. meta: An R package for meta-analysis. R News. 2007;7:40–5.
9. R Core Team. R: a language and environment for statistical computing. R Foundation for Statistical Computing, Vienna, Austria. 2017. https://www.R-project.org/. Accessed 29 June 2018.
10. Alibay Y, Beauchet A, El Mahmoud R, Schmitta C, Brun-Neyd D, Benoite M, et al. Plasma N-terminal pro-brain natriuretic peptide and brain natriuretic peptide in assessment of acute dyspnea. Biomed Pharmacother. 2005;59:20–4.
11. Arques S, Roux E, Sbragia P, Gelisse R, Ambrosi P, Pieri B, et al. Comparative accuracy of color M-mode and tissue Doppler echocardiography in the emergency diagnosis of congestive heart failure in chronic hypertensive patients with normal left ventricular ejection fraction. Am J Cardiol. 2005;96:1456–9.
12. Arques S, Roux E, Sbragia P, Pieri B, Gelisse R, Luccioni R, et al. Usefulness of bedside tissue Doppler echocardiography and B-type natriuretic peptide (BNP) in differentiating congestive heart failure from noncardiac cause of acute dyspnea in elderly patients with a normal left ventricular ejection fraction and permanent, nonvalvular atrial fibrillation: insights from a prospective, monocenter study. Echocardiography. 2007;24:499–507.
13. Barcarse E, Kazanegra R, Chen A, Chiu A, Clopton P, Maisel A. Combination of B-type natriuretic peptide levels and non-invasive hemodynamic parameters in diagnosing congestive heart failure in the emergency department. Congest Heart Fail. 2004;10:171–6.
14. Blonde-Cynober F, Morineau G, Estrugo B, Fillie E, Aussel C, Vincent J-P. Diagnostic and prognostic value of brain natriuretic peptide (BNP) concentrations in very elderly heart disease

patients: specific geriatric cut-off and impacts of age, gender, renal dysfunction, and nutritional status. Arch Gerontol Geriatr. 2011;52:106–10.

15. Chenevier-Gobeaux C, Guerin S, Andre S, Ray P, Cynober L, Gestin S, et al. Midregional pro-atrial natriuretic peptide for the diagnosis of cardiac-related dyspnea according to renal function in the emergency department: a comparison with B-type natriuretic peptide (BNP) and N-terminal proBNP. Clin Chem. 2010;56:1708–17.
16. Chung T, Sindone A, Foo F, Dwyer A, Paoloni R, Janu MR, et al. Influence of history of heart failure on diagnostic performance and utility of B-type natriuretic peptide testing for acute dyspnea in the emergency department. Am Heart J. 2006;152:949–55.
17. Dao Q, Krishnaswamy P, Kazanegra R, Harrison A, Amirnovin R, Lenert L, et al. Utility of B-type natriuretic peptide in the diagnosis of congestive heart failure in an urgent-care setting. J Am Coll Cardiol. 2001;37:379–85.
18. Davis M, Espiner E, Richards G, Billings J, Town I, Neill A, et al. Plasma brain natriuretic peptide in assessment of acute dyspnoea. Lancet. 1994;343:440–4.
19. Dokainish H, Zoghbi WA, Lakkis NM, Quinones MA, Nagueh SF. Comparative accuracy of B-type natriuretic peptide and tissue Doppler echocardiography in the diagnosis of congestive heart failure. Am J Cardiol. 2004;93:1130–5.
20. Fleischer D, Espiner EA, Yandle TG, Livesey JH, Billings J, Town I, et al. Rapid assay of plasma brain natriuretic peptide in the assessment of acute dyspnoea. N Z Med J. 1997;110:71–4.
21. Gorissen C, Baumgarten R, de Groot M, van Haren E, Kragten H, Leers M. Analytical and clinical performance of three natriuretic peptide tests in the emergency room. Clin Chem Lab Med. 2007;45:678–84.
22. Karmpaliotis D, Kirtane AJ, Ruisi CP, Polonsky T, Malhotra A, Talmor D, et al. Diagnostic and prognostic utility of brain natriuretic Peptide in subjects admitted to the ICU with hypoxic respiratory failure due to noncardiogenic and cardiogenic pulmonary edema. Chest. 2007;131:964–71.
23. Lainchbury JG, Campbell E, Frampton CM, Yandle TG, Nicholls MG, Richards AM. Brain natriuretic peptide and n-terminal brain natriuretic peptide in the diagnosis of heart failure in patients with acute shortness of breath. J Am Coll Cardiol. 2003;42:728–35.
24. Logeart D, Saudubray C, Beyne P, Thabut G, Ennezat PV, Chavelas C, et al. Comparative value of Doppler echocardiography and B-type natriuretic peptide assay in the etiologic diagnosis of acute dyspnea. J Am Coll Cardiol. 2002;40:1794–800.
25. Lokuge A, Lam L, Cameron P, Krum H, de Villiers S, Bystrzycki A, et al. B-type natriuretic peptide testing and the accuracy of heart failure diagnosis in the emergency department. Circ Heart Fail. 2010;3:104–10.
26. Maisel AS, Krishnaswamy P, Nowak RM, McCord J, Hollander JE, Duc P, et al. Rapid measurement of B-type natriuretic peptide in the emergency diagnosis of heart failure. N Engl J Med. 2002;347:161–7.
27. Maisel A, Mueller C, Nowak R, Peacock WF, Landsberg JW, Ponikowski P, et al. Mid-region pro-hormone markers for diagnosis and prognosis in acute dyspnea: results from the BACH (Biomarkers in Acute Heart Failure) trial. J Am Coll Cardiol. 2010;55:2062–76.
28. Mueller T, Gegenhuber A, Poelz W, Haltmayer M. Diagnostic accuracy of B type natriuretic peptide and amino terminal proBNP in the emergency diagnosis of heart failure. Heart. 2005;91:606–12.
29. Parab R, Vasudevan A, Brensilver J, Gitler B. Utility of brain natriuretic peptide as a diagnostic tool for congestive heart failure in the elderly. Crit Pathw Cardiol. 2005;4:140–4.
30. Ray P, Arthaud M, Lefort Y, Birolleau S, Beigelman C, Riou B, et al. Usefulness of B-type natriuretic peptide in elderly patients with acute dyspnea. Intensive Care Med. 2004;30:2230–6.
31. Kevin Rogers R, Stehlik J, Stoddard GJ, Greene T, Collins SP, Peacock WF, et al. Adjusting for clinical covariates improves the ability of B-type natriuretic peptide to distinguish cardiac from non-cardiac dyspnoea: a sub-study of HEARD-IT. Eur J Heart Fail. 2009;11:1043–9.

32. Sanz MP, Borque L, Rus A, Vicente B, Ramirez Y, Lasa L. Comparison of BNP and NT-proBNP assays in the approach to the emergency diagnosis of acute dyspnea. J Clin Lab Anal. 2006;20:227–32.
33. Villacorta H, Duarte A, Duarte NM, Carrano A, Mesquita ET, Dohmann HJ, et al. The role of B-type natriuretic peptide in the diagnosis of congestive heart failure in patients presenting to an emergency department with dyspnea. Arq Bras Cardiol. 2002;79:569–72.
34. Wang HK, Tsai MS, Chang JH, Wang TD, Chen WJ, Huang CH. Cardiac ultrasound helps for differentiating the causes of acute dyspnea with available B-type natriuretic peptide tests. Am J Emerg Med. 2010;28:987–93.
35. Lijmer JG, Bossuyt PM, Heisterkamp SH. Exploring sources of heterogeneity in systematic reviews of diagnostic tests. Stat Med. 2002;21:1525–37.
36. Whiting P, Rutjes AWS, Reitsma JB, Glas AS, Bossuyt PMM, Kleijnen J. Sources of variation and bias in studies of diagnostic accuracy. Ann Intern Med. 2004;140:189–202.
37. Whiting PF, Rutjes AWS, Westwood ME, Mallett S, Deeks JJ, Reitsma JB, et al. QUADAS-2: A revised tool for the quality assessment of diagnostic accuracy studies. Ann Intern Med. 2011;155:529–36.
38. Whiting P, Rutjes AWS, Reitsma JB, Bossuyt PMM, Kleijnen J. The development of QUADAS: a tool for the quality assessment of studies of diagnostic accuracy included in systematic reviews. BMC Med Res Methodol. 2003;3:25.
39. Rutjes AW, Reitsma JB, Di Nisio M, Smidt N, van Rijn JC, Bossuyt PM. Evidence of bias and variation in diagnostic accuracy studies. CMAJ. 2006;174:469–76.
40. Song JW, Kim HM, Bellfi LT, Chung KC. The effect of study design biases on the diagnostic accuracy of magnetic resonance imaging for detecting silicone breast implant ruptures: a meta-analysis. Plast Reconstr Surg. 2011;127:1029–44.
41. Parker LA, Saez NG, Porta M, Hernández-Aguado I, Lumbreras B. The impact of including different study designs in meta-analyses of diagnostic accuracy studies. Eur J Epidemiol. 2013;28:713–20.
42. Leeflang MM, Rutjes AW, Reitsma JB, Hooft L, Bossuyt PM. Variation of a test's sensitivity and specificity with disease prevalence. CMAJ. 2013;185:E537–44.
43. Ochodo EA, van Enst WA, Naaktgeboren CA, de Groot JAH, Hooft L, Moons KGM, et al. Incorporating quality assessments of primary studies in the conclusions of diagnostic accuracy reviews: a cross-sectional study. BMC Med Res Methodol. 2014;14:33.
44. Cohen JF, Korevaar DA, Wang J, Leeflang MM, Bossuyt PM. Meta-epidemiologic study showed frequent time trends in summary estimates from meta-analyses of diagnostic accuracy studies. J Clin Epidemiol. 2016;77:60–7.
45. Moses LE, Shapiro DE, Littenberg B. Combining independent studies of a diagnostic tests into a summary ROC curve: Data-analytic approaches and some additional considerations. Stat Med. 1993;12:1293–316.
46. Leeflang MMG, Deeks JJ, Rutjes AWS, Reitsma JB, Bossuyt PMM. Bivariate meta-analysis of predictive values of diagnostic tests can be an alternative to bivariate meta-analysis of sensitivity and specificity. J Clin Epidemiol. 2012;65:1088–97.
47. Phillips B, Stewart LA, Sutton AJ. 'Cross hairs' plots for diagnostic meta-analysis. Res Synth Methods. 2010;1:308–15.
48. Light RJ, Pillemer DB. Summing up: the science of reviewing research. Cambridge, Massachusetts: Harvard University Press; 1984.
49. Song F, Khan KS, Dinnes J, Sutton AJ. Asymmetric funnel plots and publication bias in meta-analyses of diagnostic accuracy. Int J Epidemiol. 2002;31:88–95.
50. Deeks JJ, Macaskill P, Irwig L. The performance of tests of publication bias and other sample size effects in systematic reviews of diagnostic test accuracy was assessed. J Clin Epidemiol. 2005;58:882–93.
51. Glas AS, Lijmer JG, Prins MH, Bonsel GJ, Bossuyt PM. The diagnostic odds ratio: a single indicator of test performance. J Clin Epidemiol. 2003;56:1129–35.

52. Jackson D, White IR, Thompson SG. Extending DerSimonian and Laird's methodology to perform multivariate random effects meta-analyses. Stat Med. 2010;29:1282–97.
53. Higgins JPT, Thompson SG. Quantifying heterogeneity in a meta-analysis. Stat Med. 2002;21:1539–58.
54. Ioannidis JP. Interpretation of tests of heterogeneity and bias in meta-analysis. J Eval Clin Pract. 2008;14:951–7.
55. Egger M, Davey Smith G, Schneider M, Minder C. Bias in meta-analysis detected by a simple, graphical test. BMJ. 1997;315:629–34.
56. Macaskill P, Walter SD, Irwig L. A comparison of methods to detect publication bias in meta-analysis. Stat Med. 2001;20:641–54.
57. Begg CB, Mazumdar M. Operating characteristics of a rank correlation test for publication bias. Biometrics. 1994;50:1088–101.
58. Bürkner PC, Doebler P. Testing for publication bias in diagnostic meta-analysis: a simulation study. Stat Med. 2014;33:3061–77.
59. Youden WJ. Index for rating diagnostic tests. Cancer. 1950;3:32–5.
60. Le CT. A solution for the most basic optimization problem associated with an ROC curve. Stat Methods Med Res. 2006;15:571–84.
61. Duval S, Tweedie R. A nonparametric 'Trim and Fill' method of accounting for publication bias in meta-analysis. JASA. 2000;95:89–98.
62. Higgins JP, Thompson SG, Deeks JJ, Altman DG. Measuring inconsistency in meta-analyses. BMJ. 2003;327:557–60.
63. Deeks JJ, Higgins JPT, Altman DG, editors. Analysing data and undertaking meta-analyses. In: Higgins JPT, Green S, editors. Cochrane handbook for systematic reviews of interventions version 5.1.0 (updated March 2011). The Cochrane Collaboration, 2011. www.handbook.cochrane.org. Accessed 29 June 2018.
64. Gatsonis C, Paliwal P. Meta-analysis of diagnostic and screening test accuracy evaluations: methodologic primer. AJR Am J Roentgenol. 2006;187:271–81.
65. Jackson D, White IR, Riley RD. Quantifying the impact of between-study heterogeneity in multivariate meta-analyses. Stat Med. 2012;31:3805–20.
66. Zhou Y, Dendukuri N. Statistics for quantifying heterogeneity in univariate and bivariate meta-analyses of binary data: The case of meta-analyses of diagnostic accuracy. Stat Med. 2014;33:2701–17.
67. Rücker G, Schwarzer G, Carpenter JR, Schumacher M. Undue reliance on I2 in assessing heterogeneity may mislead. BMC Med Res Methodol. 2008;8:79.
68. Borenstein M, Higgins JP, Hedges LV, Rothstein HR. Basics of meta-analysis: I2 is not an absolute measure of heterogeneity. Res Synth Methods. 2017;8:5–18.
69. Böhning D, Malzahn U, Dietz E, Schlattmann P, Viwatwongkasem C, Biggeri A. Some general points in estimating heterogeneity variance with the DerSimonian-Laird estimator. Biostatistics. 2002;3:445–57.
70. Jackson D, White IR, Riley RD. A matrix-based method of moments for fitting the multivariate random effects model for meta-analysis and meta-regression. Biom J. 2013;55:231–45.
71. Ohle R, McIsaac SM, Woo MY, Perry JJ. Sonography of the optic nerve sheath diameter for detection of raised intracranial pressure compared to computed tomography: a systematic review and meta-analysis. J Ultrasound Med. 2015;34:1285–94.
72. Leeflang MM, Moons KG, Reitsma JB, Zwinderman AH. Bias in sensitivity and specificity caused by data-driven selection of optimal cutoff values: mechanisms, magnitude, and solutions. Clin Chem. 2008;54:729–37.
73. Rücker G, Schumacher M. Letter to the editor. Biostatistics. 2009;10:806–7.
74. Janda S, Swiston J. Diagnostic accuracy of pleural fluid NT-pro-BNP for pleural effusions of cardiac origin: a systematic review and meta-analysis. BMC Pulm Med. 2010;10:58.
75. Trikalinos TA, Balion CM, Coleman CI, Griffith L, Santaguida PL, Vandermeer B, et al. Chapter 8: meta-analysis of test performance when there is a 'gold standard'. J Gen Intern Med. 2012;27:S56–66.

76. GRADE Working Group. Grading quality of evidence and strength of recommendations. BMJ. 2004;328:1490.
77. Schünemann HJ, Oxman AD, Brozek J, Glasziou P, Jaeschke R, Vist GE, et al. Rating quality of evidence and strength of recommendations–GRADE: grading quality of evidence and strength of recommendations for diagnostic tests and strategies. BMJ. 2008;336:1106–10.
78. Reitsma JB, Glas AS, Rutjes AW, Scholten RJ, Bossuyt PM, Zwinderman AH. Bivariate analysis of sensitivity and specificity produces informative summary measures in diagnostic reviews. J Clin Epidemiol. 2005;58:982–90.
79. Littenberg B, Moses LE. Estimating diagnostic accuracy from multiple conflicting reports: a new meta-analytic method. Med Decis Mak. 1993;13:313–21.
80. Rutter CM, Gatsonis CA. A hierarchical regression approach to meta-analysis of diagnostic test accuracy evaluations. Stat Med. 2001;20:2865–84.
81. Lee J, Kim KW, Choi SH, Huh J, Park SH. Systematic review and meta-analysis of studies evaluating diagnostic test accuracy: a practical review for clinical researchers-Part II. Statistical methods of meta-analysis. Korean J Radiol. 2015;16:1188–96.
82. Harbord RM, Deeks JJ, Egger M, Whiting P, Sterne JA. A unification of models for meta-analysis of diagnostic accuracy studies. Biostatistics. 2007;8:239–51.
83. Arends LR, Hamza TH, van Houwelingen JC, Heijenbrok-Kal MH, Hunink MG, Stijnen T. Bivariate random effects meta-analysis of ROC curves. Med Decis Mak. 2008;28:621–38.
84. Harbord RM, Whiting P, Sterne JA, Egger M, Deeks JJ, Shang A, et al. An empirical comparison of methods for meta-analysis of diagnostic accuracy showed hierarchical models are necessary. J Clin Epidemiol. 2008;61:1095–103.
85. Sutton AJ, Higgins JP. Recent developments in meta-analysis. Stat Med. 2008;27:625–50.
86. Chen Y, Liu Y, Ning J, Nie L, Zhu H, Chu H. A composite likelihood method for bivariate meta-analysis in diagnostic systematic reviews. Stat Methods Med Res. 2014;26:914–30.
87. Chen Y, Hong C, Ning Y, Su X. Meta-analysis of studies with bivariate binary outcomes: a marginal beta-binomial model approach. Stat Med. 2016;35:21–40.
88. Guolo A. A double SIMEX approach for bivariate random-effects meta-analysis of diagnostic accuracy studies. BMC Med Res Methodol. 2017;17:6.
89. Rücker G, Schumacher M. Summary ROC curve based on a weighted Youden index for selecting an optimal cutpoint in meta-analysis of diagnostic accuracy. Stat Med. 2010;29:3069–78.
90. Doebler P, Holling H, Böhning D. A mixed model approach to meta-analysis of diagnostic studies with binary test outcome. Psychol Methods. 2012;17:418–36.
91. Holling H, Böhning W, Böhning D. Meta-analysis of diagnostic studies based upon SROC-curves: a mixed model approach using the Lehmann family. Stat Model. 2012;12:347–75.
92. Charoensawat S, Böhning W, Böhning D, Holling H. Meta-analysis and meta-modelling for diagnostic problems. BMC Med Res Methodol. 2014;14:56.
93. Doebler P, Holling H. Meta-analysis of Diagnostic Accuracy and ROC Curves with Covariate Adjusted Semiparametric mixtures. Psychometrika. 2015;80:1084–104.
94. Schlattmann P, Verba M, Dewey M, Walther M. Mixture models in diagnostic meta-analyses—clustering summary receiver operating characteristic curves accounted for heterogeneity and correlation. J Clin Epidemiol. 2015;68:61–72.
95. Menke J. Bayesian bivariate meta-analysis of sensitivity and specificity: summary of quantitative findings in 50 meta-analyses. J Eval Clin Pract. 2014;20:844–52.
96. Dahabreh IJ, Trikalinos TA, Lau J, Schmid C. An empirical assessment of bivariate methods for meta-analysis of test accuracy. Methods Research Reports; Agency for Healthcare Research and Quality (US). 2012;12(13)-EHC136-EF.
97. Novielli N, Cooper NJ, Sutton AJ, Abrams KR. Bayesian model selection for meta-analysis of diagnostic test accuracy data: Application to Ddimer for deep vein thrombosis. Res Synth Methods. 2010;1:226–38.
98. Dukic V, Gatsonis C. Meta-analysis of diagnostic test accuracy assessment studies with varying number of thresholds. Biometrics. 2003;59:936–46.
99. Putter H, Fiocco M, Stijnen T. Meta-analysis of diagnostic test accuracy studies with multiple thresholds using survival methods. Biom J. 2010;52:95–110.

100. Poon WY. A latent normal distribution model for analysing ordinal responses with applications in meta-analysis. Stat Med. 2004;23:2155–72.
101. Bipat S, Zwinderman AH, Bossuyt PMM, Stoker J. Multivariate random-effects approach: for meta-analysis of cancer staging studies. Acad Radiol. 2007;14:974–84.
102. Hamza TH, Arends LR, van Houwelingen HC, Stijnen T. Multivariate random effects meta-analysis of diagnostic tests with multiple thresholds. BMC Med Res Methodol. 2009;9:73.
103. Riley RD, Takwoingi Y, Trikalinos T, Guha A, Biswas A, Ensor J, et al. Meta-analysis of test accuracy studies with multiple and missing thresholds: a multivariate-normal model. J Biomet Biostat. 2014;5:196.
104. Steinhauser S, Schumacher M, Rücker G. Modelling multiple thresholds in meta-analysis of diagnostic test accuracy studies. BMC Med Res Methodol. 2016;16:97.
105. Martínez-Camblor P. Fully non-parametric receiver operating characteristic curve estimation for random-effects meta-analysis. Stat Methods Med Res. 2017;26:5–20.
106. Hoyer A, Hirt S, Kuss O. Meta-analysis of full ROC curves using bivariate time-to-event models for interval-censored data. Res Syn Meth. 2018;9:62–72.
107. Chen S, Watson P, Parmigiani G. Accuracy of MSI testing in predicting germline mutations of MSH2 and MLH1: a case study in Bayesian meta-analysis of diagnostic tests without a gold standard. Biostatistics. 2005;6:450–64.
108. Chu H, Nie L, Cole S, Poole C. Meta-analysis of diagnostic accuracy studies accounting for disease prevalence: alternative parameterizations and model selection. Stat Med. 2009;28:2384–99.
109. Dendukuri N, Schiller I, Joseph L, Pai M. Bayesian meta-analysis of the accuracy of a test for *Tuberculous pleuritis* in the absence of a gold standard reference. Biometrics. 2012;68:1285–93.
110. Liu Y, Chen Y, Chu H. A unification of models for meta-analysis of diagnostic accuracy studies without a gold standard. Biometrics. 2015;71:538–47.
111. De Groot JA, Dendukuri N, Janssen KJ, Reitsma JB, Brophy J, Joseph L, et al. Adjusting for partial verification or workup bias in meta-analyses of diagnostic accuracy studies. Am J Epidemiol. 2012;175:847–53.
112. Begg CB, Greenes RA. Assessment of diagnostic tests when disease verification is subject to selection bias. Biometrics. 1983;39:207–15.
113. Menten J, Boelaert M, Lesaffre E. Bayesian meta-analysis of diagnostic tests allowing for imperfect reference standards. Stat Med. 2013;32:5398–413.
114. Ma X, Chen Y, Cole SR, Chu H. A Hybrid Bayesian Hierarchical Model Combining Cohort and Case-control Studies for Meta-analysis of Diagnostic Tests: Accounting for Partial Verification Bias. Stat Methods Med Res. 2016;25:3015–37.
115. Li J, Fine JP. Assessing the dependence of sensitivity and specificity on prevalence in meta-analysis. Biostatistics. 2011;12:710–22.
116. Chen Y, Liu Y, Chu H, Ting Lee ML, Schmid CH. A simple and robust method for multivariate meta-analysis of diagnostic test accuracy. Stat Med. 2017;36:105–21.
117. Hoyer A, Kuss O. Meta-analysis of diagnostic tests accounting for disease prevalence: a new model using trivariate copulas. Stat Med. 2015;34:1912–24.
118. Takwoingi Y, Guo B, Riley RD, Deeks JJ. Performance of methods for meta-analysis of diagnostic test accuracy with few studies or sparse data. Stat Methods Med Res. 2017;26:1896–911.
119. Riley RD, Dodd SR, Craig JV, Thompson JR, Williamson PR. Meta-analysis of diagnostic test studies using individual patient data and aggregate data. Stat Med. 2008;27:6111–36.
120. Ter Riet G, Bachmann LM, Kessels AG, Khan KS. Individual patient data meta-analysis of diagnostic studies: opportunities and challenges. Evid Based Med. 2013;18:165–9.
121. Begg CB, Greenes RA, Iglewicz B. The influence of uninterpretability on the assessment of diagnostic tests. J Chronic Dis. 1986;39:575–84.
122. Schütz GM, Schlattmann P. Use of 3×2 tables with an intention to diagnose approach to assess clinical performance of diagnostic tests: meta-analytical evaluation of coronary ct angiography studies. BMJ. 2012;345:e6717.

123. Menke J, Kowalski J. Diagnostic accuracy and utility of coronary CT angiography with consideration of unevaluable results: a systematic review and multivariate Bayesian random-effects meta-analysis with intention to diagnose. Eur Radiol. 2016;26:451–8.
124. Ma X, Suri MF, Chu H. A trivariate meta-analysis of diagnostic studies accounting for prevalence and non-evaluable subjects: re-evaluation of the meta-analysis of coronary CT angiography studies. BMC Med Res Methodol. 2014;14:128.
125. McClish DK. Combining and comparing area estimates across studies or strata. Med Decis Mak. 1992;12:274–9.
126. Kester AD, Buntinx F. Meta-analysis of ROC curves. Med Decis Mak. 2000;20:430–9.
127. Zwinderman AH, Bossuyt PM. We should not pool diagnostic likelihood ratios in systematic reviews. Stat Med. 2008;27:687–97.

Statistical Packages for Diagnostic Meta-Analysis and Their Application

12

Philipp Doebler, Paul-Christian Bürkner, and Gerta Rücker

12.1 Introduction

The vast majority of meta-analytic approaches are intended for the analysis of univariate effect-size measures. As a consequence, most software packages focus on meta-analytic techniques for univariate data, e.g., tools like RevMan [1] or R-packages like meta [2]. However, the accuracy of a diagnostic test is typically evaluated in a positive and a negative arm relative to a gold standard (Chap. 3) and thus produces two end points, the sensitivity and false-positive rate (Chap. 11) calculated from a 2 × 2 table. While such a table can be boiled down to a univariate effect size and meta-analyzed (e.g., [3]), it is recommended to employ the Reitsma et al. [4] bivariate model that simultaneously analyzes the reported pairs of sensitivity and false-positive rate [5, 6]. Alternatively, the HSROC model of Rutter and Gatsonis [7] can be used, which is equivalent to the bivariate model in the absence of covariates [8]. Regardless whether the bivariate model of the HSROC model is employed, complex iterative algorithms are needed, so in contrast to, say, a DerSimonian and Laird [9] meta-analysis, a spreadsheet program is not an option.

P. Doebler (✉)
Department of Statistics, TU Dortmund University, Dortmund, Germany
e-mail: doebler@statistik.tu-dortmund.de

P.-C. Bürkner
Institute of Psychology, Faculty of Psychology and Sport Sciences, University of Münster, Münster, Germany
e-mail: paul.buerkner@uni-muenster.de

G. Rücker
Faculty of Medicine, Institute for Medical Biometry and Statistics, Medical Center – University of Freiburg, Freiburg im Breisgau, Germany
e-mail: ruecker@imbi.uni-freiburg.de

G. Biondi-Zoccai (ed.), *Diagnostic Meta-Analysis*,
https://doi.org/10.1007/978-3-319-78966-8_12

As a consequence, the meta-analysis of diagnostic test accuracy (DTA) requires specialized packages. Another reason to employ such packages is powerful graphical techniques like summary receiver operating characteristic (SROC) curves (Chap. 11), which add substantially to a diagnostic meta-analysis in the presence of different (implicit or explicit) cutoff values. Note that packages for bivariate and multivariate meta-analyses such as the R-packages `metafor` [10] or `mvmeta` [11] do not include functionality to produce SROC curves.

The aim of this chapter is to inform the diagnostic meta-analyst of software options and to present a workflow in R [12] with some detail including computer code. Others have recently contributed similar work to aid DTA meta-analysts in the analysis stage: A book chapter by Schwarzer et al. [13] discusses in detail how to perform an analysis in R, and several recent tutorials and/or reviews exist in the medical literature of Liu et al. [14]; Kim et al. [15]; and Lee et al. [16]. The contribution by Macaskill et al. [6] is worth mentioning for authors of Cochrane Reviews.

The remainder of this chapter is structured as follows: After an overview of existing packages and short discussion of their strength and weaknesses, techniques are presented for descriptive statistics in Sect. 12.2 and the fitting of the bivariate model in Sect. 12.3, including the calculation and plotting for SROC curves. A brief discussion wraps up the chapter and hints at computer code for advanced methods.

12.1.1 Overview of Software Packages

Table 12.1 contains an overview of software packages for diagnostic meta-analysis. The selection is based on packages that allow to fit the bivariate model and includes specialized packages for meta-analysis of DTA as well as general packages with capabilities for multivariate meta-analysis. The table omits discontinued packages and those only suited for outdated approaches like the Moses-Littenberg SROC curve (e.g., RevMan,[1] MetaDiSc). In addition to the packages found in Table 12.1, there are other packages that allow to fit generalized linear models (and hence the bivariate model as a special case), but we omit them as we are not aware that they have been referenced for this purpose in the literature. In addition, there are (R-) packages for special variants of the bivariate models not listed here [17–19].

We caution the reader that all general packages will require more effort in implementing the bivariate model and producing output specific for the DTA context such as SROC curves. There is hence a trade-off between extensibility of the software and convenient use. Clearly, the diagnostic meta-analyst will have to balance these two factors, as extensibility comes with more time and effort in implementation or even requires programming skills. In the Discussion, we reference packages and computer code for some specialized analysis methods.

[1] We mention in passing that RevMan can plot SROC curves if suitable output is supplied from other packages.

Table 12.1 Current software packages for diagnostic meta-analysis that include the bivariate model

Statistical Framework	Package/macro	Features and notes	Reference(s)
Open-source software			
BUGS language	WinBUGS, OpenBUGS	General statistical package, Bayesian, extensible, programming needed	[20, 21]
	jags, rjags	General statistical package, Bayesian, extensible, programming needed	[22]
R	brms	General mixed model package, Bayesian, extensible, implementation needed	[23]
	lme4	General mixed model package, extensible, implementation needed	[24]
	mada	Specialized package for DTA meta-analysis, LMM approximation to bivariate model, graphical methods	[25]
	meta4diag	Specialized package for DTA meta-analysis, Bayesian, graphical methods	[26]
	metafor	General univariate and multivariate meta-analysis package, implementation needed	[10]
	Metatron	Specialized package for DTA meta-analysis, multinomial processing tree models for imperfect gold standards	[27, 28]
	mvmeta	General multivariate meta-analysis package, implementation needed	[11]
Proprietary software			
MLwiN	–	General mixed model package	[29]
SAS	Proc NLMIXED	General mixed model functions, implementation needed	[30, 31]
	Proc GLIMMIX	General mixed model functions, implementation needed	[32]
	METADAS	Specialized package for DTA meta-analysis	[33]
Stata	glamm	General mixed model package, implementation needed	[34]
	metandi	Specialized package for DTA meta-analysis, graphical methods	[35]
	meqrlogit (xtmelogit)	General binary mixed model package, implementation needed	[36]
	midas	Specialized package for DTA meta-analysis, graphical methods	[37]

12.2 Sample Workflow in R

Since all three authors of this chapter are biased toward R, we present a fairly detailed worked example with R code in the following section.[2] For this

[2] Example code for other packages can typically be found in the references in Table 12.1 or in the technical documentation.

purpose, we mainly use the R-package mada [25], a specialized package for DTA meta-analysis.[3]

We begin by advising on the first steps of an analysis of DTA meta-analysis data. We show ways to import data and then demonstrate descriptive techniques that might be useful prior to an analysis with the bivariate model. We use selected variables from a dataset originally reported in Patrick et al. [38] on the diagnostic accuracy of interviewer or self-administered questionnaires to detect smoking relative to biochemical gold standards.

12.2.1 Importing Data Into R

After coding data (Chap. 8), the analyst obtains a raw data file. Importing data into R is often made easier by employing graphical user interfaces (GUIs) like RStudio. Depending on the source of the data, the preinstalled R-package foreign can be helpful (say to read SPSS files) or the R-package readxl (for Microsoft Excelfiles; [39]). Typically a data.frame is obtained, i.e., an R-object containing data of different types (especially numerical and categorical data).

Some rows of the Patrick et al. [38] smoking data are shown in Table 12.2. From some of the original primary studies, more than one 2 × 2-table could be reasonably coded, since authors reported results for multiple samples, multiple

Table 12.2 Selected rows of the Patrick et al. [38] smoking data

Row	Author	Study_id	Type	TP	FN	FP	TN	Population
1	Bauman and Dent (1982)	1	SAQ	21	15	28	324	S
2	Bauman and Dent (1982)	1	SAQ	90	10	120	969	S
3	Bauman and Dent (1982)	1	SAQ	104	8	26	232	G
4	Bauman and Dent (1982)	1	SAQ	332	18	92	673	G
5	Bauman et al. (1982)	2	SAQ	3	0	2	77	S
6	Bauman and Koch (1983)	3	SAQ	437	23	78	901	G
⋮	⋮	⋮	⋮	⋮	⋮	⋮	⋮	⋮
46	Vogt et al. (1977)	23	IAQ	83	2	11	43	G
47	Vogt et al. (1977)	23	IAQ	71	3	7	42	G
48	Vogt et al. (1977)	23	IAQ	76	3	18	42	G
49	Wagenknecht et al. (1990)	24	IAQ	1357	185	68	3322	G
50	Wald et al. (1981)	25	IAQ	1649	17	423	6632	G
51	Williams et al. (1979)	26	SAQ	19	2	1	96	S

Note: *SAQ* self-administered questionnaire, *IAQ* interviewer-administered questionnaire, *S* student, *G* general

[3]The package can be installed by typing install.packages("mada") at an R-prompt. After this, the package only needs to load once in an R session with library(mada). The most current (development) version of mada is found at http://r-forge.r-project.org/projects/mada/. Some additional functionality of mada is explained in the package vignette that is automatically installed with the package and can be accessed by typing vignette("mada") at an R-prompt.

screening tests, or multiple gold standards. This corresponds to more than one row for some studies. Also, the dataset does not contain the sensitivities and false-positive rates originally reported in some studies but the (reconstructed) frequencies from the underlying 2 × 2-table. The chapter by (Chap. 8) discusses how to obtain them during coding. In the following, we will assume that at least the four columns TP, FN, FP, and TN are present in the data, corresponding to the frequencies of true positives, false negatives, false positives, and true negatives, respectively.

12.2.2 Calculating Summary Statistics for Each Study

Chapter 11 discusses a range of useful summary statistics of diagnostic accuracy. The `madad` function can be conveniently used to calculate these. Note that by default a continuity correction of 0.5 is added to all cells, in case there is a zero cell in any 2 × 2-table. Confidence intervals are Wilson score intervals.

```
library (mada) # load the mada package for this session
# In this example, an example data.frame named smoking
# with several variables used.
data (smoking) # make data available
# Many of the following commands assume that
# the data.frame contains variables for the
# frequencies named TP,FN,FP and TN. If not,
# the syntax has to be modified (see the manual).
descr <- madad (smoking) # includes continuity correction!
print (descr, digits = 2 ) # print lengthy results
```

```
## Descriptive summary of smoking with 51 primary studies.
## Confidence level for all calculations set to 95
## Using a continuity correction of 0.5 if applicable
##
## Diagnostic accuracies
```

	sens	2.5%	97.5%	spec	2.5%	97.5%
[1,]	0.58	0.42	0.72	0.92	0.89	0.94
[2,]	0.90	0.82	0.94	0.89	0.87	0.91
[3,]	0.92	0.86	0.96	0.90	0.85	0.93

```
## ...
## Test for equality of sensitivities:
## X-squared = 1569.401, df = 50, p-value = <2e-16
## Test for equality of specificities:
## X-squared = 1320.466, df = 50, p-value = <2e-16
##
```

```
## Diagnostic OR and likelihood ratios
```

	DOR	2.5%	97.5%	posLR	2.5%	97.5%	negLR	2.5%	97.5%
[1,]	15.79	7.41	33.67	7.20	4.61	11.24	0.46	0.31	0.67
[2,]	69.35	35.61	135.04	8.11	6.76	9.71	0.12	0.07	0.21
[3,]	107.86	48.16	241.58	9.04	6.28	13.01	0.08	0.04	0.16

```
## ...
## Correlation of sensitivities and false positive rates:
```

rho	2.5 %	97.5 %
0.27	0.00	0.51

Note that in addition to the sensitivity and specificity, χ^2-tests of equality are calculated: The null hypothesis is that all (true but unobservable) sensitivities are identical and similar for the specificities. These tests typically confirm the presence of substantial heterogeneity in DTA meta-analysis data. We omit the discussion of the diagnostic odds ratios and the positive and negative likelihood ratios also resulting from a madad call and refer to (Chap. 11) of this volume for details on these statistics. Sometimes it is convenient to use output of R-functions in subsequent calculations:

```
# if you need to work with (part of) the output,
# check the structure:
str(descr)
## List of 17
## $ sens                :List of 2
## ..$ sens    : num [1:51] 0.581 0.896 0.925 0.947 0.875 ...
## ..$ sens.ci: num [1:51, 1:2] 0.422 0.821 0.861 0.919 0.396 ...
## .. ..- attr( * , "dimnames")=List of 2
## .. .. ..$   : NULL
## .. .. ..$   : chr [1:2] "2.5%" "97.5%"
## [...]
# From the structure, we see the list-structure
# and can use it to extract parts of the output:
descr$sens$sens # extract vector of sensitivities
## [1] 0.58108108 0.89603960 0.92477876 0.94729345 0.87500000
## [...]
# redo calculations without continuity correction:
descr0 <- madad(smoking, correction = 0) # output omitted
```

The last line shows how to omit the continuity correction if desired (e.g., to reproduce original results).

12.2.3 Graphical Techniques

Patterns can often be much more easily recognized from graphical representations of data than from tables. Pairs of sensitivity and false-positive rate should be plotted at some point of the analysis. In addition to the point estimates, their uncertainty is of interest. Especially outliers with large standard errors might otherwise influence the perception of the data.

Next we show how to produce a paired forest plot as well as a "cross hairs" plot [40] and a plot with confidence ellipses. To prevent large and/or cluttered plots, we use an (essentially arbitrary) subset of the smoking data here for didactic purposes.[4]

```
# First reduce to a subset of with independent 2x2-tables:
smoking1 <- subset(smoking, result_id == 1)
# Reduce further to a random (and essentially arbitray) subset of
# ten studies to prevent a cluttered plot:
set.seed(12345) # fix random number seed for reproducibilty
smoking1 <- smoking1[sample(1:nrow(smoking1), 10), ]
smoking1 <- smoking1[order(smoking1$author), ] # reorder
# make forest plots
descr1 <- madad(smoking1) # data for forest plots
mynames <- smoking1$author # vector of names for forest plot
forest(descr1, "sens", snames = mynames, main = "Sensitivity")
forest(descr1, "spec", snames = mynames, main = "Specificity")
# make crosshair plot:
crosshair(smoking1, pch = ifelse(smoking1$type == "IAQ", 1, 2),
          col = ifelse(smoking1$population == "G", 1, 2),
          cex = 1.5)
legend("bottomright", c("IAQ", "SAQ"), pch = 1:2, cex = 1.5)
legend("topright", c("general population", "student population"),
     pch = 15, col = 1:2, cex = 1.5)
# make ROC-ellipse plot
ROCellipse(smoking1, pch = ifelse(smoking1$type == "IAQ", 1, 2),
          col = ifelse(smoking1$population == "G", 1, 2),
          cex = 1.5)
legend("bottomright", c("IAQ", "SAQ"), pch = 1:2, cex = 1.5)
legend("topright", c("general population", "student population"),
     pch = 15, col = 1:2, cex = 1.5)
```

[4] Note that the subset function is a convenient way in R to form subsets.

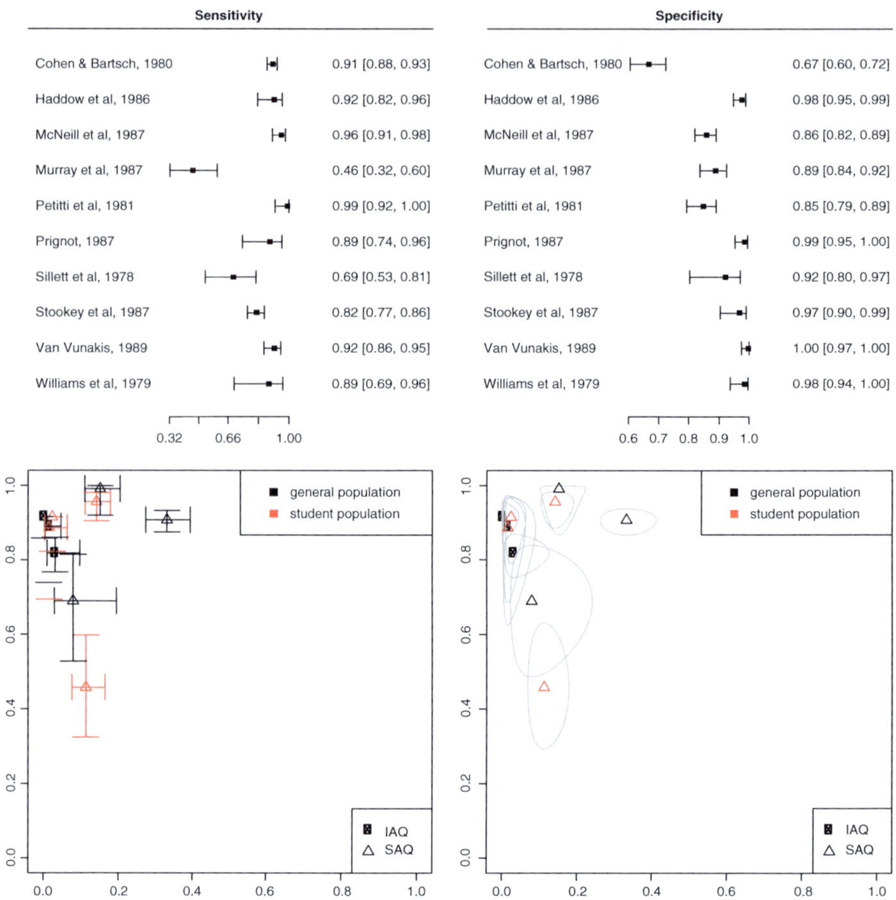

Fig. 12.1 Paired forest plots (top), "crosshairs" plot (bottom left), and confidence ellipses plot (bottom right) for a subset of the smoking data

Figure 12.1 contains the corresponding output. Note that the variable type and population have been used to set color and shape of symbols, so that trends resulting from these covariates might be recognized.

Here, one learns about outliers (easily observed in the sensitivity forest plot or in the crosshair and ellipse plots) and heterogeneity (nonintersecting confidence ellipses). Also, the use of color reveals that diagnostic accuracy is not only determined by the underlying population, while the symbols indicate that IAQs (at least in the arbitrary subset) are more accurate, since they cluster in the top-left corner.

12.2.4 Fitting the Bivariate Model

The bivariate model of Reitsma et al. [4] has been introduced in (Chaps. 10 and 11) of this volume. As the de facto standard in DTA meta-analysis, fitting it deserves special attention in this chapter. Recall that there are (in the absence of covariates)

five parameters of this model: the logit-transformed mean sensitivity and false-positive rate, their between-study variances (again on logit scale), and the between-study covariance (or equivalently the between-study correlation). The interpretation of these parameters is covered in the chapters by Chaps. 10 and 11. All packages mentioned in Table 12.1 can estimate these parameters, with a variety of algorithms. Roughly, the algorithms can be subdivided into frequentist algorithms, which are typically based on the maximum likelihood principle, and Bayesian approaches, which entail Markov-Chain-Monte-Carlo (MCMC) techniques. In this section, we provide examples of software using both types of algorithms without going into their technical foundations.

The bivariate model assumes that independent 2 × 2-tables are available. Since there are multiple rows for some of the studies in the smoking dataset, we only analyze the very first 2 × 2-table from each study subsequently but hint how to overcome this restriction at the end of this section. Also, we reduce the dataset further to include only the self-administered questionnaire (SAQ) data.

12.2.5 Fitting the Bivariate Model Without Covariates

We now show two ways to fit the bivariate model in R. The reitsma function from the R-package mada implements a linear mixed model approximation to the bivariate model, which parallels the implementation with SAS Proc MIXED by Reitsma et al. [4] with restricted maximum likelihood estimation (REML). Chu and Cole [30] caution that this approximation is slightly biased. It can be improved upon by fitting a generalized linear mixed model, a point made more precise in the recent simulation study of Vogelsang et al. [41]. In R, the fit.bivar function from the R-package Metatron, which implements the generalized linear mixed model version of the bivariate model, gives similar results as SAS Proc NLMIXED. Both R-functions discussed here need data from 2 × 2-tables as in Table 12.2. After fitting the model, a summary is produced, which we annotate:

```
# smoking2 is to contain only data for the SAQs from
# independent 2x2-tables:
smoking2 <- subset(smoking, result_id == 1 & type == "SAQ")
library(mada) # LMM-approximation to the bivariate model
# if the dataset contains columns names TP,FN,FP and TN, use
fit1 <- reitsma(smoking2)
summary(fit1) # detailed output
## Call: reitsma.default(data = smoking2)
##
## Bivariate diagnostic random-effects meta-analysis
## Estimation method: REML
```

First, we learn what the input was (which is more useful if covariates are added to the model) and that REML estimation was performed (by default, some other estimators are available). We then see estimates of the fixed effects of the model, which are the logit-transformed sensitivity and false-positive rate:

```
## Fixed-effects coefficients
##                  Estimate Std. Error z Pr(>|z|) 95%ci.lb 95%ci.ub
##
## Fixed-effects coefficients
```

	Estimate Std.	Error	z	Pr(>lzl)	95%ci.lb	95%ci.ub
tsens.(Intercept)	1.68	0.47	3.56	0.00	0.76	2.61
tfpr.(Intercept)	-2.46	0.24	-10.27	0.00	-2.93	-1.99
sensitivity	0.84	-	-	-	0.68	0.93
false pos. rate	0.08	-	-	-	0.05	0.12

```
##
## tsens.(Intercept) ***
## tfpr.(Intercept) ***
## sensitivity
## false pos. rate
## ---
## Signif. codes: 0 ' *** ' 0.001 ' ** ' 0.01 ' * ' 0.05 '.'
0.1 ' ' 1
```

Confidence intervals and asymptotic Wald tests indicate here that the logit-transformed accuracy parameters are significantly different from 0, which means the pooled sensitivity and false-positive rate are significantly different from 0.50. These backtransformed estimates are available in two extra lines. Note that for reasons of formatting, the significance codes for the fixed effects occupy four additional lines in this output, where the three stars for sensitivity and false-positive rate indicate $p < 0.001$ and the backtransformed parameters do not have any stars, as no inference is performed. The output then contains the standard deviations of the random effects and an estimate of the correlation (0.50 here), followed by the log-likelihood and fit measures:

```
## Variance components: between-studies Std. Dev and correlation
matrix
##          Std. Dev   tsens   tfpr
## tsens        1.80    1.00      .
## tfpr         0.90    0.50   1.00
##
## logLik   AIC     BIC
## 32.82 -55.64 -48.31
```

Note that the log-likelihood includes terms for the Jacobian of the logit transformation, which might differ from implementations with SAS Proc MIXED. For further details see Doebler et al. [42]. The remainder of the output contains an estimate of the area under the SROC curve (AUC) with a value of 0.949, which is close to optimal (though the partial AUC of 0.869 is a bit more modest). More details on SROC curves follow in the next section. The SROC curve is calculated based on the parametrization of the HSROC model, and the parameters of this model are also given:

```
## AUC: 0.949
## Partial AUC (restricted to observed FPRs and normalized): 0.869
##
## HSROC parameters
```

Theta	Lambda	beta	sigma2theta	sigma2alpha
-1.14	4.67	-0.69	1.21	1.62

In sum, all parameters of the bivariate model are found in the output of summary(fit1): The pooled logit-transformed sensitivity and false-positive rate are found in the Estimate column. For convenience, also the backtransformed values are given (0.84 and 0.08 here). The between-study standard deviations of the random effects follow (1.80 and 0.90 here) together with their correlation (0.50 here), from which the covariance can be computed if necessary.

12.2.6 SROC Curves

In the majority of areas of application of DTA meta-analysis, explicit or implicit cutoff values are used to dichotomize the result of the screening test. Authors of primary studies choose cutoff values to compromise between false-positive rate and sensitivity. On the level of the primary studies, the curve representing the different trade-offs of false-positive rate versus sensitivity is known as the receiver operating characteristic (ROC) curve.

Variation in the cutoff leads to different pairs of false-positive rate and sensitivity, even if the primary studies were otherwise equal and hence to (apparent) heterogeneity on the meta-analytic level. As a consequence summary ROC (SROC) curves are of special interest in DTA meta-analyses. From the parameters of the bivariate model, SROC curves can be computed. As a default, we recommend the SROC curve suggested by Rutter and Gatsonis [7] for the HSROC model. A straightforward way to plot this SROC curve in R is a simple call of plot: If fit1 is an object produced by the reitsma function, then plot(fit1, predict = TRUE) produces the SROC curve and a prediction region.

Figure 12.2 displays the output of the call to plot: We see the pair of pooled accuracies together with a 95%-confidence region, the analogon of a 95%-confidence interval in the bivariate case. Also, a 95%-prediction region is displayed (dashed line). This can be interpreted as follows: If a new study was to be performed, its pair of sensitivity and false-positive rate would end up in the prediction region with a probability of 95%.

Next to the SROC curve discussed here, other SROC models exist. We will come back to software packages for older and more current models in the Discussion.

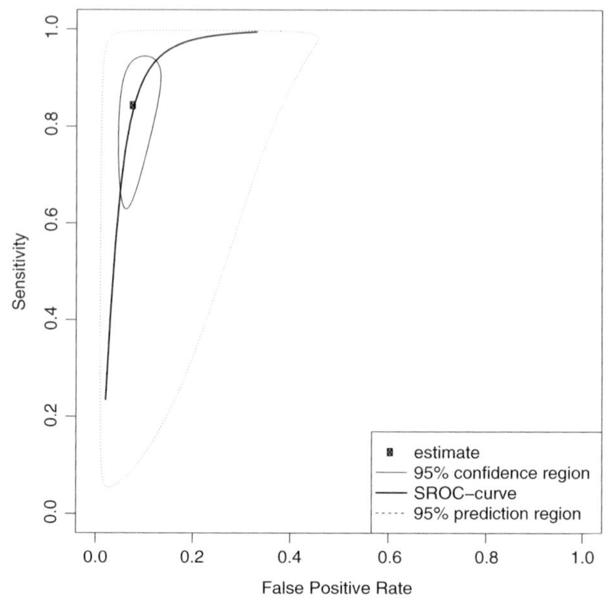

Fig. 12.2 Graphical representation of a bivariate model fit

12.2.7 The Bivariate Model with Covariates

If the DTA meta-analyst's interest is in the influence of a covariate on the diagnostic accuracy, an extension of the bivariate model is needed. We use the general term covariate here to include the categorical case and the continuous case. Examples of categorical covariates include screening test type and population (sub-)type, while mean age and publication year are typically treated as continuous covariates.

Chapter 11 should be consulted for a detailed specification of the technical details of the extension by covariates. In a nutshell, a regression of the logit-transformed sensitivity and/or false-positive rate on the covariate(s) is added to the model. Estimating such a model results in separate (fixed) regression coefficients for sensitivity and false-positive rate. Significance tests for the regression coefficients are a useful by-product. Some expertise with regression modeling is helpful when conducting a DTA meta-analysis with covariates, and in fact, the bivariate model with covariates is an example of a multivariate meta-regression.

Note that the multivariate meta-regression discussed here, similar to its univariate counterpart, assumes that the between-study covariance of the random effect is the same for all combinations of the covariates. For the case of a single categorical covariate, i.e., subgroups, this implies that the between-study covariance is identical in all subgroups. This assumption can be relaxed with subgroup-specific between-study covariance, but we do not discuss this case here.

All packages in Table 12.1 are capable of fitting the bivariate model with covariates. A relatively compact syntax can be used in R, so we demonstrate this for the smoking data. We use the categorical moderator questionnaire type with levels interviewer-administered and self-administered (IAQ and SAQ), so that differences in diagnostic accuracy for these two types of screening measures can be studied.

```
# smoking3 is a subset of the smoking data
# with independent 2x2-tables:
smoking3 <- subset(smoking, smoking$result_id == 1)
fit_type1 <- reitsma(smoking3, formula = cbind(tsens,tfpr) ~ type)
```

Again, fitting does not produce output right away, but a detailed summary is produced by calling summary:

```
summary(fit_type1)
## Call: reitsma.default(data = smoking3,
##                       formula = cbind(tsens, tfpr) ~ type)
##
## Bivariate diagnostic random-effects meta-analysis
## Estimation method: REML
```

Again we learn what the input was and that REML estimation was performed (by default). The output continues by estimates of the logit-transformed sensitivity for the IAQ studies (which are represented by the model's intercept term), and the regression coefficients for SAQ are then interpreted as log odds ratios. The DTA meta-analyst could consider to backtransform the log odds ratios for readers more familiar with odds ratios, say as in the regressions tabulated by Karrasch et al. [43].

```
## Fixed-effects coefficients
```

	Estimate	Std. Err.	Z	Pr(>|z|)	95%ci.lb	95%ci.ub
tsens.(Intercept)	2.81	0.49	5.74	0.00	1.85	3.78
tsens.typeSAQ	-1.17	0.63	-1.84	0.07	-2.41	0.08
tfpr.(Intercept)	-3.34	0.31	-10.73	0.00	-3.95	-2.73
tfpr.typeSAQ	0.88	0.39	2.27	0.02	0.12	1.65

```
##
## tsens.(Intercept) ***
## tsens.typeSAQ .
## tfpr.(Intercept) ***
## tfpr.typeSAQ *
## ---
## Signif. codes: 0 ' *** ' 0.001 ' ** ' 0.01 ' * ' 0.05 '.' 0.1 '
' 1
```

The covariance matrix of the random effects on fit measures then follows, similar to the case without covariates. Note that no parameters of an SROC curve are reported, as there is, at least in general, not a unique curve in models with covariates[5]:

```
## Variance components: between-studies Std. Dev and correlation
## matrix
##         Std. Dev  tsens   tfpr
## tsens    1.508   1.000      .
## tfpr     0.875   0.551  1.000
##
## logLik       AIC        BIC
## 70.721  -127.441  -113.783
```

12.2.8 Fitting Strategies for Advanced Models

The bivariate model is a special case of a generalized linear mixed model (GLMM; e.g., [44, 45]), a type of regression model that includes fixed and random effects. From the GLMM perspective, a range of extensions of the bivariate model are possible, including multiple cutoff values per study (Chap. 11) or trivariate extensions including the observed prevalence [46–48]. As a discussion of all extensions is beyond the scope of this chapter, only an example implementation of the bivariate model as a GLMM is provided.

The multipurpose R-package brms is used in our sample implementation, as it is a (relatively) convenient open-source alternative to commercial packages for GLMMs [23] and also because its Bayesian approach to parameter estimation allows to include prior information, which is in contrast to frequentist packages like lme4 [49]. The following code presents an example of an analysis of the smoking data in brms with and without covariates.[6]

First, the data is rearranged, so that each study fills two rows: one for the positive arm of the study (i.e., condition = "yes") and the other for the negative arm. Many GLMM packages expect data arranged in this fashion:

```
nstudy <- nrow(smoking3)
# convert data to long format:
smoking3_long <- with(smoking3,
     data.frame(P = c(TP, FP), N = c(FN, TN),
          condition = rep(c("yes", "no"), each = nstudy),
```

[5]Note that for special cases like a binary covariate, plotting SROC curves for the parameters corresponding to each of both levels of the covariates is meaningful. For an example, see Meyer, Frings, Rücker, and Hellwig [68].

[6]Note that brms's syntax is very similar to lme4's so that the sample code below can be adapted. For similar lme4 code, also consult Partlett and Takwoingi [24].

```
          type = rep(type, 2),
          study = rep(1:nstudy, 2))
)
smoking3_long$total <- with(smoking3_long, P + N)
```

Next we load the package, and the bivariate model is fitted with and without the type covariate.

```
library(brms) # load brms package
# fit a GLMM corresponding to the bivariate model
fit <- brm(P | trials(total) ~ 0 + condition +
            (0 + condition | study),
          data = smoking3_long, family = binomial())
summary(fit) # obtain model parameters
# produce plot of marginal effects:
marginal_effects(fit, conditions = list(total = 1))
# add study type as a covariate (IAQ vs. SAQ)
fit_type <- brm(P | trials(total) ~ 0 + condition +
            condition:type +(0 + condition | study),
          data = smoking3_long, family = binomial())
summary(fit_type) # check influence of covariate
# plot marginal effects for type:
marginal_effects(fit_type, "condition:type",
          conditions = list(total = 1))
```

Parameter estimates similar to mada's result (not shown), and the discrepancies are a consequence of brms' Bayesian approach and, more importantly, the fact that mada uses a linear approximation to a GLMM. The marginal_effects function produces a graphical display of the estimated pooled sensitivities and false-positive rates (we omit the output for space constraints). Further details are found in the documentation of brms and in Bürkner [23].

12.3 Discussion

We have discussed software options for DTA meta-analysis and, given the space constraint of a single chapter, could not cover everything in detail. Hints at software packages for some additional aspects are provided as part of the discussion.

12.3.1 SROC Models

12.3.1.1 Moses-Littenberg SROC Approach

The Moses-Littenberg SROC curve [50] might be convenient for exploratory purposes, though it might lead to a curve with negative slope if thresholds are similar in all studies. We do not reiterate the theory behind these curves here as (Chap. 10) covers them. The Moses-Littenberg SROC curve can be produced with the help of RevMan or mada. Hand calculation with any statistical package is feasible but typically inconvenient.

12.3.1.2 Software for Current SROC Approaches

Recently, several models featuring educated guesses for the ROC curves at the primary study level have been proposed in the literature. All models mentioned in this paragraph are complementary to the bivariate model, as they produce additional insight into the distribution and especially the heterogeneity of the underlying ROC curves (Chap. 11).

Holling et al. [51] propose an adjusted profile maximum likelihood estimator (APMLE) for the so-called Lehmann family of (S)ROC curves. This estimator is available in mada in the phm function. The Lehmann family approach has inspired several other methods: Holling et al. [52] cluster the Lehmann family curves with semiparametric mixtures, and the approach could be implemented in R using the R-package CAMAN[7] [53], though no convenient off-the-shelf implementation is available. In a similar fashion, the covariate-adjusted mixtures employing t_α-(S) ROC curves instead of Lehmann curves proposed by Doebler and Holling [54] could be implemented, again with some programming on the side of the user. The variant of Charoensawat et al. [55] can be used with any package for univariate meta-analysis, say with meta or metafor in R. Another line of SROC models starts with the weighted Youden index models of Rücker and Schumacher [56], implemented in mada in the rsSROC function. An extension of this approach by Steinhauser et al. [57] is discussed in the subsequent section of models for multiple thresholds.

12.3.2 Multiple Thresholds

If 2 × 2-tables for more than one cutoff value are available from some of the primary studies (say from ROC curves in the primary studies), one has to be careful not to treat them as independent estimates. Also, the diagnostic meta-analyst might want to obtain pairs of pooled sensitivity and false-positive rate for common cutoff values. In this situation, the diagnostic meta-analyst could consider to reduce the coded data in several ways: A reduction of the data could be to select a single 2 × 2-table per study, which clearly entails a loss of information, or to form subsets of the data for each threshold. Subsetting the data in this fashion is only advisable if enough studies end up in each subset, so it might not be possible in some DTA meta-analyses; also see the discussion by Macaskill et al. [6] and empirical work on the introduced bias by Levis et al. [58]. This problem has led to special models for this situation.

[7] CAMAN is also the backbone for the implementation of the semiparametric mixture approach of Schlattmann, Verba, Dewey, and Walther [69], which extends the bivariate model.

We mention some of the existing models for multiple thresholds and what kind of code they supply for fitting the models. Dukic and Gatsonis [59], generalizing the HSROC model of Rutter and Gatsonis [7], propose a Bayesian approach for which code in the BUGS language is available.[8] Implementing the approach in full will require some additional programming.

Hamza et al. [60] extend the bivariate model of Reitsma et al. [4] in a hierarchical fashion and obtain a multivariate random effects model. Code for SAS NLMIXED is supplied in the paper, but the approach is known to be prone to convergence problems and assumes that 2 × 2-tables for the same set of cutoff values can be coded for each study. Putter et al. [61] instead argue in favor of an approach based on survival methods, for which R code is available as supporting information. The survival approach was not convincing enough in a simulation study of Simoneau et al. [62] compared to an approach with the bivariate model.

Riley et al. [63] propose a model that handles missing cutoff values. Code in Stata is available as an additional file on the journal's website. Steinhauser et al. [57] build on ideas of Rücker and Schumacher [56] to present a model that handles multiple thresholds per study to estimate pooled sensitivity and false-positive rate as well as an SROC curve. R code for this approach is part of the supplementary files for this paper. Hoyer et al. [64] propose an approach for meta-analysis of full ROC curves based on information from all thresholds by using bivariate time-to-event models for interval-censored data with random effects. They supply SAS code for their approach. For some additional current approaches [65, 66], we are not aware of readily available implementations.

12.3.3 The Right Tool for the Job

The diagnostic meta-analyst is advised to select the appropriate software package at the planning stage of the meta-analysis, when it is decided which analyses are to be carried out. Preferably, the meta-analysis follows a protocol ((Chap. 11); [67]), similar to that of a randomized clinical trial, and so software should be part of this protocol. From our experience, an early decision will help to organize the coding process and data preparation, as it is clear which form the data file must have to be amenable for the statistical analyses. Regardless of the chosen analysis methods, analysts can choose from a range of algorithms, several Bayesian and many frequentist, and software packages (open source and proprietary). Depending on programming skills and prior experience with mixed regression models and time budget, the meta-analyst is advised to compromise between flexibility and extensibility of the package on the one hand and ease of use on the other hand.

Key Messages

- A number of statistical packages allow to fit the bivariate model.

[8] At the time of writing, code is found on V. Dukic's homepage: http://amath.colorado.edu/faculty/vdukic/software/ROC.html

- Specialized packages for DTA meta-analysis include convenient options for plotting SROC curves.
- Currently, familiarity with more general packages is needed for special models, including those for multiple thresholds.

References

1. The Nordic Cochrane Centre. Review manager (RevMan) [Computer Program], version 5.3. The Cochrane Collaboration, Copenhagen; 2014.
2. Schwarzer G. meta: an R package for meta-analysis. R News. 2007;7:40–5.
3. Glas A, Lijmer J, Prins M, Bonsel G, Bossuyt P. The diagnostic odds ratio: a single indicator of test performance. J Clin Epidemiol. 2003;56:1129–35.
4. Reitsma J, Glas A, Rutjes A, Scholten R, Bossuyt P, Zwinderman A. Bivariate analysis of sensitivity and specificity produces informative summary measures in diagnostic reviews. J Clin Epidemiol. 2005;58:982–90.
5. Leeflang M, Deeks J, Gatsonis C, Bossuyt P. Systematic reviews of diagnostic test accuracy. Ann Intern Med. 2008;149:889–97.
6. Macaskill P, Gatsonis C, Deeks J, Harbord R, Takwoingi Y. Chapter 10: analysing and presenting results. In: Deeks J, Bossuyt P, Gatsonis C, editors. Cochrane handbook for systematic reviews of diagnostic test accuracy version 1.0. The Cochrane Collaboration; 2010. Available from http://srdta.cochrane.org/. Accessed 29 June 2018.
7. Rutter C, Gatsonis C. A hierarchical regression approach to meta-analysis of diagnostic test accuracy evaluations. Stat Med. 2001;20:2865–84.
8. Harbord R, Deeks J, Egger M, Whiting P, Sterne J. A unification of models for meta-analysis of diagnostic accuracy studies. Biostatistics. 2007;8:239–51.
9. DerSimonian R, Laird N. Meta-analysis in clinical trials. Control Clin Trials. 1986;7:177–88.
10. Viechtbauer W. Conducting meta-analyses in R with the metafor package. J Stat Softw. 2010;36:1–48. Available from http://www.jstatsoft.org/v36/i03/. Accessed 29 June 2018.
11. Gasparrini A, Armstrong B, Kenward M. Multivariate meta-analysis for non-linear and other multi-parameter associations. Stat Med. 2012;31:3821–39.
12. R Core Team. R: a language and environment for statistical computing. Vienna: R Foundation for Statistical Computing; 2017. Available from https://www.R-project.org/. Accessed 29 June 2018.
13. Schwarzer G, Carpenter J, Rücker G. Meta-analysis with r. New York: Springer; 2015. UseR!
14. Liu Z, Yao Z, Li C, Liu X, Chen H, Gao C. A step-by-step guide to the systematic review and meta-analysis of diagnostic and prognostic test accuracy evaluations. Br J Cancer. 2013;108:2299–303.
15. Kim K, Lee J, Choi S, Huh J, Park S. Systematic review and meta-analysis of studies evaluating diagnostic test accuracy: a practical review for clinical researchers-part I. General guidance and tips. Korean J Radiol. 2015;16:1175–87.
16. Lee J, Kim K, Choi S, Huh J, Park S. Systematic review and meta-analysis of studies evaluating diagnostic test accuracy: a practical review for clinical researchers-part II. Statistical methods of meta-analysis. Korean J Radiol. 2015;16:1188–96.
17. Nikoloulopoulos A. CopulaREMADA: copula mixed effect models for bivariate and trivariate meta-analysis of diagnostic test accuracy studies. R package version 1.0. 2016. Available from https://CRAN.R-project.org/package=CopulaREMADA. Accessed 29 June 2018.
18. Schiller I, Dendukuri N. HSROC: joint meta-analysis of diagnostic test sensitivity and specificity with or without a gold standard reference test. R package version 2.1.8; 2015.
19. Verde PE. bamdit: bayesian meta-analysis of diagnostic test data. R package version 3.1.0. 2017. Available from https://CRAN.R-project.org/package=bamdit. Accessed 29 June 2018.

20. Lunn D, Thomas A, Best N, Spiegelhalter D. WinBUGS—a Bayesian modelling framework: concepts, structure, and extensibility. Stat Comput. 2000;10:325–37.
21. Lunn D, Spiegelhalter D, Thomas A, Best N. The BUGS project: evolution, critique and future directions. Stat Med. 2009;28:3049–67.
22. Plummer M. rjags: Bayesian graphical models using MCMC. R package version 4-6. 2016. Retrieved from https://CRAN.R-project.org/package=rjags. Accessed 29 June 2018.
23. Bürkner P-C. brms: an R package for Bayesian multilevel models using Stan. J Stat Softw. 2017;80:1–28.
24. Partlett C, Takwoingi Y. Meta-analysis of test accuracy studies in R: a summary of user-written programs and step-by-step guide to using glmer. Version 1.0. 2016. Available from http://methods.cochrane.org/sdt/. Accessed 29 June 2018.
25. Doebler P. mada: meta-analysis of diagnostic accuracy. R package version 0.5.7. 2015. Available from https://CRAN.R-project.org/package=mada. Accessed 29 June 2018.
26. Guo J, Riebler A. meta4diag: meta-analysis for diagnostic test studies. R package version 2.0.5. 2016. Available from https://CRAN.R-project.org/package=meta4diag. Accessed 29 June 2018.
27. Huang H. Metatron: meta-analysis for classification data and correction to imperfect reference. R package version 0.1-1. 2014. Available from https://CRAN.R-project.org/package=Metatron. Accessed 29 June 2018.
28. Botella J, Huang H, Suero M. Multinomial tree models for assessing the status of the reference in studies of the accuracy of tools for binary classification. Front Psychol. 2013;4:694.
29. Charlton C, Rasbash J, Browne W, Healy M, Cameron, B. Mlwin [computer program] version 3.00. Centre for Multilevel Modelling, University of Bristol; 2017.
30. Chu H, Cole S. Bivariate meta-analysis of sensitivity and specificity with sparse data: a generalized linear mixed model approach. J Clin Epidemiol. 2006;59:1331–2.
31. Arends L, Hamza T, Van Houwelingen J, Heijenbrok-Kal M, Hunink M, Stijnen T. Bivariate random effects meta-analysis of ROC curves. Med Decis Mak. 2008;28:621–38.
32. Menke J. Bivariate random-effects meta-analysis of sensitivity and specificity with sas proc glimmix. Methods Inf Med. 2010;49:54–64.
33. Takwoingi Y, Deeks J. METADAS: an SAS macro for meta-analysis of diagnostic accuracy studies, version 1.3. Computer program; 2011.
34. Rabe-Hesketh S, Skrondal A, Pickles A. Generalized multilevel structural equation modeling. Psychometrika. 2004;69:167–90.
35. Harbord R, Whiting P. Metandi: meta-analysis of diagnostic accuracy using hierarchical logistic regression. Stata J. 2010;9:211–29.
36. Takwoingi Y. Meta-analysis of test accuracy studies in Stata: a bivariate model approach. Version 1.1. 2016. Available from http://methods.cochrane.org/sdt/. Accessed 29 June 2018.
37. Dwamena B. midas: Stata module for meta-analytical integration of diagnostic accuracy studies. 2007. Available from: http://econpapers.repec.org/software/bocbocode/s456880.htm. Accessed 29 June 2018.
38. Patrick D, Cheadle A, Thompson D, Diehr P, Koepsell T, Kinne S. The validity of self-reported smoking: a review and meta-analysis. Am J Public Health. 1994;84:1086–93.
39. Wickham H, Bryan J. readxl: read excel files. R package version 1.0.0. 2017. Available from https://CRAN.R-project.org/package=readxl. Accessed 29 June 2018.
40. Phillips B, Stewart L, Sutton A. 'cross hairs' plots for diagnostic meta-analysis. Res Synth Methods. 2010;1:308–15.
41. Vogelgesang F, Schlattmann P, Dewey M. The evaluation of bivariate mixed models in meta-analyses of diagnostic accuracy studies with SAS, Stata and R. Methods Inf Med. 2018;57:111–9.
42. Doebler P, Holling H, Böhning D. A mixed model approach to meta-analysis of diagnostic studies with binary test outcome. Psychol Methods. 2012;17:418–36.
43. Karrasch S, Linde K, Rücker G, Sommer H, Karsch-Völk M, Kleijnen J, et al. Accuracy of FENO for diagnosing asthma: a systematic review. Thorax. 2017;72:109–16.

44. Brown H, Prescott R. Applied mixed models in medicine. 3rd ed. Hoboken: John Wiley & Sons; 2015.
45. Demidenko E. Mixed models: theory and applications. Hoboken: John Wiley & Sons; 2013.
46. Chu H, Nie L, Cole S, Poole C. Meta-analysis of diagnostic accuracy studies accounting for disease prevalence: alternative parameterizations and model selection. Stat Med. 2009;28:2384–99.
47. Hoyer A, Kuss O. Meta-analysis of diagnostic tests accounting for disease prevalence: a new model using trivariate copulas. Stat Med. 2015;34:1912–24.
48. Nikoloulopoulos A. A vine copula mixed effect model for trivariate meta-analysis of diagnostic test accuracy studies accounting for disease prevalence. Stat Methods Med Res. 2017;26:2270–86.
49. Bates D, Mächler M, Bolker B, Walker S. Fitting linear mixed-effects models using lme4. J Stat Softw. 2015;67:1–48.
50. Moses L, Shapiro D, Littenberg B. Combining independent studies of a diagnostic test into a summary ROC curve: data-analytic approaches and some additional considerations. Stat Med. 1993;12:1293–316.
51. Holling H, Böhning W, Böhning D. Meta-analysis of diagnostic studies based upon SROC-curves: a mixed model approach using the Lehmann family. Stat Model. 2012;12:347–75.
52. Holling H, Böhning W, Böhning D. Likelihood-based clustering of meta-analytic SROC curves. Psychometrika. 2012;77:106–26.
53. Schlattmann P, Höhne J, Verba M. CAMAN: finite mixture models and meta-analysis tools–based on C.A.MAN. R package version 0.74. 2016. Available from https://CRAN.R-project.org/package=CAMAN. Accessed 29 June 2018.
54. Doebler P, Holling H. Meta-analysis of diagnostic accuracy and ROC curves with covariate adjusted semiparametric mixtures. Psychometrika. 2015;80:1084–104.
55. Charoensawat S, Böhning W, Böhning D, Holling H. Meta-analysis and meta-modelling for diagnostic problems. BMC Med Res Methodol. 2014;14:56.
56. Rücker G, Schumacher M. Summary ROC curve based on a weighted Youden index for selecting an optimal cut point in meta-analysis of diagnostic accuracy. Stat Med. 2010;29:3069–78.
57. Steinhauser S, Schumacher M, Rücker G. Modelling multiple thresholds in meta-analysis of diagnostic test accuracy studies. BMC Med Res Methodol. 2016;16:97.
58. Levis B, Benedetti A, Levis A, Ioannidis J, Shrier I, Cuijpers P, et al. Selective cutoff reporting in studies of diagnostic test accuracy: a comparison of conventional and individual-patient-data meta-analyses of the Patient Health Questionnaire-9 depression screening tool. Am J Epidemiol. 2017;185:954–64.
59. Dukic V, Gatsonis C. Meta-analysis of diagnostic test accuracy assessment studies with varying number of thresholds. Biometrics. 2003;59:936–46.
60. Hamza T, Arends L, van Houwelingen H, Stijnen T. Multivariate random effects meta-analysis of diagnostic tests with multiple thresholds. BMC Med Res Methodol. 2009;9:73.
61. Putter H, Fiocco M, Stijnen T. Meta-analysis of diagnostic test accuracy studies with multiple thresholds using survival methods. Biom J. 2010;52:95–110.
62. Simoneau G, Levis B, Cuijpers P, Ioannidis J, Patten S, Shrier I, et al. A comparison of bivariate, multivariate random-effects, and Poisson correlated gamma-frailty models to meta-analyze individual patient data of ordinal scale diagnostic tests. Biom J. 2017;59:1317.
63. Riley R, Ahmed I, Ensor J, Takwoingi Y, Kirkham A, Morris R, et al. Meta-analysis of test accuracy studies: an exploratory method for investigating the impact of missing thresholds. Syst Rev. 2015;4:12.
64. Hoyer A, Hirt S, Kuss O. Meta-analysis of full ROC curves using bivariate time-to-event models for interval-censored data. Res Synth Methods. 2018;9:62–72.
65. Martínez-Camblor P. Fully non-parametric receiver operating characteristic curve estimation for random-effects meta-analysis. Stat Methods Med Res. 2017;26:5–20.
66. Riley R, Takwoingi Y, Trikalinos T, Guha A, Biswas A, Ensor J, et al. Meta-analysis of test accuracy studies with multiple and missing thresholds: a multivariate-normal model. J Biomet Biostat. 2014;5:196.

67. Deeks J, Wisniewski S, Davenport C. Chapter 4: guide to the contents of a Cochrane Diagnostic Test Accuracy Protocol. In: Deeks J, Bossuyt P, Gatsonis C, editors Cochrane handbook for systematic reviews of diagnostic test accuracy version 1.0.0. 2013. Available from http://srdta.cochrane.org/. Accessed 29 June 2018.
68. Meyer P, Frings L, Rücker G, Hellwig S. 18F-FDG PET in parkinsonism: differential diagnosis and cognitive impairment in Parkinson's disease. J Nucl Med. 2017;58:1888.
69. Schlattmann P, Verba M, Dewey M, Walther M. Mixture models in diagnostic meta-analyses—clustering summary receiver operating characteristic curves accounted for heterogeneity and correlation. J Clin Epidemiol. 2015;68:61–72.

Network Meta-Analysis of Diagnostic Test Accuracy Studies

13

Gerta Rücker

13.1 Introduction

In this chapter, we consider the situation that a number of diagnostic accuracy studies evaluated multiple (i.e., two or more) diagnostic tests for a given medical condition, where different studies may have evaluated/compared different tests. Network meta-analysis of diagnostic test accuracy studies aims at comparing all these tests in a meta-analysis. To introduce network meta-analysis of diagnostic test accuracy studies, in Sect. 13.1.1 we first address network meta-analysis of interventional studies, which is a more familiar and well-developed topic. We then recapitulate meta-analysis of diagnostic test accuracy studies, already introduced in Chap. 10 of this book, and ask how this may be extended to network meta-analysis in Sect. 13.1.2. As we will see and extend in Sect. 13.2, there is an important difference between both areas of application, which requires the development of special methodology. In Sect 13.3, we will briefly comment on some common, but less appropriate approaches. A number of recently published advanced methods will be treated in more detail in Sect. 13.4. The chapter ends with a discussion in Sect. 13.5.

13.1.1 Network Meta-Analysis

Network meta-analysis (NMA) is an extension of pairwise meta-analysis, mainly applied to compare interventions in healthcare [1]. A question naturally leading to NMA of interventions is: "Which of a number of available interventions (i.e., drugs, surgical procedures, or psychological interventions) is the best for patients with the

G. Rücker
Institute of Medical Biometry and Statistics, Faculty of Medicine,
Medical Center—University of Freiburg, Freiburg, Germany
e-mail: ruecker@imbi.uni-freiburg.de

G. Biondi-Zoccai (ed.), *Diagnostic Meta-Analysis*,
https://doi.org/10.1007/978-3-319-78966-8_13

given medical condition?" To answer this question, one usually conducts a comprehensive literature search to look for existing comparisons (studies) among eligible treatments for the condition at hand. In most applications, NMA is based on randomized studies comparing two or (often) more interventions for the same medical condition. If there are at least three interventions (treatments), these build a network where the nodes are the treatments and connections between nodes represent direct comparisons between treatments that were directly compared in studies. Usually, the network is not complete, as in most cases not all possible comparisons have been investigated in a study. For those treatments that have not been directly compared in a study, we must rely on indirect evidence from the network. As an example, in Fig. 13.1 we present a network of antidepressants analyzed by Cipriani et al. [2]. Here we see, e.g., that there was no study directly comparing mirtazapine and reboxetine.

To combine direct and indirect evidence, it is assumed that the studies are independent, that the interventions groups within each study are independent, that missing comparisons are missing at random, and that the patient populations of different studies are comparable. Further, if multi-arm studies are included, this must be adjusted for. The simplest models also assume that the underlying effects are consistent, and differences between them are only due to random error. For estimation, Bayesian or frequentist methods (weighted least squares regression) can be applied

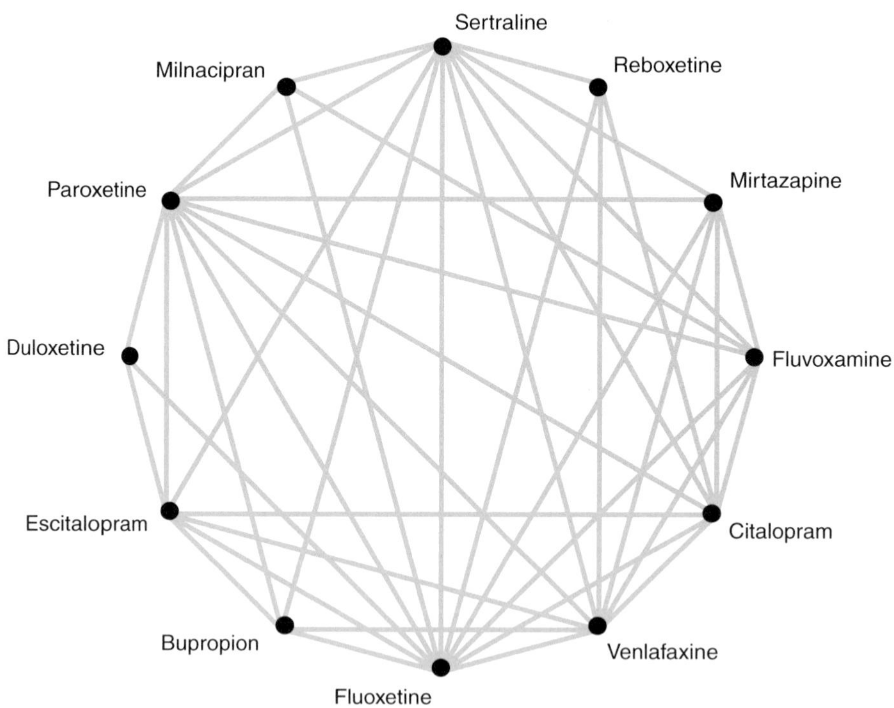

Fig. 13.1 A network of interventions [2]

while adjusting for multi-arm studies. Like in pairwise meta-analysis, fixed and random effects models may be used, and heterogeneity should be explored. For further reading, see [3] or the book [4].

13.1.2 Diagnostic Test Accuracy Studies

As described in Chaps. 10 and 11, the research question of standard meta-analysis of diagnostic test accuracy (DTA) studies is the same as that of a DTA study: to evaluate the diagnostic accuracy of a (single) diagnostic test, where we assume the existence of a reference standard ("gold standard"). An overview of existing methods for meta-analysis of diagnostic accuracy studies is given in [5]. These can be generalized in several respects. Here, we focus on the generalization to multiple tests.

The aim of a study may be to compare the accuracy of two or more diagnostic tests for the same medical condition, with or without an existing gold standard. Note that there is an important difference between interventional and diagnostic studies: Whereas in interventional research different treatments are usually compared between different groups of patients (preferably allocated in a randomized manner), in diagnostic research tests usually are evaluated in the same individuals, with or without the target condition. In interventional research, intraindividual treatment comparisons (e.g., crossover studies) are an exception rather than a rule. This means that in diagnostic research we have correlated observations, in contrast to most interventional studies, where the treatment arms are independent. It follows that methods of NMA of interventions cannot be readily translated to NMA of DTA studies.

13.2 Network Meta-Analysis: Differences Between Diagnostic Tests and Interventions

Thinking of NMA of DTA studies leads to two possible perspectives, a diagnostic perspective and a prognostic perspective. Here, we present an overview over possible connections between NMA and meta-analysis of DTA studies and potential generalizations of standard methodology.

13.2.1 Diagnostic Perspective: NMA of DTA Studies as Pairwise Multivariate Meta-Analysis

As noted in the preceding section, when evaluating/comparing $K \geq 1$ diagnostic tests, this means that each study in a meta-analysis has performed a subset (i.e., one or more) of these tests, usually in the same groups of individuals with or without the target condition. The result of each test (positive or negative) is a binary outcome. Thus, in total we consider a multi($2K$)variate outcome with mostly unknown correlation structure. In

Table 13.1 Diagnostic perspective: pairwise meta-analysis of interventions with a binary outcome vs meta-analysis of DTA studies

		Interventions	Diagnostic tests
	Aim	Compare two treatments	Discriminate two groups
Pairwise meta-analysis	Groups	Two interventions	With/without target condition
	Outcome	Event yes/no	Test positive/negative
	Proportions	r_1, r_0	Sens, 1 − Spec
	Effect measures	$\mathrm{RD} = r_1 - r_0$	$J = \mathrm{Sens} + \mathrm{Spec} - 1$
		$\mathrm{OR} = \dfrac{r_1(1-r_0)}{r_0(1-r_1)}$	$\mathrm{DOR} = \dfrac{\mathrm{Sens}^*\mathrm{Spec}}{(1-\mathrm{Sens})(1-\mathrm{Spec})}$
	Modeling	Univariate model, contrast-based	Bivariate model, arm-based
Multivariate pairwise meta-analysis	Groups	Two interventions	With/without target condition
	Outcome	$K \geq 2$ outcomes	$K \geq 2$ tests
	Measures	Pairs of proportions	Pairs of accuracy measures
		$(r_{1k}, r_{0k}),\ \ k = 1, \ldots, K$	$(\mathrm{Sens}_k, 1 - \mathrm{Spec}_k)$, $k = 1, \ldots, K$
	Effect measures	$\mathrm{RD}_k,\ \ k = 1, \ldots, K$	$J_k,\ \ k = 1, \ldots, K$
		$\mathrm{OR}_k,\ \ k = 1, \ldots, K$	$\mathrm{DOR}_k,\ \ k = 1, \ldots, K$
	Modeling	Multi(K)variate model	Multi($2K$)variate model

RD risk difference, *OR* odds ratio, *DOR* diagnostic odds ratio, *J* Youden index

Chap. 10, the special case of $K = 1$ was considered, which led to the bivariate model ($2K = 2$), as we consider two groups of individuals [6, 7]. More generally, comparing $K \geq 2$ tests corresponds to a ($2K$)variate or a pairwise multivariate meta-analysis. Table 13.1 illustrates this perspective. While the left column represents the standard situation in meta-analysis of interventions with a binary outcome, the right column translates this to meta-analysis of DTA studies. The upper part of the table represents the case of one (binary) outcome (in the diagnostic situation, this is a test). We note that in meta-analysis of interventions, contrast-based models are common. For a binary outcome, these models are based on effect measures such as the relative risk (RR), the odds ratio (OR), or the risk difference (RD). They are less common and also not recommended in the diagnostic setting. Here, we are interested in estimating both sensitivity and specificity; hence the bivariate model is preferred. The bottom part of Table 13.1 shows the generalization to a multivariate outcome, i.e., two or more tests. In the diagnostic context, this leads to a multi($2K$)variate outcome.

13.2.2 Prognostic Perspective: NMA of DTA Studies as NMA of Diagnostic Odds Ratios

An alternative perspective is to consider the diagnostic tests as $K \geq 2$ test covariates to predict the true status of an individual as a binary outcome (with/without the target condition, according to the reference standard). Within a study, this could be

Table 13.2 Prognostic perspective: NMA of DTA studies as NMA of diagnostic odds ratios

		Interventions	Diagnostic tests
	Aim	Compare treatments	Compare tests
Pairwise meta-analysis	Groups	Two interventions	Test positive/negative
	Outcome	Event yes/no	With/without target condition
	Proportions	r_1	PPV
		r_0	1 − NPV
	Effect measures	RD = $r_1 - r_0$	J^* = PPV + NPV − 1
		$\text{OR} = \frac{r_1(1-r_0)}{r_0(1-r_1)}$	$\text{DOR} = \frac{\text{Sens}^*\text{Spec}}{(1-\text{Sens})(1-\text{Spec})}$
	Modeling	Univariate model, contrast-based,	Bivariate model, arm-based,
		models binary outcome	models truth (gold standard)
Network meta-analysis	Groups	$K \geq 2$ interventions	$K \geq 2$ diagnostic tests
	Outcome	Event yes/no	With/without target condition
	Proportions	$\begin{pmatrix} r_{11} & r_{10} \\ \vdots & \vdots \\ r_{K1} & r_{K0} \end{pmatrix}$	
	Modeling	Multivariate model, contrast-based models binary outcome	Multivariate model Models truth (gold standard), given results of K diagnostic tests

RD risk difference, *OR* odds ratio, *DOR* diagnostic odds ratio, *PPV* positive predictive value, *NPV* negative predictive value

analyzed using logistic regression. For each test investigated in a study, this provides a regression coefficient that estimates the test's study-specific log diagnostic odds ratio (logDOR). If the reference standard is identical across studies, logDORs from different tests may be compared in a NMA. This perspective is illustrated in Table 13.2. Again, the left-hand side of the table refers to meta-analysis of interventions, whereas the right-hand side refers to the diagnostic setting. We note that in this table group and outcome have changed their role, corresponding to the change of perspective: from modeling the test result (as in Table 13.1) to predicting the true status of the individual, based on the test(s). The bottom row refers to the situation with more than two interventions (left) or tests (right), respectively. If the test populations for each test were independent in all studies that investigated the test, this could be analyzed like NMA of interventions. However, this situation does not seem to occur frequently in practice, as tests, in contrast to treatments, are mostly compared intraindividually. An exception is the meta-analysis by Patrick et al. (1994) [8] who compared self-administered and interviewer-administered questionnaires for smoking behavior, where each primary study used only one kind of questionnaire.

In the remainder of this chapter, we will leave the prognostic perspective and focus on the diagnostic perspective, as described in Sect. 13.2.1, where we aim to model sensitivity and specificity as distinct outcomes for each test.

13.3 Approaches for Comparing Multiple Diagnostic Tests

In this section we briefly mention possible approaches for comparing multiple diagnostic tests that take the diagnostic perspective in the sense of Sect. 13.2.1. The starting point is the bivariate model [6, 7].

13.3.1 Separate Meta-Analyses

Let us consider the case of n studies, each of which compared a subset of K diagnostic tests for the same target condition. Instead of considering a complex multi($2K$) variate model (Table 13.1, bottom right), often K separate bivariate models are analyzed. Without doubt, this is the easiest way of analyzing these data. However, the between-test correlations within individuals in the same study are ignored; in fact they are often not reported in primary studies. For example, Roberts et al. separately investigated three natriuretic peptides (plasma B-type natriuretic peptide, NTproBNP, and MRproANP) for diagnosis of heart failure [9].

13.3.1.1 Special Case: Separate Meta-Analyses for Multiple Thresholds

The review by Roberts et al. [9] is also a good example for a situation reviewers are often confronted with when extracting data for meta-analysis of a single diagnostic test: the primary studies reported various sets of different multiple thresholds for each of the peptides. Often, like here, a diagnostic test is based on a biomarker, or a questionnaire, or a psychological or other score. In this case, to define a test, a threshold must be selected which separates the population with the target condition ("diseased") from the population without the target condition ("non-diseased"). Then sensitivity and specificity depend on the threshold that is chosen to decide whether the test is positive or negative. If large values suggest that the individual has the target condition, specificity increases and sensitivity decreases with increasing threshold. Different studies may have selected different thresholds or may present results based on several thresholds. One motivation is to use different thresholds for "ruling out" and "ruling in" the target condition.

The Cochrane Handbook for DTA Reviews recommends conducting separate meta-analyses (based on the bivariate model) for each threshold (or a subset of thresholds) found in the primary studies [10]. The results may be put together to obtain a pooled sensitivity/specificity for each threshold or to compare sensitivity and specificity between tests based on different thresholds. Again, this method does not account for the intraindividual correlation that arises because part of the data do not only come from the same individuals but also from the same measurements.

This has motivated researchers to develop more advanced methods that account for this complex correlation structure [11–18].

13.3.2 Meta-Regression with Type of Test as a Covariate

Software implementations of the standard bivariate model allow incorporating covariates. Therefore one way to analyze data from multiple tests is to include the type of test as a categorical covariate into the bivariate model. This analysis is appropriate if the type of test is a study-level covariate, i.e., each study uses only one of a number of tests, as in the abovementioned meta-analysis of smoking questionnaires [8, 19]. It would be also suitable if the individuals undergoing the different tests were independent subgroups within each study and were separately reported. In most cases, however, all individuals in a study are subject to all tests compared in that study, and their results are correlated. Then the type of test is not a study-level, not even an individual-level covariate, but a repeated measurement at the individual level, and meta-regression is not applicable.

13.3.3 Multivariate Meta-Analysis: Contrast-Based vs Arm-Based Approach

The appropriate method to analyze multiple tests DTA data is multivariate meta-analysis, as indicated in Table 13.1. Before going into details of existing approaches, we want to mention a certain consequence of the difference between (network) meta-analysis of interventions and meta-analysis of DTA tests. In meta-analysis of interventions, mostly based on randomized controlled trials, traditionally a contrast-based approach has been used. This means, contrasts (i.e., within-study treatment effect differences) are calculated between each pair of treatments within each study. These form, together with their standard errors, the basis for modeling. This has led to some debate [20, 21].

Contrary to meta-analysis of interventions, in standard meta-analysis of DTA studies, simple contrast-based approaches are thought insufficient by most researchers due to the bivariate character of the outcome (sensitivity and specificity). Nevertheless, they were occasionally proposed, for example, using the diagnostic odds ratio [22] or a proportional hazards measure [23]. One could also think of the Youden index or the area under the curve (AUC) as a univariate outcome.

If DTA studies have investigated more than one test, the question of a contrast-based approach again comes up, but in a different sense. In the context of comparing multiple tests, we may look at differences of (transformed) sensitivities/specificities between different tests within a study in the same individuals, rather than contrasts between treatment groups or groups by health status (such as the diagnostic odds ratio). To be appropriate, contrast-based approaches have to model contrasts of sensitivities and specificities as bivariate outcomes. Clearly, this leads to a different and more complicated data structure than we have in NMA of interventions. We come back to this issue in Sects. 13.4.3 and 13.4.6.

13.4 Existing Approaches to Meta-Analysis of Multiple DTA Studies

In this section we describe a number of existing approaches to NMA of diagnostic accuracy studies. After having a look into the Cochrane Handbook for DTA Reviews [10], we discuss the models proposed by Trikalinos et al. (2014), Menten and Lesaffre (2015), Dimou et al. (2016), Hoyer and Kuss (2016), and Nyaga et al. (2016) [5, 24–28].

13.4.1 The Cochrane Handbook for DTA Reviews

In the Cochrane Handbook for DTA Reviews ([10], Section 10.5.4), two settings for comparing the diagnostic accuracy of two tests are discussed.

13.4.1.1 Comparing Two Tests Between Studies

If most studies evaluate only one of the tests of interest, the data from both tests can be seen as independent, and the type of test is a study-level covariate as described in Sect. 13.3.2 above. In case of tests based on a biomarker, this approach is recommended only if all studies used similar thresholds. It is also important to adjust for further important confounders because studies evaluating different tests are expected to differ also in their spectrum of patients and other covariates.

13.4.1.2 Comparing Two Tests Within Studies

Studies comparing two tests could either apply both tests to each individual or randomize each individual to one of the tests, in both cases using a common reference test for all individuals. The data must be analyzed within study, using a binary covariate for the type of test. The authors of the Cochrane Handbook mention that there are often only two 2 × 2 tables given, without information on paired results at the individual patient level. Then an approach using the two tables effectively assumes a randomized design, which they say represents a conservative approach. They do not go into detail for models that truly account for tests compared at the individual level but mention that such models would require a cross classification of test results within both the diseased and non-diseased groups for all available studies. Such approaches exist, as we will see in Sects. 13.4.2 and 13.4.4.

13.4.2 The Approach by Trikalinos et al.

Trikalinos et al. (2014) were among the first authors who pointed to the problem that conducting separate meta-analyses for different tests is inappropriate if the tests were applied to the same individuals [28]. They investigated models for the joint meta-analysis of studies comparing multiple index tests on the same participants in paired designs in a Bayesian setting. In their paper, they stepwise generalized the model, starting from the standard bivariate model ("the case of a single test").

13.4.2.1 The Case of Two Tests

The combination of two tests in a single combination leads to four possible combinations of positive and negative results with different probabilities for individuals with or without the target condition, that is, the eight combinations presented as probabilities in ([28], Table 5). The authors consider for each study $i = 1, \ldots, n$ and each test $k = 1, 2$ the logit-transformed true-positive rate η_{ik} (i.e., η_{i1} and η_{i2}), the logit-transformed false-positive rate ξ_{ik} (ξ_{i1} and ξ_{i2}), the "joint true-positive rate" η_i^*, and the "joint false-positive rate" ξ_i^*, both corresponding to the proportion of results that are positive for both tests. For these 6 parameters per study, the authors discuss 2 variance-covariance matrices, an unstructured version with 6*7/2 = 21 parameters and, setting variances and correlations of both tests equal, a structured version with 12 parameters. Generalizing the binomial within-study model used in the standard case to a multinomial model, they use Bayesian methods to estimate the parameters.

13.4.2.2 The Case of Three or More Tests

Trikalinos et al. [28] only very briefly discuss that their approach may be generalized to the case of more than two tests but mention that their parameterization leads to a very large number of parameters and problems with estimation.

13.4.3 The Approach by Menten and Lesaffre

Menten and Lesaffre (2015) present a general framework for comparative meta-analysis of diagnostic studies in a Bayesian setting [25]. They list five models ([25], Table 13.2) (three assuming a perfect reference standard, two assuming an imperfect reference standard) and explain ways of estimation, partly also including indirect comparisons and based on methods from NMA. In case of an imperfect reference standard (models 4 and 5), they consider latent class models. All models have in common that they (1) consider the (standard) case of one pair of sensitivity and specificity per test and study, (2) model transformed (e.g., logit) sensitivity and specificity (models 1 and 4) or differences (contrasts) of them between different tests (models 2, 3, and 5), and (3) use Markov chain Monte Carlo (MCMC) methods for estimation. We briefly discuss the five models.

13.4.3.1 Model 1: Standard Bivariate Model

Model 1 is the standard bivariate model. Results for each test are pooled separately across all studies that used the test. The within-study correlation between tests is ignored. As the authors remark [25], "the results may be biased by study characteristics."

13.4.3.2 Model 2: Meta-Analysis Based on Direct Comparisons

Like the standard bivariate model, model 2 is a two-level model. It is limited to two tests and uses only studies that compared the tests directly. The transformed (e.g., logit-transformed) sensitivities and specificities are modeled under the assumption of study-specific differences between them. In the second stage, these differences are modeled under the assumption that they follow a bivariate normal distribution. It is not distinguished between tests that were applied to the same individuals and tests that were randomized between individuals in the same study.

13.4.3.3 Model 3: Meta-Analysis Based on Direct and Indirect Comparisons

Models 3–5 are hierarchical models to compare $K \geq 2$ tests. Model 3 (also described in [26]) is a generalization of model 2 and models the contrasts between transformed sensitivities and specificities, using one test as a baseline. Thus model 3 allows modeling indirect comparisons between tests that were not directly compared in a study via common comparators. However, as the authors note, specification and estimation of the variance-covariance matrix are complicated.

13.4.3.4 Models 4 and 5

Models 4 and 5 are latent class models that can be applied if no perfect reference standard is available. While model 4 ignores the correlation between tests from the same study, model 5, like model 3, is based on contrasts between tests.

13.4.4 The Approach by Dimou et al.

Like Trikalinos et al. (2014) [28], Dimou et al. (2016) focus on the case of two diagnostic tests [5]. The authors introduce their notation for the case of two tests ([5], Table I), leading to eight possible combinations as in ([28], Table 5). The observed numbers are then presented in a second table ([5], Table II) as marginal sums of the numbers in the first table ([5], Table I). From these, for each study i the estimated study-specific logit-transformed true-positive rates TPR and false-positive rates FPR for test 1 (denoted $\hat{y}_{1i}, \hat{y}_{2i}$) and test 2 $\left(\hat{y}_{3i}, \hat{y}_{4i}\right)$ and their estimated variances are derived. The parameters $(\beta_1, \beta_2, \beta_3, \beta_4)$ correspond to the parameters $(\eta_1, \xi_1, \eta_2, \xi_2)$ introduced in [28]. In generalization of the standard bivariate model, the vector $\left(\hat{y}_{1\cdot}, \hat{y}_{2\cdot}, \hat{y}_{3\cdot}, \hat{y}_{4\cdot}\right)^T$ is modeled using a multivariate normal distribution with a study-specific mean vector and a within-study covariance matrix that is observable. The between-study model is of the same but unstructured type.

In contrast to Trikalinos et al. [28], who modeled the “joint true-positive rate” and the “joint false-positive rate” based on the observations (see Sect. 13.4.2), Dimou et al. use this information (from their Table I) to inform the within-study covariance matrix, which thus is assumed as known and fixed. As they state ([5], p. 3519), “the key point of this method is that the within-studies covariances can be calculated via a closed form expression.” With respect to three or more diagnostic tests, they briefly note “A direct extension of the method for more than two diagnostic tests is straightforward” ([5], p. 3513); however, they do not make explicit how to calculate the multiple correlations in the general case.

In contrast to other approaches discussed here, the model by Dimou et al. can be fitted by standard frequentist software used for multivariate meta-analysis. It also allows determining further standard measures such as the diagnostic odds ratio, a summary receiver operating characteristic (SROC) curve and the area under the curve (AUC).

13.4.5 The Approach by Hoyer and Kuss

Hoyer and Kuss (2016) propose, in generalization of the bivariate model, a quadrivariate logistic regression model for comparing two index tests with a common reference standard within studies [24]. At the study level, they model the number of true-positives and true-negatives of test k $(k = 1, 2)$ within study i $(i = 1, \ldots, n)$ following binomial distributions, given the study-specific true sensitivities and specificities for both tests. At the meta-analysis level, the mean parameters are μ_1, μ_2 (logit sensitivities of tests 1 and 2) and ν_1, ν_2 (logit specificities of tests 1 and 2), with the random study effects modeled by a quadrivariate normal distribution with an unstructured variance-covariance matrix. Estimation is possible using standard software for generalized linear mixed models. Again, the parameters are closely related to those in the approaches by Trikalinos et al. [28] and Dimou et al. [5], with the only difference that not the false-positives, but specificities are modeled. Moreover, the analysis is based on two 2 × 2 tables per study and thus (as the authors admit) does not account for potential within-individual correlation. The authors also present a generalization accounting for multiple thresholds. In addition, they give a concise overview over existing methods.

13.4.6 Two Approaches by Nyaga et al.

Nyaga et al. (2016) published two papers, beginning with a discussion of the contrast-based versus the arm-based approach [26], arguing that the contrast-based models lead to problems with model identifiability and variance estimation. Therefore they suggest arm-based approaches.

13.4.6.1 Two-Stage Model Based on Logit Transformation

The arm-based two-stage Bayesian approach in the first paper is based on the logit-transformed sensitivities and specificities, as in the standard bivariate model. The model is described as follows. Denote the groups $j = 0, 1$ where 0 means without the target condition ("without disease") and 1 means with the target condition ("diseased"). Further, let us have $i = 1, \ldots, n$ studies, each comparing a subset of K diagnostic tests for the target condition ($k = 1, \ldots, K$). Let π_{ijk} be the true probability of a correct result (i.e., sensitivity or specificity) for an individual in group j of study i with respect to test k. Then logit(π_{ijk}) is modeled as

$$\text{logit}\left(\pi_{ijk}\right) = \mu_{jk} + \eta_{ij} + \delta_{ijk}$$

where μ_{jk} is the true mean logit-transformed sensitivity ($j = 1$) or specificity ($j = 0$) of test k over all studies, $\eta_{ij}(j = 0, 1)$ are group-specific random study effects, and δ_{ijk} are random errors. For the study effects we assume

$$\begin{pmatrix} \eta_{i1} \\ \eta_{i0} \end{pmatrix} \sim N\left(\begin{pmatrix} 0 \\ 0 \end{pmatrix}, \begin{pmatrix} \sigma_1^2 & \rho\sigma_1\sigma_0 \\ \rho\sigma_1\sigma_0 & \sigma_0^2 \end{pmatrix}\right)$$

with variances σ_1, σ_0 and across-study correlation ρ. The random errors δ_{ijk} are assumed to be normally distributed with mean 0 and conditionally independent, given a study i, with variances $(\tau_{j1}, \ldots, \tau_{jK})$ that are constant across studies, but depending on the test and the group. The model is enriched with covariate information. Estimation of marginal sensitivity and specificity uses Bayesian methods.

13.4.6.2 Beta-Binomial Model

In their second paper, Nyaga et al. consider a one-stage approach based on a copula model [27]. The bivariate joint distribution of sensitivity and specificity is modeled using the marginal distributions with a so-called copula that describes the dependence between both. Instead of modeling the latent sensitivities and specificities in the studies via the logit transformation and assuming normal distribution, the sensitivities and specificities were directly modeled using a beta-binomial model [29]. The beta distribution family consists of an infinite number of two-parameter distributions defined on the interval [0,1]. The special parameterization in the paper is very flexible and captures the mean sensitivity and specificity for each of K tests, their association, and two sources of overdispersion due to repeated tests in a study. Estimation is again based on Bayesian methods.

13.4.7 Multivariate Meta-Analysis

As we have seen, (network) meta-analysis of diagnostic accuracy data is a special case of multivariate meta-analysis. Therefore it would at first seem obvious to look at existing approaches to multivariate NMA that were not particularly designed for diagnostic accuracy data, however may be applied to these.

There are some approaches to network meta-analysis of multiple correlated outcomes. Mavridis and Salanti (2013) mentioned meta-analysis of DTA studies in the context of multivariate meta-analysis but only described the standard bivariate model [30]. Riley et al. (2014) used multivariate random effects meta-analysis models to treat multiple prognostic effect estimates due to multiple methods of measurement within the same study, taking the prognostic perspective (see Sect. 13.2.2) [17]. Achana et al. (2014) and Efthimiou and colleagues (2014, 2015) considered multiple outcomes in networks of interventions [31–33]. However, none of these papers addressed the special situation of a bivariate outcome (sensitivity/specificity) in a network of correlated tests.

13.4.8 Other Potential Research Questions

The standard bivariate model is designed for meta-analysis of studies that consider a single test. The methods discussed in this chapter generalize the bivariate model with respect to the number of diagnostic tests compared. Of course, there are other aspects that may be generalized.

First, already mentioned in Sect. 13.3.1.1, the index test may rely on a measurement and a threshold which separates the population with the target condition ("diseased") from the population without the target condition ("non-diseased").

Secondly, a single test may be developed for differentiating between more than two conditions, e.g., identifying different stages or subclassifications of a disease. For instance, Mitchell (2009) published a meta-analysis of the accuracy of the mini-mental state examination in the detection of dementia and mild cognitive impairment, compared to healthy persons [34]. For this setting, a (bivariate) standard network meta-analysis would be appropriate for comparing the test accuracy between the independent conditions.

Finally, at least theoretically, all these aspects could be combined to a very complex meta-analysis of multiple tests with multiple thresholds, applied in various studies to individuals with multiple different health conditions. A model perfectly suitable to evaluate such data would need individual patient data from all studies.

13.5 Discussion

While the standard bivariate model meta-analysis of DTA studies is appropriate to synthesize evidence on the accuracy of a single diagnostic test, in this chapter we collected approaches for generalizing the model to the case of multiple diagnostic tests.

For investigating possible designs and analysis strategies, both a diagnostic and a prognostic perspective are possible. We found arm-based and contrast-based approaches. Most approaches use Bayesian methodology and seem to be computationally demanding. Exceptions are the models by Dimou et al. (2016) and Kuss and Hoyer (2016) that can be fitted using standard frequentist software [5, 29]. As all approaches are quite novel, we expect that there will be more research in this field. Also, methodological reviews comparing different approaches in simulations have to be awaited before recommendations for their use in practice can be made.

Like this chapter, some of these approaches are titled "network meta-analysis of diagnostic accuracy tests." As we have seen, however, this may be misleading because of the difference between NMA of interventions and NMA of diagnostic tests: Interventions are usually compared between independent groups, while diagnostic tests are compared within the same individuals. Hence, networks of diagnostic tests have a structure quite different from networks of interventions, and the statistical analysis must account for this. We therefore would like to put it up for discussion whether the term "network meta-analysis" for meta-analysis of DTA studies is appropriate or should be avoided.

Key Messages

- For meta-analysis of DTA studies of a single test, the standard bivariate model is appropriate.
- Meta-analysis of DTA studies comparing multiple tests differs from network meta-analysis of interventions, as tests, unlike interventions, usually are compared within individuals.
- For comparing multiple diagnostic tests in a meta-analysis, methods of multivariate meta-analysis are needed.
- Existing approaches differ in their methods (arm-based vs contrast-based, frequentist vs Bayesian, specification of correlations).

Acknowledgments The author gratefully thanks Philipp Doebler, Paul-Christian Bürkner, and Martin Schumacher for valuable hints and comments.

References

1. Rücker G. Network meta-analysis. Wiley StatsRef: Statistics Reference Online; 2016. p. 1–8. http://onlinelibrary.wiley.com/doi/10.1002/9781118445112.stat07909/abstract. Stat07909. Accessed 29 June 2018.
2. Cipriani A, Furukawa TA, Salanti G, Geddes J, Higgins J, Churchill R, Watanabe N, Nakagawa A, Omori I, McGuire H, Tansella M, Barbui C. Comparative efficacy and acceptability of 12 new-generation antidepressants: a multiple-treatments meta-analysis. Lancet. 2009;373:746–58.
3. Salanti G. Indirect and mixed-treatment comparison, network, or multiple-treatments meta-analysis: many names, many benefits, many concerns for the next generation evidence synthesis tool. Res Synth Methods. 2012;3:80–97.
4. Biondi-Zoccai G, editor. Network meta-analysis: evidence synthesis with mixed treatment comparison. Hauppauge: Nova Science Publishers Inc.; 2014.
5. Dimou NL, Adam M, Bagos PG. A multivariate method for meta-analysis and comparison of diagnostic tests. Stat Med. 2016;35:3509–23.
6. Chu H, Cole SR. Bivariate meta-analysis of sensitivity and specificity with sparse data: a generalized linear mixed approach. J Clin Epidemiol. 2006;59:1331–3.
7. Reitsma J, Glas A, Rutjes A, Scholten R, Bossuyt P, Zwinderman A. Bivariate analysis of sensitivity and specificity produces informative summary measures in diagnostic reviews. J Clin Epidemiol. 2005;58:982–90.
8. Patrick D, Cheadle A, Thompson D, Diehr P, Koepsell T, Kinne S. The validity of self-reported smoking: a review and meta-analysis. Am J Public Health. 1994;84:1086–93.
9. Roberts E, Ludman A, Dworzynski K, Al-Mohammad A, Cowie M, McMurray J, Mant J, On behalf of the NICE Guideline Development Group for Acute Heart Failure. The diagnostic accuracy of the natriuretic peptides in heart failure: systematic review and diagnostic meta-analysis in the acute care setting. BMJ. 2015;350:h910.
10. Cochrane Methods Screening and Diagnostic Tests: Handbook for DTA Reviews; 2016. http://methods.cochrane.org/sdt/handbook-dta-reviews. Accessed 29 June 2018.
11. Dukic V, Gatsonis C. Meta-analysis of diagnostic test accuracy assessment studies with varying number of thresholds. Biometrics. 2003;59:936–46.
12. Hamza TH, Arends LR, van Houwelingen HC, Stijnen T. Multivariate random effects meta-analysis of diagnostic tests with multiple thresholds. BMC Med Res Methodol. 2009;9:73.

13. Putter H, Fiocco M, Stijnen T. Meta-analysis of diagnostic test accuracy studies with multiple thresholds using survival methods. Biom J. 2010;52:95–110.
14. Martínez-Camblor P. Fully non-parametric receiver operating characteristic curve estimation for random-effects meta-analysis. Stat Methods Med Res. 2014;26:5.
15. Riley RD, Takwoingi Y, Trikalinos T, Guha A, Biswas A, Ensor J, Morris RK, Deeks JJ. Meta-analysis of test accuracy studies with multiple and missing thresholds: a multivariate-normal model. J Biomet Biostat. 2014;5:196.
16. Riley RD, Ahmed I, Ensor J, Takwoingi Y, Kirkham A, Morris RK, Noordzij JP, Deeks JJ. Meta-analysis of test accuracy studies: an exploratory method for investigating the impact of missing thresholds. Syst Rev. 2015;4:12.
17. Riley RD, Elia EG, Malin G, Hemming K, Price MP. Multivariate meta-analysis of prognostic factor studies with multiple cut-points and/or methods of measurement. Stat Med. 2015;34:2481–96.
18. Steinhauser S, Schumacher M, Rücker G. Modelling multiple thresholds in meta-analysis of diagnostic test accuracy studies. BMC Med Res Methodol. 2016;16:97.
19. Doebler P, Holling H, Böhning D. A mixed model approach to meta-analysis of diagnostic studies with binary test outcome. Psychol Methods. 2012;17:418–36.
20. Dias S, Ades AE. Absolute or relative effects? Arm-based synthesis of trial data. Res Synth Methods. 2016;7:23–8.
21. Hawkins N, Scott D, Woods B. 'arm-based' parameterization for network meta-analysis. Res Synth Methods. 2016;7:306–13.
22. Glas AS, Lijmer J, Prins M, Bonsel G, Bossuyt PM. The diagnostic odds ratio: a single indicator of test performance. J Clin Epidemiol. 2003;56:1129–35.
23. Charoensawat S, Böhning W, Böhning D, Holling H. Meta-analysis and meta-modelling for diagnostic problems. BMC Med Res Methodol. 2014;14:56.
24. Hoyer A, Kuss O. Meta-analysis for the comparison of two diagnostic tests to a common gold standard: a generalized linear mixed model approach. Stat Methods Med Res. 2018;27:1410–21.
25. Menten J, Lesaffre E. A general framework for comparative Bayesian meta-analysis of diagnostic studies. BMC Med Res Methodol. 2015;15:70.
26. Nyaga VN, Aerts M, Arbyn M. ANOVA model for network meta-analysis of diagnostic test accuracy data. Stat Methods Med Res. 2018;27:1766–84.
27. Nyaga VN, Arbyn M, Aerts M. Beta-binomial analysis of variance model for network meta-analysis of diagnostic test accuracy data. Stat Methods Med Res. 2016. https://doi.org/10.1177/0962280216682532. Accessed 29 June 2018.
28. Trikalinos TA, Hoaglin DC, Small KM, Terrin N, Schmid C. Methods for the joint meta-analysis of multiple tests. Res Synth Methods. 2014;5:294–312.
29. Kuss O, Hoyer A, Solms A. Meta-analysis for diagnostic accuracy studies: a new statistical model using beta-binomial distributions and bivariate copulas. Stat Med. 2013;33:17.
30. Mavridis D, Salanti G. A practical introduction to multivariate meta-analysis. Stat Methods Med Res. 2013;22:133–58.
31. Achana FA, Cooper NJ, Bujkiewicz S, Hubbard SJ, Kendrick D, Jones DR, Sutton AJ. Network meta-analysis of multiple outcome measures accounting for borrowing of information across outcomes. BMC Med Res Methodol. 2014;14:92.
32. Efthimiou O, Mavridis D, Cipriani A, Leucht S, Bagos P, Salanti G. An approach for modelling multiple correlated outcomes in a network of interventions using odds ratios. Stat Med. 2014;33:2275–87.
33. Efthimiou O, Mavridis D, Riley RD, Cipriani A, Salanti G. Joint synthesis of multiple correlated outcomes in networks of interventions. Biostatistics. 2015;16:84–97.
34. Mitchell A. A meta-analysis of the accuracy of the mini-mental state examination in the detection of dementia and mild cognitive impairment. J Psychiatr Res. 2009;43:411–31.

Transition to Intervention Meta-Analysis 14

Umberto Benedetto and Colin Ng

14.1 Introduction

Medical treatment for diseases ("intervention") has been developing faster than ever in the last few decades. New drugs are tested and approved every day for many diseases that were previously thought incurable. Cancer research is an example of an especially rapidly advancing field—antibody therapies are being developed to control both solid-organ and blood tumors [1]. New procedures and surgical techniques are being developed, fueled by the exchange of ideas at nowadays popular conferences and meetings. A major focus today is the use of minimally invasive techniques to minimize the risks of open surgery such as wound infection and bleeding and to enable faster recovery times [2].

As such, the onus is on clinicians to be up to date with the latest evidence so that their patients receive fair and appropriate treatment. As our reader might recall from earlier chapters, a meta-analysis of randomized controlled trials provides for top quality evidence, and indeed, these are the studies experts look for when designing clinical practice guidelines at major conferences and meetings of societies. Even our patients are getting up to date with the advances in medical care as the internet provides ample information to anyone who is keen to look. The rise in complexity of medicolegal cases means that doctors cannot be too careful when counseling a patient of the risks and benefits of treatment before starting it [3]. A good understanding of how outcomes are reported and analyzed enables the clinician to counsel patients about an intervention more accurately.

As soon as a new intervention is developed for a medical condition, its creators are quick to scientifically test it, performing studies to show efficacy as well as

U. Benedetto (✉)
Bristol Heart Institute, University of Bristol, Bristol, UK

C. Ng
Singapore General Hospital, Singapore, Singapore

G. Biondi-Zoccai (ed.), *Diagnostic Meta-Analysis*,
https://doi.org/10.1007/978-3-319-78966-8_14

safety. A major treatment is typically tested more than once, and a meta-analysis is thereby useful in statistically combining the results of these studies, synthesizing a "big picture" out of the many trials.

14.2 Trials and Their Outcomes

For an intervention to be considered useful in the treatment of a medical condition, it has to show not only effectiveness in treating or curing the disease but also safety. The gold standard for investigating such intervention is the conduct of a randomized controlled trial (RCT). In such a study, participants are randomly assigned into groups—at least one with the new or proposed treatment that is being studied and at least one to be the control group. The control need not be a "no-treatment" or placebo group; it can be the previous gold standard in the treatment of the particular disease. There can be more than one treatment group in the trial, for example, when testing different doses of a particular drug.

There are other study designs, such as retrospective or non-randomized trials. However, the use of data from such studies weakens the quality of the evidence, as there are inherent limitations such as selection bias in a retrospective cohort study [4]. As such, it is recommended that a meta-analysis should only include randomized trials.

One emerging technique that is increasingly applied to intervention studies is the use of propensity score matching to create "matched pairs" of equal baseline characteristics (e.g., age, gender, weight, etc.). Such a technique is applied to retrospectively reviewed data that may be valuable, yet overcomes the limitation of not having a fully planned prospective study done years ago at the start of the use of the intervention. Studies that report propensity score-matched data can be relied upon as evidence where RCTs are not available [5] and can be considered in meta-analyses as well.

Trials on intervention will have to report the outcomes of efficacy and safety, which are typically decided on before the start of the trial (i.e., prospective study design). These are sometimes called *endpoints*. Examples of efficacy endpoints include cure rate, freedom from disease at specified intervals after the administration of treatment, while typical safety endpoints include measures such as mortality and incidence of known or expected side effects of treatment. These endpoints vary greatly depending on the type of disease in question, and an exhaustive list of such outcomes is impractical in this present literature.

Outcomes may be reported as continuous variables or rates of discrete events. For example, in a study investigating the effects of anticoagulation with a vitamin K antagonist, an outcome that is a continuous variable would be the international normalized ratio (INR)—it can take on any numerical value. An example of a discrete variable would be the rate of stroke—either a subject has experienced a stroke or not; there are only two possible scenarios. A useful way of reporting the incidence would be a percentage of subjects who experienced a stroke in the study or follow-up period. An example of some commonly encountered discrete and continuous variables is listed in Table 14.1.

Consequently, when performing a meta-analysis, it is important to identify the relevant outcomes and the format in which it is reported as the mode of analysis is

Table 14.1 A list of commonly reported outcomes of treatment in medical literature—some examples of continuous variables that may be reported as rates of a defined event are listed; example of units by which the continuous variable is measured in is included in brackets

Discrete variable	Continuous variable
Rate of death	Patient satisfaction scores (numerical scale)
Rate of recurrence of a disease at a specified time period	Days before the recurrence of a particular condition (days)
Rate of major bleeding during a surgical procedure[a]	Amount of blood loss in a surgical procedure (milliliters)
Rate of reduction in systolic blood pressure by at least 5 mmHg	Blood pressure (mmHg)
Rate of cure[b]	Time taken to complete a surgical procedure (minutes)

[a]The criteria "major bleeding" would have to be defined by the author or adapted from a universally accepted definition by a consensus body

[b]The definition of cure would have to be explained by the author and is specific to each medical condition

different between them. The software Review Manager [6] readily analyzes dichotomous or discrete and continuous variables as described above. To analyze discrete outcomes, the number of participants in the control and experimental group with the specified event and the total number in each group are needed. To analyze continuous variables, the mean, standard deviation, and number of participants in each group will be needed.

Generally, when selecting outcomes, the researcher chooses the outcomes that matter—i.e., those that are relevant in assessing the utility of the intervention, but at times there is frustration in finding that not all the outcomes of interest are universally reported by the different trials. It is helpful at times to look in the supplementary appendices of the included studies or even contact the authors to request for additional data not reported in the main text of the published study. Having mentioned that, one can usually find key outcomes reported in most of the studies worth their salt. There may be studies that enthusiastically report many other outcomes that may not be reported by other studies, hence unsuitable for numerical statistical analysis, but can make for qualitative analyses in a systematic review.

It is important to note that different studies may report outcomes at different time periods—the *follow-up* after performing the intervention. Larger, well-funded prospective studies may follow up with patients for years, allowing for insight into the long-term effects of the intervention. When performing a meta-analysis, it is ideal to choose outcomes reported at follow-up times common to all the included studies. This allows for uniform synthesis and comparison at a particular time point following the intervention.

14.3 Making Sense of the Data

It is important not only to perform your own meta-analysis but also to understand how to appreciate the works of others, aprising them critically for quality and finding information that would be relevant in clinical work—such as when counseling for an intervention.

The most important information one would be looking for in a meta-analysis on an intervention would usually be the efficacy endpoints. In an intervention that is designed to cure a disease, the rate of cure at the end of the follow-up period would be relevant. Another way by which data may be reported would be the freedom from disease at specific time points in the follow-up period. The combined rates are usually reported as odds ratios, which are measures of association between an exposure and an outcome [6]. In interventions designed to treat specifically measureable endpoints, such as for lowering blood pressure or serum cholesterol, the amount of lowering would be a numerical value. As discussed earlier, safety endpoints are also important to consider, when presenting risks of the intervention to patients.

In evaluating results, the 95% confidence interval statistic is crucial, because it gives information on whether the final calculated result is statistically significant and on the precision of the result. A common way of representing the analyzed data is on a forest plot. Visual inspection of the forest plot can easily show if the 95% confidence interval falls entirely on the same side of the plot as the calculated result. Another way of representing a statistically significant result is to use the *p*-value. A *p*-value of less than 0.05 is generally considered statistically significant.

In the event that the result is not statistically significant, a definite conclusion cannot be drawn about the effect of the treatment. Otherwise in cases, where there is a clear effect, there is a statistical technique of removing individual studies from the analysis to check if the other remaining studies still consistently produce a statistically significant result. The use of such techniques tells the reader that the design of the meta-analysis has been rigorous and there is usually little doubt about the result.

Another consideration in meta-analyses is the evaluation of the risk of bias in the included studies. The Cochrane Handbook [4] provides a comprehensive instruction on the assessment of bias. The risk of bias is usually presented as a table in the text, showing the risks for each study across the different types of bias. A meta-analysis that includes studies with high risks of bias in different categories may raise suspicion that the primary evidence is not of good quality, which may in turn affect the final results of the analysis. Caution should be exercised when the trials are largely heavily funded by private companies or if the authors have conflicts of interest at the time of publishing the studies.

Finally, it is unwise to get caught up with numbers and statistics without appreciating a manuscript as a whole. Any intervention is bound to have its side effects, and as discussed earlier, there are instances where few of the included studies publish all the safety endpoints. This may result in certain crucial information not being subjected to a mathematical analysis. The *discussion* and *limitations* sections of any meta-analysis may contain key information and qualitative analysis of the intervention and most certainly should not be neglected. The author may also state suggestions for future research directions.

Conclusion

There is tremendous utility for meta-analyses in the investigation of intervention. Such research is the basis for the creation of guidelines that would direct therapy across the world.

It is important to select good-quality primary evidence (randomized controlled trials) to include in the analysis. The outcomes of interests are analyzed, and common follow-up time points are ideally chosen. Bias should be evaluated as not all studies are equally rigorous.

When reading meta-analyses on interventions, the focus is on the key outcomes in effect and safety of the treatment. Attention should be paid to the summaries in the text that may give important information on certain outcomes unsuitable for a numerical analysis.

At the top of the hierarchy of evidence, meta-analysis is a practical tool in clinical decision-making, and utmost care should be taken to always conduct a thorough and statistically sound one.

References

1. Scott A, Wolchok J, Old L. Antibody therapy of cancer. Nat Rev Cancer. 2012;12:278–87.
2. Mohiuddin K, Swanson S. Maximizing the benefit of minimally invasive surgery. J Surg Oncol. 2013;108:315–9.
3. Abbott R, Cohen M. Medico-legal issues in cardiology. Cardiol Rev. 2013;21:222–8.
4. Higgins JPT, Green S, editors. Cochrane handbook for systematic reviews of interventions version 5.1.0 [updated March 2011]. The Cochrane Collaboration; 2011. www.handbook.cochrane.org. Accessed 29 June 2018.
5. Lonjon G, Boutron I, Trinquart L, Ahmad N, Aim F, Nizard R, Ravaud P. Comparison of treatment effect estimates from prospective nonrandomized studies with propensity score analysis and randomized controlled trials of surgical procedures. Ann Surg. 2014;259:18–25.
6. Sedgwick P. Odds and odds ratios. BMJ. 2013;347:f5067.

Updating Diagnostic Test Accuracy Systematic Reviews: Which, When, and How Should They Be Updated?

15

Ersilia Lucenteforte, Alessandra Bettiol, Salvatore De Masi, and Gianni Virgili

15.1 Introduction

The number of diagnostic test accuracy (DTA) studies has rapidly increased, especially over the last 5 years. A quick PubMed search (sensitivity[tiab] or specificity[tiab] or accuracy[tiab], filters: humans) revealed there were 15,772 published studies in 2000; 20,916 in 2005 (5144 more than 2000); 28,723 in 2010 (7807 more than 2005); and 39,110 in 2015 (10,387 more than 2010).

Systematic reviews (SRs) represent a very useful tool to synthesize the most relevant findings from different studies regarding a specific DTA question, as well as to investigate the possible reasons for discrepancies among studies and to assess the efficacy and clinical impact of new tests [1].

In the diagnostic field, assessing the impact of a new test is particularly critical and much more complicated than assessing the impact of new treatments. In fact, differently from new therapies, which are directly connected to clinical outcomes (either therapeutic effect or adverse event), the relationship between a new

E. Lucenteforte (✉)
Department of Clinical and Experimental Medicine, University of Pisa, Pisa, Italy
e-mail: ersilia.lucenteforte@unipi.it

A. Bettiol
Department of Neurosciences, Psychology, Drug Research and Child Health (NEUROFARBA), University of Florence, Florence, Italy
e-mail: alessandra.bettiol@unifi.it

S. De Masi
Clinical Trial Office, University Hospital "Azienda Ospedaliero-Universitaria Meyer", Florence, Italy
e-mail: salvatore.demasi@meyer.it

G. Virgili
Department of Surgery and Translational Medicine (DCMT), University of Florence, Florence, Italy
e-mail: gianni.virgili@unifi.it

G. Biondi-Zoccai (ed.), *Diagnostic Meta-Analysis*,
https://doi.org/10.1007/978-3-319-78966-8_15

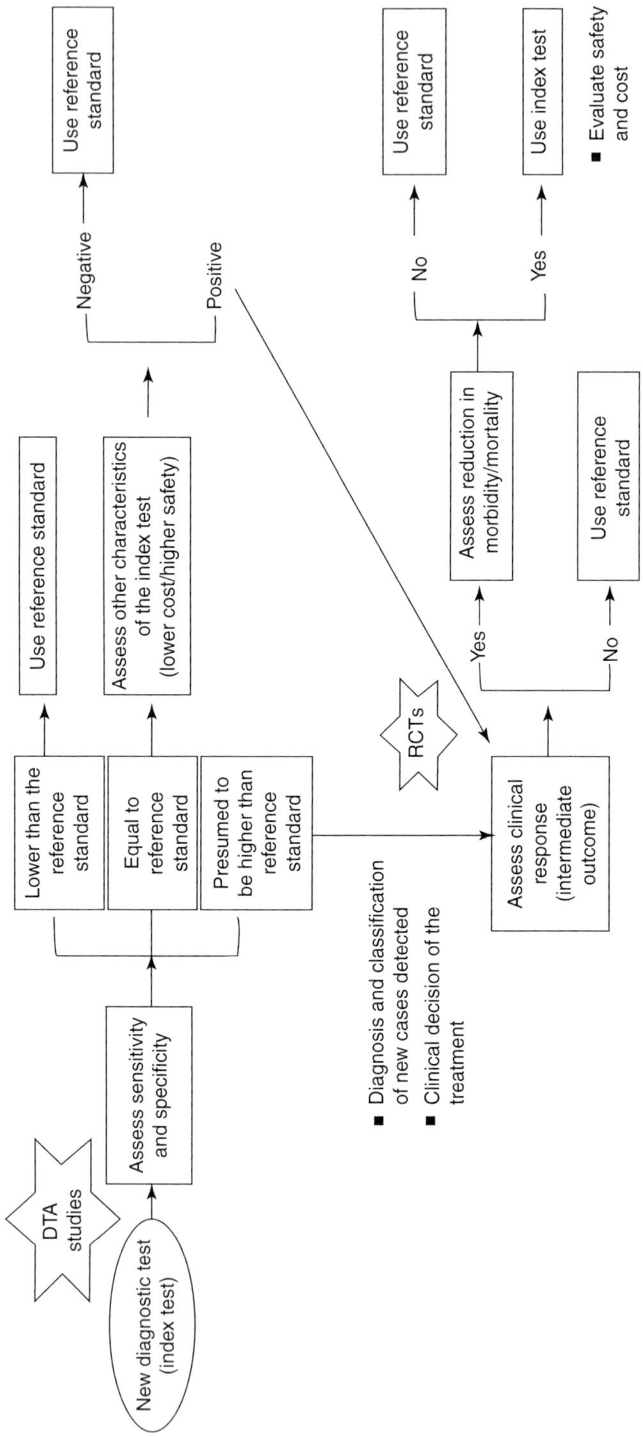

Fig. 15.1 Testing the impact of a new diagnostic test

diagnostic test and the final clinical outcome is much more complex and indirect [2] (Fig. 15.1). In light of this, studies on new tests naturally tend to concentrate more on the performance of the test alone (sensitivity, specificity, safety, and costs), rather than on its overall possible clinical impact, with DTA studies measuring only sensitivity and specificity (such as cross-sectional studies) being more common than randomized clinical trials (RCTs). In diagnostic fields, in fact, RCTs are not required for marketing approval, and new diagnostic tests often enter clinical practice without having their impact tested on patient outcomes [3]. All this makes it particularly complex to write a DTA SR and summarize evidence on the clinical impact of a new test. Moreover, it is time- and labor-consuming to write a DTA SR and evaluate and re-elaborate the latest and most interesting works concerning the topic of interest.

Despite the effort, SRs in general are destined to become "out of date" due to ongoing progress and newly published works. In fact, new studies may contain relevant elements of novelty which could significantly affect the conclusions and validity of the previous review, making it not only incomplete but also misleading. This is particularly true in the field of DTA, given the high rate of development of new diagnostic tools, ongoing changes in current reference techniques, and clinical pathways.

Therefore, when elements of novelty are available, systematic reviews need to be either completely rewritten or updated. Updating a SR is a new version of a previously published review with novelties in terms of data, methods, or analyses compared to the previous edition, as defined by the international panel for updating guidance for systematic review (PUGs) organized by Cochrane [4]. Compared to an ex novo edition, an update presents significant advantages, since it is generally more efficient and time-saving. However, the decision whether to update or completely rewrite a new review should be based on the quality of the already existing review. In fact, if the SR was imprecisely conducted using unsound methods (e.g., vague inclusion criteria, poorly developed outcomes, etc.), then starting all over again is probably the best choice. AMSTAR (a measurement tool to assess systematic reviews) is an example of a useful instrument that can be adopted to assess the overall quality of a SR [5], while PRISMA (Preferred Reporting Items for Systematic reviews and Meta-analyses) is useful to check reporting [6]. If updating is more convenient than rewriting, authors need to choose the review to update and when.

15.2 Which SR Should Be Updated?

Updating a SR is a challenging process, and its real worth must be well-balanced in order to channel the efforts into those areas where new evidence is crucial [4]. Therefore, choosing which reviews should be updated is a central problem. The systematic approach used to prioritize which SR to update may vary among guideline panels and review groups. However, some elements are common key points in the decisional approach (Fig. 15.2).

Among them, **currency** of a systematic review is essential. In fact, only reviews addressing questions of current interest can be considered worthy of being updated. This is particularly true in the field of DTA, where diagnostic tests are rapidly and easily exceeded by more modern diagnostic techniques (particularly in the field of imaging).

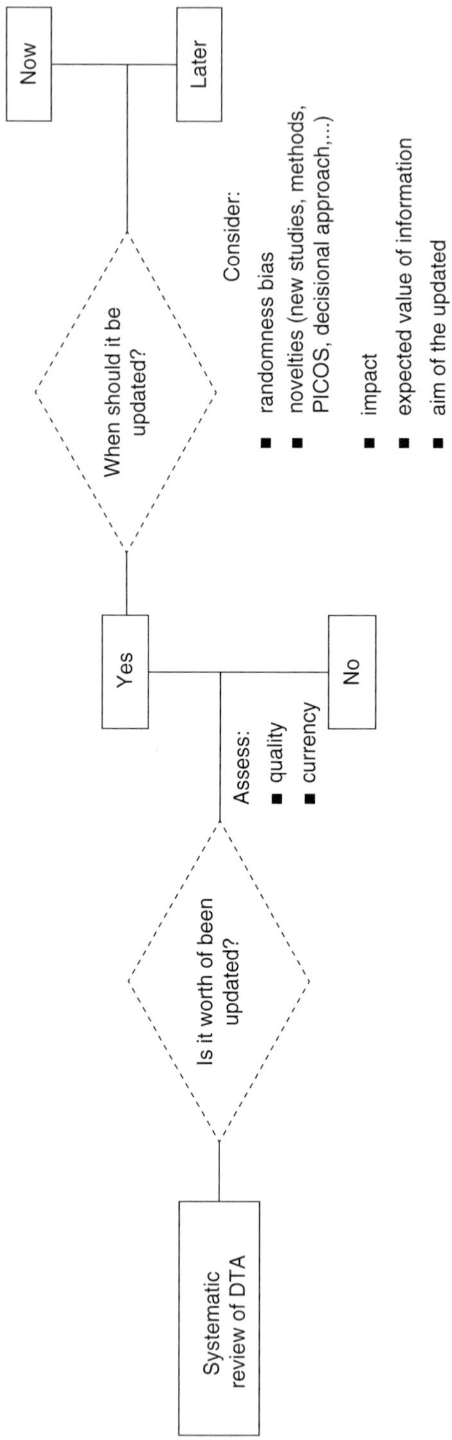

Fig. 15.2 Which and when SRs should be updated

To estimate the currency of a DTA SR, different strategies can be used. Among them, analysis of diagnostic approaches adopted in clinical practice is fundamental. In fact, reviews on diagnostic tests no longer used in routine diagnosis are probably out of date and unworthy of being updated.

Another valid strategy to assess currency is to evaluate whether the systematic review under consideration and/or other studies surrounding the DTA of interest receive good access, estimated through metrics for citations and downloads. In fact, widely cited or downloaded articles probably refer to topics of current interest, whereas reviews that are no longer cited or read probably refer to out-of-date diagnostic tools. In the latter case, updating of the review is generally considered unwarranted.

Even when currency is verified, the decision to update a SR must be based on the **quality** of the review itself; as reported above, when a SR addresses a question of current interest but is of poor quality, starting a completely new SR is the best choice.

15.3 When Should a SR Be Updated?

After having evaluated whether a review is worth being updated, choosing when to update it is a crucial point [4] (Fig. 15.2).

Theoretically, SRs should always be kept updated with the newest available evidence in order to avoid healthcare decisions being made on out-of-date or even misleading information. However, updating a SR every time a new study is published is both a utopian and methodologically incorrect approach. In fact, in addition to being extremely time-consuming, a "too-frequent" or "too-soon" update might lead to **randomness bias** since evidence from a single newer trial might completely modify the previous conclusions of the review. This is particularly true in light of the fact that studies with significant and particularly interesting results are more likely to be published and more quickly.

Some review groups arbitrarily decide to update the most relevant reviews with a fixed frequency (the Cochrane Library) [7], whereas others decide to update them according to the availability of elements of novelty [8] or to several other factors such as public health importance, rapidity of scientific developments, or nature of the health condition in question (AHRQ—Agency for Healthcare Research and Quality) [9].

To assess when to update, routine surveillance for **newly published studies** around the topic of interest should be performed. Novelties in studies not only include completely original works but also follow-up results of already included studies (although follow-up studies are uncommon in the diagnostic field since the majority of studies on diagnostic tests are designed as cross-sectional or observational studies).

Given the high rate of publication of DTA studies, a systematic approach is often useful for an exhaustive literature screening. Adopted approaches may vary among groups and are often based on the use of full or abbreviated search strategies, focusing on the review of either the overall literature or of selected groups of core journals in the field of interest [10]. Two valid search approaches are the RAND and Ottawa methods [11–13]. Together with the GRADE approach [14], with statistical prediction tools and value of information analysis (described below), these methods also represent valid tools to estimate how relevant new studies can be in changing or confirming the conclusions of a review.

The RAND method [11] performs an abbreviated search in five major journals to find new studies. Following this first step, the method abstracts the results of relevant articles and qualitatively assesses whether the new findings change or confirm the conclusion of the previous review. The RAND method also includes a subsequent step of consultation of the US Food and Drug Administration website and of external expert judgments to evaluate the currency and possible impact of these findings. Based on this approach, one of four levels indicating update necessity is attributed to the review: (1) original conclusion is still valid, and this portion of the original report does not need updating; (2) original conclusion is possibly out of date, and this portion of the original report may need updating; (3) original conclusion is probably out of date, and this portion of the original report may need updating; and (4) original conclusion is out of date.

On the other hand, the Ottawa method [12] is a full-search approach that uses a PubMed search to identify new studies around a selected topic. If new studies are detected, this method performs quantitative and qualitative analysis to evaluate the possible impact of these findings on the conclusions of the review, without involving an expert judgment.

In addition to availability of newly published studies, **novelties in methodology** can affect the decision of when to update a review. Changes in methods are particularly important in the field of DTA SRs, where marked inhomogeneity in results of DTA studies often occurs due to differences in the applied methods [15].

Methodological changes usually involve one or more of the parameters considered in the PICO(S) tool (i.e., population, intervention, comparison, outcomes, and study design of an article) or in the SPIDER tool (i.e., sample, phenomenon of interest, design, evaluation, and research type of quantitative or mixed-method studies) [16].

However, methodological novelties may also involve routine approaches and procedures adopted in clinical practice. In diagnostic fields, **changes in the decisional approach** in which the diagnostic test of interest is inserted could significantly affect the conclusions and level of certainty of a review. Therefore, an update of a DTA SR should be considered every time the decisional tree undergoes modifications.

Similarly, changes in the **standards of quality** requested for studies included in the SR could occur as well. In fact, removal of some studies included in the previous version of the review, due to a reclassification as "poor-quality studies" following variations in the reference standards, may lead to significant variations in the overall conclusions.

When elements of novelty have been found, assessing the possible **impact** of novelties on the conclusions and certainty of a systematic review is a crucial step in the decision of whether or not to update a review. Experts in the diagnostic field of interest, as well as editors or referees, can often provide an informed and critical estimate of this impact [11] (RAND method).

However, the consensus of experts is often limitative and not objective. Therefore, different tools have been developed to estimate the impact of an update. A possible approach is GRADE [14], which is based on the assessment of the level of certainty of the evidence reported in a review. According to this approach, the highest assigned level is the certainty of outcomes reported in the review, with the lowest referring to the probability that results from new not-yet-included studies will affect the conclusions of the review.

Assessment of the impact of a review cannot be considered only in terms of gains in scientific knowledge. In fact, the strongest is evidence reported in a review, and the highest will be its probability of influencing the clinical practice, leading to both social and economic consequences.

In light of this consideration, also a **value of information analysis** should be performed before starting a review update [17]. This statistical prediction method allows calculation of the gain in terms of reduction of losses related to uncertainty compared to the cost measured in days required to update the SR. Those with significantly positive estimated value of information are worthy of being updated soon due to their probable relevant implications in clinical practice.

Along with the abovementioned considerations, the moment of updating a review may also be influenced by the **aim** of the update itself. In fact, the objective of systematic reviews can go beyond a simple synthesis of evidence, aiming to estimate a ROC curve or to summarize evidence on the validity of a certain test in a specific setting (such as for a particular clinical condition or in a particular range of values) [1].

15.4 How Should a SR Be Updated?

If a review has been judged as worthy of updating, authors should carefully plan the work according to these points suggested by the International PUGs [4]:

1. Authorship must be updated: if authors differ from those of the first review, then the previous author team should be acknowledged in the update.
2. State of the art must be refreshed, including all background information and evidence already known about the topic.
3. The aim of the previous review should be reconsidered to evaluate if it is still relevant to patients and clinical practice. If so, the question of the previous review can be readdressed; otherwise a new question of current relevance should be formulated.
4. Inclusion criteria should be revisited: not all previously included studies should be included in the new edition. When better-quality and larger studies are published, previously included weaker and smaller studies should be excluded from the update. Similarly, studies comparing the test of interest with obsolete or no longer commonly used tests should be removed.

5. Methods should be revisited: authors are advised to use the latest and most accurate accepted methods, eventually repeating the whole data extraction for all studies.
6. A search for newly published studies should be started, taking into account the new inclusion criteria and aims of the update; thus, search strategies may vary compared to the previous version of the review.
7. A clear description of novelties, in terms of search strategy or methods, must be provided and well-documented to assure replicability. Moreover, given that newly included studies can partially or radically change the overall conclusions of the review, it is crucial to clearly and attractively present the new findings, highlighting and discussing the differences compared to the previous edition. Users of reviews greatly benefit from a concise and easy-to-read synthesis of results and novelties, with possible explanations for changes. A valid choice is to use a stand-alone concise summary composed mainly of tables and figures providing a full report with a detailed description of all data and results, especially for those who need more accurate information on the topic [18].
8. Updating can be conducted manually; however this is both time-consuming and poorly efficient; various technological innovations have been developed to increase both the rapidity and efficacy of an update [4]. The implementation of the speed and rapidity of the update process through the already-existing and the underdevelopment tools aims to allow, in a near future, the real-time update of knowledge with the results from new studies [4, 19].

15.5 Case Study

In order to assess the impact of updating DTA SRs, we searched Cochrane reviews reporting the terms "accuracy" or "sensitivity" or "specificity" in the title or abstract and labeled as updated by a "new search" in the Cochrane Library (Table 15.1). We found four SRs which fulfilled these requirements:

1. Galactomannan detection for invasive aspergillosis in immunocompromised patients [20, 21]
2. Optical coherence tomography (OCT) for detection of macular edema in patients with diabetic retinopathy [22, 23]
3. The diagnostic accuracy of the GenoType® MTBDRsl assay for the detection of resistance to second-line antituberculosis drugs [24, 25]
4. Diagnostic accuracy of laparoscopy following computed tomography (CT) scanning for assessing the resectability with curative intent in pancreatic and periampullary cancer [26, 27]

We assessed the following features: months since the original and the updated search and number of new studies found; any change in review objectives in the main text, including PICO, clinical pathway, and test role; conclusions as presented

Table 15.1 Comparison of four SRs and their corresponding updates published in the Cochrane Library

	First version of SR	Update of SR
Title of first version: Galactomannan Detection for Invasive Aspergillosis in Immunocompromised Patients [20, 21]		
Years	August 2005–April 2007	February 2014
N. studies	42 (of whom 30 included in the meta-analysis), 6792 subjects	54 (of whom 50 included in the meta-analysis), 8305 subjects
Objectives	Assess the diagnostic accuracy of galactomannan detection in serum for the diagnosis of invasive aspergillosis in immunocompromised patients, at different cutoff values for test positivity	Same
Pathway	There is substantial variation in the way the galactomannan ELISA is currently used in the clinic: – Some clinicians do not use it at all – Others use the galactomannan ELISA as a screening tool, to monitor whether patients at risk develop invasive aspergillosis (IA) or not. In those cases, serum is tested for IA once or twice every week – Sometimes the galactomannan ELISA is used to test for IA in BAL fluid when IA is already suspected, and in those situations, the test is only used in serum when there is no BAL fluid – In most situations, the galactomannan ELISA is used as a triage test: if the ELISA is positive, patients will be referred for further diagnostic testing – The test is also used in the definition of proven, probable, or possible IA or as final decision-making tool to start antifungal therapy	Same In addition: further diagnostic testing may involve either laboratory testing of BAL fluid, CT scanning or radiography, or a combination of tests. Patients may also be referred for further diagnostic work-up on the basis of clinical signs and symptoms
Index	Two commercially available assays for the detection of galactomannan: – The Pastorex© latex agglutination test: rarely used – The Platelia© sandwich ELISA test: mostly used for the detection of antigen in serum and in fluid that is obtained via bronchoalveolar lavage (BAL). Other specimens in which the test can also be used are cerebrospinal fluid (CSF) or urine The SR focused on the ELISA test in serum	Same

(continued)

Table 15.1 (continued)

	First version of SR	Update of SR
Reference	The following reference standards can be used to define the target condition: – Autopsy (gold standard combined with a positive culture of *Aspergillus* species from the autopsy specimens or with histopathological evidence of *Aspergillus*; however autopsy is rarely reported) – The criteria of the EORTC/MSG (reference standard in the SR) – The demonstration of hyphal invasion in biopsies, combined with a positive culture for *Aspergillus* species from the same specimens The criteria of the EORTC/MSG divide the patient population into four categories: patients with proven IA, patients who probably have IA, patients who possibly have IA, and patients without IA Clinical studies have shown that these criteria do not match autopsy results perfectly. This is especially true for the possible category. For clinical trials investigating the effect of treatment, for example, it is recommended that only the proven and probable categories are used	Same In addition: the exclusion of patients with "possible" invasive aspergillosis, which can be regarded as group of "difficult or atypical" patients, is likely to affect the observed diagnostic accuracy of a test. Also, the exclusion of any other of the reference standard groups may affect the accuracy of the index test. We therefore excluded studies explicitly excluding one of the four categories of patients from the review, as well as studies in which it is not clear how many patients with proven, probable, possible, or no invasive aspergillosis had positive or negative index test results
Heterogeneity	Three sources of heterogeneity: effect of cutoff value, effect of the reference standard, and existence of clinical subgroups	Same
Conclusions (taken from the Abstract)	Using the test at a cutoff value 0.5 ODI in a population with a disease prevalence of 8% (overall median prevalence): – Sensitivity 78%, 22% false negatives – Specificity of 81%, 19% false negatives Using the test at cutoff value 1.5 in the same population: – Sensitivity 64%, 36% false negatives – Specificity of 95%, 5% false negatives These numbers should however be interpreted with caution, because the results were very heterogeneous	Using the test at a cutoff value 0.5 ODI in a population with a disease prevalence of 9% (overall median prevalence): – Sensitivity 82%, 18% false negatives – Specificity 81%, 19% false negatives Using the test at cutoff value 1.5 in the same population: – Sensitivity 61%, 39% false negatives – Specificity 93%, 7% false negatives These numbers should, however, be interpreted with caution because the results were very heterogeneous

Table 15.1 (continued)

	First version of SR	Update of SR
Bias	QUADAS	QUADAS 2
Summary of findings (SoF)	Yes	Yes
Title of first version: Optical Coherence Tomography (OCT) for Detection of Macular Oedema in Patients with Diabetic Retinopathy [22, 23]		
Years	May 2011	June 2013
N. studies	9, 768 subjects, 1325 eyes	10, 830 subjects, 1387 eyes
Objective	To determine the diagnostic accuracy of OCT for detecting diabetic macular edema (DMO) and clinically significant macular edema (CSMO), defined according to ETDRS 1985	To determine the diagnostic accuracy of OCT for detecting DMO and clinically significant macular edema (CSMO), defined according to ETDRS 1985, in patients referred to ophthalmologists after DR is detected. In the update of this review, we also aimed to assess whether OCT might be considered the new reference standard for detecting DMO
Pathway and role	Measurements of retinal thickness may be obtained directly from the tomograms either by manually measuring the distance between the inner and outer retinal boundaries or by using computer image-processing techniques OCT is increasingly used for detecting macular edema in people with DR because it is an objective and reliable tool. Furthermore, OCT allows a quantitative follow-up of the effects of treatment. However, purchasing an OCT machine is costly, and personnel are needed to use it OCT is unlikely to be used by primary care professionals as a triage test to detect DMO; OCT is mainly used by secondary care professionals to further investigate patients who are suspected of having macular edema. As such it would be used by an ophthalmologist as an add-on test, to assess the need for laser treatment by recording macular thickness	In the updated version of this review, we acknowledge that the clinical pathway of patients with DMO is unclear and probably dependent on the country and setting. Thus, the applicability of the results of the review will depend on patient selection in included studies, such as inclusion criteria and results of prior testing

(continued)

Table 15.1 (continued)

	First version of SR	Update of SR
Index	The index test was OCT, regardless of the generation of development of the instrument (low- or high-resolution, three-dimensional, or spectral-domain OCTs)	The index test was OCT, regardless of the generation development of the instrument (low- or high-resolution, three-dimensional, or spectral-domain OCTs). Despite the fact that retinal thickness measurements with OCT have been compared to those obtained with the retinal thickness analyzer in at least one study, based on their best knowledge, authors believed that such a comparison is no longer of interest given the dominant use of OCT devices. Authors were not aware of any other instruments that can be compared to OCT
Reference	In the ETDRS study, DMO was defined on the basis of stereoscopic fundus photography (ETDRS 1985). This technique is complicated and difficult to use in a clinical setting. It was replaced by contact fundus biomicroscopy, which was found to be in close agreement with stereophotography, particularly for CSMO. Noncontact fundus biomicroscopy is more commonly used, since sophisticated fundus lenses have been proposed for binocular fundus observation during the past two decades, yet it has been shown to be slightly less sensitive than contact fundus biomicroscopy Finally, valid reference tests considered in this review were stereoscopic fundus photography and contact lens or noncontact lens biomicroscopy of the fundus	Same In addition: In the update of this review, authors acknowledge that OCT is increasingly thought of as a new reference standard for DMO and will not update the review further Although the American Academy of Ophthalmology's Preferred Practice Patterns (AAO PPP 2012) still considers clinical examination as the current recommendation for routine diagnosis of DMO, Schneider (2013) found that the use of OCT has greatly increased for patients with neovascular age-related macular degeneration or DMO in recent years, while that of fluorescein angiography or fundus photography has decreased

Table 15.1 (continued)

	First version of SR	Update of SR
Heterogeneity	Heterogeneity related to retinal thickness cutoff, to index test, to reference standard, to characteristics of the study population, and to methodological study quality items of the QUADAS checklist	Same
Conclusions	Central retinal thickness measured with OCT cannot be used as a stand-alone test to diagnose the central type of CSMO and decide on the use of laser photocoagulation in patients who are referred to retina clinics. In fact, there is a substantial disagreement of OCT with the ETDRS definition of CSMO based on clinical examination. Some researchers have observed that OCT can detect macular thickening earlier than clinical examination but also found that such cases did not necessarily progress to CSMO and need photocoagulation Care should be taken in applying the conclusions of this review to other test-treatment pathways. In fact, OCT will become an essential tool to manage antiangiogenic therapy, an expanding therapeutic option for patients with macular edema due to DR, because OCT is a component of the diagnostic algorithms of studies on this new treatment	Using retinal thickness thresholds lower than 300 μm and ophthalmologist's fundus assessment as reference standard, central retinal thickness measured with OCT was not sufficiently accurate to diagnose the central type of CSMO in patients with DR referred to retina clinics. However, at least OCT false positives are generally cases of subclinical DMO that cannot be detected clinically but still suffer from increased risk of disease progression. Therefore, the increasing availability of OCT devices, together with their precision and the ability to inform on retinal layer structure, now makes OCT widely recognized as the new reference standard for assessment of DMO, even in some screening settings. Thus, this review will not be updated further
Bias	QUADAS	QUADAS 2
SoF	Yes	Yes
Title of first version: The Diagnostic Accuracy of the Genotype® MTBDRsl Assay for the Detection of Resistance to Second-Line Anti-tuberculosis Drugs [24, 25]		
Years	January 2014	September 2015
N. studies	21	27

(continued)

Table 15.1 (continued)

	First version of SR	Update of SR
Objective and role	• Primary objectives: – To assess and compare the diagnostic accuracy of MTBDR*sl* for the detection of resistance to fluoroquinolones (FQs) in patient specimens (using direct testing) and culture isolates (using indirect testing) confirmed as tuberculosis (TB) positive – To assess and compare the diagnostic accuracy of MTBDR*sl* for the detection of resistance to second-line injectable drugs (SLIDs) in patient specimens (using direct testing) and culture isolates (using indirect testing) confirmed as TB positive – To assess and compare the diagnostic accuracy of MTBDR*sl* for the detection of extensively drug-resistant TB (XDR-TB) in patient specimens (using direct testing) and culture isolates (using indirect testing) confirmed as TB positive • Secondary objectives: – To investigate heterogeneity in relation to the reference standard (culture-based drug susceptibility testing (DST) compared with: 1. Genetic sequencing 2. Culture-based DST and genetic sequencing 3. Culture-based DST followed by genetic sequencing with discordant results) and individual drugs within a drug class (e.g., ofloxacin and moxifloxacin within the FQ class) Authors also prespecified in the protocol investigations of heterogeneity in relation to HIV status, condition of the specimens (fresh or frozen, volume of specimen), patient population (patients suspected of having MDR-TB or XDR-TB), and whether WHO-recommended critical drug concentrations were used for culture-based reference testing	• Primary objectives: Same In addition: the populations of interest were people with MDR-TB or rifampicin-resistant TB, which is considered a proxy for MDRTB in high-burden settings • Secondary objectives: Same In addition: Subsequent to the published protocol, we added an investigation of heterogeneity in relation to microscopy smear grade

Table 15.1 (continued)

	First version of SR	Update of SR
Pathway	Depending on the setting, DST is either performed on all patients with confirmed TB or only on patients who are clinically suspected of having DR-TB (e.g., if the patient's symptoms have failed to improve on first-line therapy or if they still have viable bacilli in their sputum after an extended period of treatment). As mentioned above, the manufacturer recommends that if the patient specimen (usually sputum) is smear positive, the assay be performed directly on the specimen (direct testing). If smear negative, it is recommended that the assay be performed on the culture isolate grown from the patient specimen (indirect testing). DST for resistance to the second-line drugs is only performed if resistance to the first-line drugs is confirmed. Where routine molecular (genotypic) testing is well established, phenotypic DST is not usually performed. However, authors expected research studies evaluating the accuracy of molecular DSTs, such as the MTBDRsl assay, to almost always include phenotypic DST as a reference standard. Furthermore, authors also expected some studies to use genetic sequencing to resolve any discordant index test-reference standard results	Depending on the setting, DST is either performed on all patients with confirmed TB or on patients who are clinically suspected of having drug-resistant TB (e.g., if the patients' symptoms have failed to improve on first-line therapy or if they still have *M. tuberculosis* bacilli in their sputum after an extended period of treatment) DST for resistance to the second-line drugs is usually only performed if resistance to the first-line drugs is confirmed. Specifically, a patient with suspected drug-resistant TB provides a specimen (usually sputum), which is examined by smear microscopy. If smear positive, MTBDR*sl* version 1.0 or version 2.0 can be performed directly on the specimen. If smear negative, MTBDR*sl* version 1.0 should not be performed directly on the specimen but rather on the culture isolate. MTBDR*sl* version 2.0 may be performed directly on a smear-negative specimen. A molecular test for first-line drug resistance (e.g., the MTBDR*plus* assay) may be performed prior to testing with MTBDR*sl* if resistance to the first-line drugs is yet to be confirmed. Phenotypic DST may still be performed on culture-positive isolates

(continued)

Table 15.1 (continued)

	First version of SR	Update of SR
Comment		This updated systematic review summarizes the current literature and includes 27 studies and integrates six new studies: five new studies for MTBDR*sl* version 1.0 identified since the original Cochrane review and one study for MTBDR*sl* version 2.0. For MTBDR*sl* version 1.0, the findings in this updated review are consistent with those reported in the previous version of the review
Index	Studies that evaluated the MTBDR*sl* assay were included MTBDR*sl* would be used as an initial test replacing phenotypic culture-based DST as the initial test	The index test was MTBDRsl version 1.0 or version 2.0 Comment: one study on version 2.0 The role of MTBDRsl would be as the initial test, replacing culture-based DST, for detecting second-line drug resistance
Reference	1. Phenotypic culture-based DST: solid culture or a commercial liquid culture system (BACTEC 460, MGIT 960, and MGIT manual system, Becton Dickinson, USA) incorporating the drug of interest. It is the conventional reference standard, but it is considered to be imperfect and is dependent on the drug concentration threshold used to define resistance 2. Genetic sequencing of the *gyrA* or *rrs* genes or both. Genetic sequencing is considered to be more accurate than phenotypic culture-based DST; however, this is only if it targets all known resistance-determining regions, which are not completely defined for the FQs and the SLIDs. Therefore, genetic sequencing can miss mutations that may cause drug resistance which fall outside of the targeted genes. Furthermore, genetic sequencing is usually applied only to culture isolates when results for the index test and the culture-based reference test do not agree. In this latter situation, there is potential for verification bias because the same reference standard is not being used to verify all index test results	1. Same 2. Sequencing of the *gyrA* or *rrs* genes (MTBDR*sl* version 1.0) or additionally the *gyrB* and *eis* promoter regions (MTBDR*sl* version 2.0). Sequencing is considered to be more accurate than culture-based DST; however, this is only if it targets all known resistance-determining regions, which are not fully known for the FQs and the SLIDs. Therefore, targeted sequencing may miss mutations that cause drug resistance 3. Same 4. Same

Table 15.1 (continued)

	First version of SR	Update of SR
	3. Two reference standards used together: phenotypic culture-based DST and genetic sequencing of the same samples. If a specimen was resistant according to phenotypic culture-based DST or had a mutation in the *gyrA* or *rrs* genes, the specimen was classified as having the target condition. If both phenotypic culture-based DST and genetic sequencing indicated susceptibility, the specimen was classified as not having the target condition 4. Two reference standards used sequentially: phenotypic culture-based DST followed by selective testing by genetic sequencing of samples with discordant results (also referred to as discrepant analysis). Discordant results may be either index test positive/phenotypic culture-based DST negative or index test negative/phenotypic culture-based DST positive	
Heterogeneity	Within each stratum (e.g., SLID resistance), heterogeneity was investigated through visual examination of forest plots of sensitivity and specificity. Then, if sufficient studies were available, we explored the possible influence of the following prespecified categorical covariates: – Reference standard (culture, genetic sequencing, culture and genetic sequencing, culture followed by genetic sequencing) – Individual drug (amikacin, kanamycin, and capreomycin)	Within each stratum (e.g., SLID resistance), heterogeneity was investigated through visual examination of forest plots of sensitivity and specificity. Then, if sufficient studies were available, we explored the possible influence of the following prespecified categorical covariates: – Reference standard (culture, genetic sequencing, culture and genetic sequencing, culture followed by genetic sequencing) – Resistance to the following drugs: ofloxacin, moxifloxacin, levofloxacin, gatifloxacin, amikacin, kanamycin, and capreomycin – Drug concentration used for culture-based DST In addition, for this updated review, authors added an investigation of heterogeneity in relation to microscopy smear grade

(continued)

Table 15.1 (continued)

	First version of SR	Update of SR
Conclusions (from the Abstract)	– A positive MTBDR*sl* result for resistance to the fluoroquinolone drugs or the second-line injectable drugs is reliable evidence that the person has drug-resistant TB and further conventional drug-resistance testing is not required – However, when the test reports a negative result, clinicians may still wish to carry out conventional testing	– In people with rifampicin-resistant or multidrug-resistant tuberculosis, MTBDRsl performed on a culture isolate or smear-positive specimen may be useful in detecting second-line drug resistance. MTBDRsl (smear-positive specimen) correctly classified around six in seven people as having fluoroquinolone or SLID resistance, although the sensitivity estimates for SLID resistance varied – However, when second-line drug resistance is not detected (MTBDRsl result is negative), conventional DST can still be used to evaluate patients for resistance to the fluoroquinolones or SLIDs – Authors recommend that future work evaluate MTBDRsl version 2.0, in particular on smear-negative specimens and in different settings to account for different resistance-causing mutations that may vary by strain – Researchers should also consider incorporating WHO-recommended critical concentrations into their culture-based reference standards

Table 15.1 (continued)

	First version of SR	Update of SR
Bias	QUADAS 2	QUADAS 2
SoF	Yes	Yes
Title of first version: Diagnostic Accuracy of Laparoscopy Following Computed Tomography (CT) Scanning for Assessing the Resectability with Curative Intent in Pancreatic and Periampullary Cancer 1 [26, 27]		
Years	September 2012	May 2016
N. studies	15, 1015 subjects	16, 1146 subjects
Objectives	• Primary objective: – To determine the diagnostic accuracy of diagnostic laparoscopy performed as an add-on test to CT scanning in the assessment of curative resectability in pancreatic and periampullary cancer • Secondary objective: Authors planned to explore the following sources of heterogeneity: 1. Studies at low risk of bias versus those at unclear or high risk of bias 2. Full-text publications versus abstracts 3. Prospective studies versus retrospective studies 4. Proportion of patients with pancreatic cancer, ampullary cancer, and bile duct cancers 5. Procedures performed under the same anesthetic versus procedures performed under a different anesthetic 6. Different definitions for resectable cancer on laparotomy 7. Additional pretests performed (besides CT scan)	Same
Pathway	There is no standard algorithm currently available for assessing the resectability of pancreatic and periampullary cancers, with different clinicians following their own algorithms based on either their clinical experience or what they were taught. Currently, almost all algorithms include a CT scan as one of the tests. CT may be the only test performed before laparotomy. Other tests such as diagnostic laparoscopy, positron-emission tomography (PET scanning), magnetic resonance imaging (MRI), or endoscopic ultrasound (EUS) may be used in addition to CT scan to assess resectability	Same

(continued)

Table 15.1 (continued)

	First version of SR	Update of SR
Index	Only diagnostic laparoscopy, in which histopathological confirmation of metastatic spread was obtained on a paraffin section, was included Diagnostic laparoscopy can be considered as an add-on test to the CT scan prior to laparotomy done with the intention of performing a potentially curative resection	Same
Reference	Confirmation of liver or peritoneal involvement by histopathological examination of suspicious (liver or peritoneal) lesions obtained at diagnostic laparoscopy or laparotomy. Authors accepted only paraffin section histology as the reference standard. In clinical practice, depending on the urgency of the results, a frozen section biopsy may be done to obtain immediate results. However, this is always confirmed by subsequent paraffin section histology (which can take several days) because frozen section biopsy is not as reliable as paraffin section histology. Authors also accepted the surgeon's judgment of unresectability at laparotomy when biopsy confirmation was not possible. For example, if the tumor has invaded the adjacent blood vessels, the surgeon may not resect the tumor because of the danger posed by resecting part of a large blood vessel, and so biopsy confirmation cannot be obtained	Same
Heterogeneity	Authors planned to explore heterogeneity by using the different sources of heterogeneity as covariate(s) in the regression model. However, this was not possible because the information was either not available or was the same in all the studies	Same
Conclusions (taken from the Abstract)	Diagnostic laparoscopy may decrease the rate of unnecessary laparotomy in patients with pancreatic and periampullary cancer found to have resectable disease on CT scan. On average, using diagnostic laparoscopy with biopsy and histopathological confirmation of suspicious lesions prior to laparotomy would avoid 23 unnecessary laparotomies in 100 patients in whom resection of cancer with curative intent is planned	Diagnostic laparoscopy may decrease the rate of unnecessary laparotomy in people with pancreatic and periampullary cancer found to have resectable disease on CT scan. On average, using diagnostic laparoscopy with biopsy and histopathological confirmation of suspicious lesions prior to laparotomy would avoid 21 unnecessary laparotomies in 100 people in whom resection of cancer with curative intent is planned
Bias	QUADAS 2	QUADAS 2
SoF	Yes	Yes

in the Abstract and implications for practice and research in the main text; and methodological tools used as risk of bias tool and summary of findings (SoF) table.

The number of studies increased from 30 to 54 in 78 months [20, 21], from 9 to 10 in 37 months [22, 23], from 21 to 27 in 18 months [24, 25], and from 15 to 16 in 32 months [26, 27].

The review objectives in the main text were unchanged or rephrased with no substantive change, in three reviews, while Virgili (2015) [23] added details on the clinical pathway and the potential for the index test to replace the reference standard. Regarding PICO components, all reviews were unchanged in terms of index and reference tests, but two reviews [23, 25] noticed that different index test versions were available. The test role was explicit in Allen (2013) and Allen (2016) [26, 27] (replacement), while other reviews referred more generically to estimating accuracy with no explicit role.

Regarding the main conclusions presented in the Abstract, Leeflang (2008) and Leeflang (2015) [20, 21] used this section to present absolute frequencies of test performance, and Allen (2013) and Allen (2014) were also unchanged with minimal rephrasing. On the other hand, Theron (2014) and Theron (2016) [24, 25] used very different wording, suggesting a change in the clinical interpretation of results. This was also the case for Virgili (2011) and Virgili (2014) [22, 23] who discussed discordances between the index and reference tests in support of the widely accepted dominance of the index test in modern clinical practice.

An update from QUADAS to QUADAS 2 was conducted in three reviews, and a summary of results or summary of findings table was present in all reviews.

This survey of four updated Cochrane DTA reviews suggests no explicit reason for updating was used apart from time since the publication of the original version, except when a change of the index test role was expected. The number of new studies in the update was quite variable, probably reflecting different phases and importance of the test development with respect to the clinical question made in the review. Updating methodological tools, such as for QUADAS checklist version, was the main structural change to the review methodology.

Conclusion

Updates of DTA SR are a precious instrument for clinical practice as well as regulatory aspects, supporting the decision-making approach based on current scientific evidence. Despite their high value, up to now, only a few updates of DTA SR have been published. However, considering that the majority of DTA studies of current relevance have been conducted in the most recent years, the number of SR will probably increase significantly in the near future as new evidence becomes available.

References

1. Leeflang MM, Deeks JJ, Gatsonis C, Bossuyt PM, Cochrane Diagnostic Test Accuracy Working Group. Systematic reviews of diagnostic test accuracy. Ann Intern Med. 2008;149:889–97.

2. Matchar DB. Chapter 1: introduction to the methods guide for medical test reviews. J Gen Intern Med. 2012;27:S4–10.
3. Lord SJ, Irwig L, Simes RJ. When is measuring sensitivity and specificity sufficient to evaluate a diagnostic test, and when do we need randomized trials? Ann Intern Med. 2006;144:850–5.
4. Garner P, Hopewell S, Chandler J, et al. When and how to update systematic reviews: consensus and checklist. BMJ. 2016;354:i3507.
5. Shea BJ, Grimshaw JM, Wells GA, et al. Development of AMSTAR: a measurement tool to assess the methodological quality of systematic reviews. BMC Med Res Methodol. 2007;7:10.
6. Stovold E, Beecher D, Foxlee R, Noel-Storr A. Study flow diagrams in Cochrane systematic review updates: an adapted PRISMA flow diagram. Syst Rev. 2014;3:54.
7. Higgins J, Green S, editors. Cochrane handbook for systematic reviews of interventions version 5.1.0 [updated March 2011]. The Cochrane Collaboration; 2011. http://handbook.cochrane.org. Accessed 29 June 2018.
8. Chalmers I, Enkin M, Keirse MJ. Preparing and updating systematic reviews of randomized controlled trials of health care. Milbank Q. 1993;71:411–37.
9. Tsertsvadze A, Maglione M, Chou R, et al. Updating comparative effectiveness reviews: current efforts in AHRQ's Effective Health Care Program. J Clin Epidemiol. 2011;64:1208–15.
10. Sagliocca L, De Masi S, Ferrigno L, Mele A, Traversa G. A pragmatic strategy for the review of clinical evidence. J Eval Clin Pract. 2013;19:689–96.
11. Shekelle P, Eccles MP, Grimshaw JM, Woolf SH. When should clinical guidelines be updated? BMJ. 2001;323:155–7.
12. Shojania KG, Sampson M, Ansari MT, Ji J, Doucette S, Moher D. How quickly do systematic reviews go out of date? A survival analysis. Ann Intern Med. 2007;147:224–33.
13. Chung M, Newberry SJ, Ansari MT, et al. Two methods provide similar signals for the need to update systematic reviews. J Clin Epidemiol. 2012;65:660–8.
14. Balshem H, Helfand M, Schunemann HJ, et al. GRADE guidelines: 3. Rating the quality of evidence. J Clin Epidemiol. 2011;64:401–6.
15. Whiting PF, Rutjes AW, Westwood ME, et al. QUADAS-2: a revised tool for the quality assessment of diagnostic accuracy studies. Ann Intern Med. 2011;155:529–36.
16. Methley AM, Campbell S, Chew-Graham C, McNally R, Cheraghi-Sohi S. PICO, PICOS and SPIDER: a comparison study of specificity and sensitivity in three search tools for qualitative systematic reviews. BMC Health Serv Res. 2014;14:579.
17. Wilson EC. A practical guide to value of information analysis. PharmacoEconomics. 2015;33:105–21.
18. Newberry SJ, Shekelle PG, Vaiana M, Motala A. Reporting the findings of updated systematic reviews of comparative effectiveness: how do users want to view new information? Rockville, MD: Agency for Healthcare Research and Quality (US); 2013.
19. Elliott JH, Turner T, Clavisi O, et al. Living systematic reviews: an emerging opportunity to narrow the evidence-practice gap. PLoS Med. 2014;11:e1001603.
20. Leeflang MM, Debets-Ossenkopp YJ, Visser CE, et al. Galactomannan detection for invasive aspergillosis in immunocompromised patients. Cochrane Database Syst Rev. 2008;(4):CD007394.
21. Leeflang MM, Debets-Ossenkopp YJ, Wang J, et al. Galactomannan detection for invasive aspergillosis in immunocompromised patients. Cochrane Database Syst Rev. 2015;(12):CD007394.
22. Virgili G, Menchini F, Murro V, Peluso E, Rosa F, Casazza G. Optical coherence tomography (OCT) for detection of macular oedema in patients with diabetic retinopathy. Cochrane Database Syst Rev. 2011;(7):CD008081.
23. Virgili G, Menchini F, Casazza G, et al. Optical coherence tomography (OCT) for detection of macular oedema in patients with diabetic retinopathy. Cochrane Database Syst Rev. 2015;1:CD008081.
24. Theron G, Peter J, Richardson M, et al. The diagnostic accuracy of the GenoType((R)) MTBDRsl assay for the detection of resistance to second-line anti-tuberculosis drugs. Cochrane Database Syst Rev. 2014;(10):CD010705.

25. Theron G, Peter J, Richardson M, Warren R, Dheda K, Steingart KR. GenoType(R) MTBDRsl assay for resistance to second-line anti-tuberculosis drugs. Cochrane Database Syst Rev. 2016;9:CD010705.
26. Allen VB, Gurusamy KS, Takwoingi Y, Kalia A, Davidson BR. Diagnostic accuracy of laparoscopy following computed tomography (CT) scanning for assessing the resectability with curative intent in pancreatic and periampullary cancer. Cochrane Database Syst Rev. 2013;(11):CD009323.
27. Allen VB, Gurusamy KS, Takwoingi Y, Kalia A, Davidson BR. Diagnostic accuracy of laparoscopy following computed tomography (CT) scanning for assessing the resectability with curative intent in pancreatic and periampullary cancer. Cochrane Database Syst Rev. 2016;7:CD009323.

Part III

16 Diagnostic Meta-Analysis: Case Study in Endocrinology

Kosma Wolinski

16.1 Introduction

The case study in endocrinology is overview of meta-analyses assessing the methods of differential diagnostics of benign and malignant thyroid lesions. Thyroid nodular goiter is a very common endocrine pathology, according to some studies present even in over a half of adult population. The risk of malignancy is assessed to be about 5%, so relatively small, however noticeable [1]. Differentiation between the lesions being at high risk of malignancy needing surgical treatment and benign ones is crucial. The main diagnostic tools are ultrasonography and fine-needle biopsy of selected nodules.

16.2 The Case Study 1: Comparison of the Diagnostic Value of Core-Needle and Fine-Needle Aspiration Biopsies of Thyroid Lesions

This chapter is based on the study "Comparison of diagnostic yield of core-needle and fine-needle aspiration biopsies of thyroid lesions: Systematic review and meta-analysis" [2].

16.2.1 Background

The cytological assessment of specimens obtained in fine-needle aspiration biopsy (FNAB) remains the most important tool in the diagnostics of sonographically suspicious thyroid lesions and presurgical assessment of the character of the lesions. Most important limitation of the method is significant proportion of nondiagnostic results.

K. Wolinski
Department of Endocrinology, Metabolism and Internal Medicine,
Poznan University of Medical Sciences, Poznań, Poland

G. Biondi-Zoccai (ed.), *Diagnostic Meta-Analysis*,
https://doi.org/10.1007/978-3-319-78966-8_16

According to numerous studies, 10–20% of biopsies gain nondiagnostic results [3–6]. Furthermore, lesions with the nondiagnostic result of the initial FNAB are at a very high risk of repetitive nondiagnostic result [7]. These diagnostic difficulties can lead on one hand to unnecessary thyroidectomies in patients with lesions finally diagnosed as benign and on the other hand to the delay of treatment in patients with thyroid malignancies. One of investigated ways to improve the cytological diagnosis is biopsy with the use of core needles (core needle biopsy (CNB))—needles with larger diameter, containing the inner stylet which can be removed just in the nodule. On the other hand, the larger diameter also favors the aspiration of liquids being under high pressure, such as blood in the arteries or liquid contained in cystic components of the lesions [7, 8]. Results of particular studies were discrepant, and CNB does not establish place in the guidelines concerning diagnostic of thyroid cancer [10].

16.2.2 Methods

The following databases had been searched: PubMed/MEDLINE, Cochrane Library, Scopus, Cinahl, Academic Search Complete, Web of Knowledge, PubMed Central, PubMed Central Canada, and ClinicalKey. The databases had been searched by two researchers independently. The search term was (("core-needle") or (core and needle)) and thyroid. We have limited our search to studies written in English and published between January 2001 and December 2014.

16.2.2.1 Inclusion and Exclusion Criteria

The most important criterion for the inclusion was comparison of the diagnostic effectiveness of FNAB and CNB; we have accepted papers with the studied group composed of subjects who underwent CNB and control group undergoing FNAB, as well as the studies in which FNAB and CNB were performed simultaneously in the same thyroid lesions (if percentage of diagnostic FNABs and CNBs was given separately). Another criterion was sonographic guidance of both types of biopsies. Exclusion criteria included studies concerned on characteristic types of thyroid lesions (e.g., follicular tumors only). All included studies were assessed using Newcastle-Ottawa scale. Studies on the topic of effectiveness of CNB but not meeting all criteria (e.g., without control group or comparing simultaneous FNAB + CNB versus the FNAB itself) were collected in separate table as part of broader systematic review of the studies.

16.2.2.2 The Data Synthesis

Results of the biopsy described as nondiagnostic or—in newer studies—Bethesda category I [3] were interpreted as nondiagnostic. Biopsies with different, particular cytological diagnoses (older studies) or Bethesda categories II–VI were interpreted as diagnostic including categories III and IV, which are inconclusive results in context of differentiation between benign and malignant lesions but assessed as adequate for cytological assessment—so apart from the clinical doubts, the quality of obtained sample is satisfying.

Risk ratios (RRs) of nondiagnostic result were meta-analyzed using random-effect model. Publication bias was assessed using Kendall's tau. We decided to perform the quantitative synthesis in steps—initially to meta-analyze results of all included studies comparing the percentage of nondiagnostic FNABs and CNBs and then to perform some analyses in subgroups—e.g., nodules with one previous nondiagnostic of FNAB.

16.2.3 Results

Eleven studies were included to the quantitative synthesis [7, 11–20]. Steps of literature selection are shown at Fig. 16.1; studies included to the meta-analysis are summarized in Table 16.1.

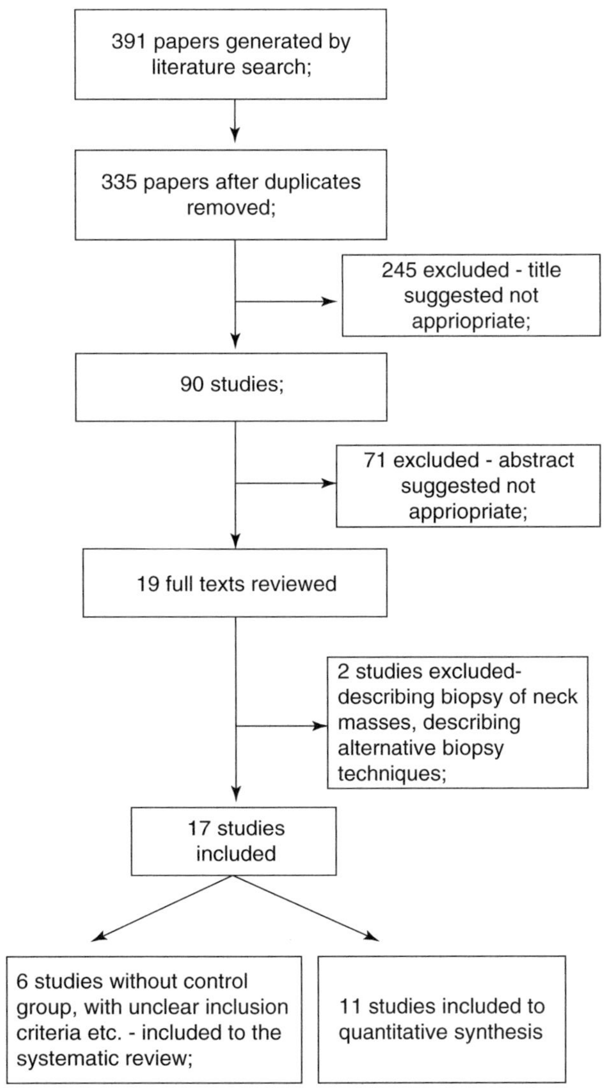

Fig. 16.1 Flowchart presenting steps of literature search and selection. Adapted from: Wolinski K et al. Comparison of diagnostic yield of core-needle and fine-needle aspiration biopsies of thyroid lesions: Systematic review and meta-analysis. Eur Radiol. 2017; 27: 431–436

Table 16.1 Studies comparing the diagnostic efficacy of CNB and FNAB in the diagnostics of thyroid lesions

Author	Year	Country	Design	Needles	FNAB – diagn.	FNAB – ndg.	CNB – diagn.	CNB – ndg.
Chen et al. [12]	2014	USA	Retrospective; no specific selection criteria—FNAB and CNB interchangeably dependent on the preference of the radiologist	FN, 25–27 G; CN, 20 G, semiautomatic biopsy device	70	26	359	6
Choi et al. [13]	2014	South Korea	Retrospective, lesions with previous ndg.	FNA, 21–23 G; CN – 18 G; automatic biopsy gun used	108	72	178	2
Lee et al. [14]	2014	South Korea	Retrospective, lesions with previous ndg.	FN, no data; CN, 18 G; automatic biopsy gun used	260	129	122	3
Stangierski et al. [7]	2013	Poland	Prospective, lesions with previous ndg.	FN, 25 G; CN, 22 G	30	29	17	13
Na et al. [15]	2012	South Korea	Prospective, FNAB and CNB simultaneously, lesions with previous ndg.	FN, 25, 23, and 21 G; CN, 18 G; automatic biopsy gun used	46	18	63	1
Samir et al. [16]	2012	USA	Retrospective, FNAB and CNB simultaneously, lesions with previous ndg.	CB, 20 G; FN, 25 G	42 (36)[a]	48 (33)[a]	69 (51)[a]	21 (18)[a]
Sung et al. [17]	2012	South Korea	Retrospective, FNAB and CNB simultaneously	CN, 18 G; FN, 21, 23, and 25 G; automatic biopsy gun used	521	34	547	8
Park et al. [18]	2011	South Korea	Retrospective, lesions with previous ndg. FNAB	CN, 18 G; FN, no data; automatic biopsy gun used	73	69	53	1
Renshaw et al. [11]	2007	USA	Retrospective, CNB and FNAB simultaneously—lesions with previous ndg. FNAB and also as first choice	FN – 25, 23 and 21 G; CN, 18, 20, 21 G	265	112	310	67

Author	Year	Country	Design	Needles	FNAB – diagn.	FNAB – ndg.	CNB – diagn.	CNB – ndg.
Strauss et al. [19]	2007	USA	CNB and FNAB—lesions with previous ndg. FNAB	CN, 20 G; FN, 22, 25 G	22	59	43	38
Karstrup et al. [20]	2001	Denmark	Palpable lesions only, FNAB and CNB simultaneously	CN, 18 G; automatic biopsy gun used; FN, 21 G	75	2	68	9

Abbreviations: *FN* fine needle, *CN* core needle, *FNAB* fine needle aspiration biopsy, *CNB* core needle biopsy, *diagn.* diagnostic results, *ndg.* nondiagnostic results

Adapted from: Wolinski K, Stangierski A, Ruchala M. Comparison of diagnostic yield of core-needle and fine-needle aspiration biopsies of thyroid lesions: Systematic review and meta-analysis. Eur Radiol. 2017; 27: 431–436

[a]Results for lesions with only one prior nondiagnostic biopsy were included

The pooled RR of gaining the nondiagnostic result using CNB was 0.27 with 95% confidence interval (CI) 0.16–0.46 ($p < 0.0001$). There was no evidence for publication bias (Kendall's tau = −0.24, two-tailed p-value = 0.31); however, heterogeneity was significant ($Q = 85.3$, df = 10, $i^2 = 88.3\%$, $p < 0.0001$). The forest plot for all studies is shown in Fig. 16.2.

Seven studies focused on lesions with one previous nondiagnostic result of FNAB [7, 13–19]. The pooled RR of gaining nondiagnostic result using CNB was 0.22 (95% CI 0.10–0.45, $p = 0.0001$). There is no evidence for publication bias (Kendall's tau = −0.33, two-tailed p-value = 0.29); however, heterogeneity was significant ($Q = 47.5$, df = 6, $i^2 = 87.37\%$, $p < 0.0001$). The forest plot is shown on Fig. 16.3.

Four studies from the same territory (South Korea) were performed with very similar methodology [13–15, 18]. Lesions with one previous nondiagnostic FNAB were included; in all studies, the same system for CNB was used. For these studies pooled RR was 0.05 (95% CI 0.02–0.10, $p < 0.0001$), without publication bias (Kendall's tau = 0.0, two-tailed p-value = 1.0) nor significant heterogeneity ($Q = 1.2$, df = 3, $i^2 = 0.0\%$, $p = 0.76$).

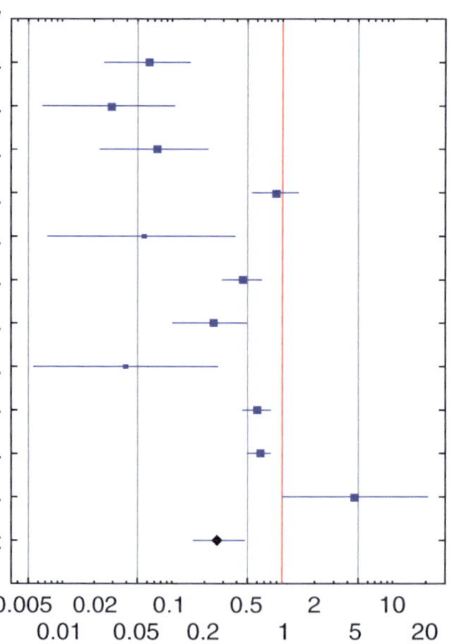

Study	RR	5%CI	95% CI	*p*-value
Chen et al.	0.06	(0.03	0.14)	0.0000
Choi et al.	0.03	(0.01	0.11)	0.0000
Lee et al.	0.07	(0.02	0.22)	0.0000
Stangierski et al.	0.88	(0.54	1.43)	0.6103
Na et al.	0.06	(0.01	0.40)	0.0043
Samir et al.	0.44	(0.29	0.67)	0.0001
Sung et al.	0.24	(0.11	0.50)	0.0002
Park et al.	0.04	(0.01	0.27)	0.0010
Renshaw et al.	0.60	(0.46	0.78)	0.0002
Strauss et al.	0.64	(0.49	0.84)	0.0012
Karstrup et al.	4.50	(1.00	20.15)	0.0493
Pool result	0.27	(0.16	0.46)	0.0000

Fig. 16.2 Forest plot presenting particular and pool results of the studies comparing the diagnostic effectiveness of core- and fine-needle aspiration biopsies. Adapted from: Wolinski K et al. Comparison of diagnostic yield of core-needle and fine-needle aspiration biopsies of thyroid lesions: Systematic review and meta-analysis. Eur Radiol. 2017; 27: 431–436

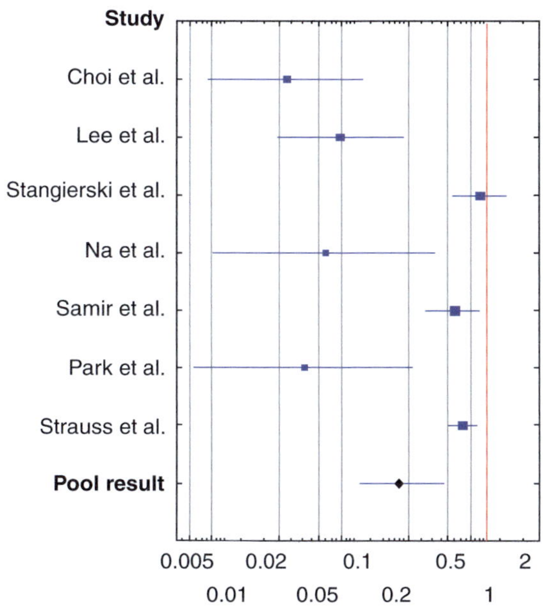

Study	RR	5%CI	95% CI	*p*-value
Choi et al.	0.03	(0.01	0.11)	0.0000
Lee et al.	0.07	(0.02	0.22)	0.0000
Stangierski et al.	0.88	(0.54	1.43)	0.6103
Na et al.	0.06	(0.01	0.40)	0.0043
Samir et al.	0.55	(0.34	0.87)	0.0110
Park et al.	0.04	(0.01	0.27)	0.0010
Strauss et al.	0.64	(0.49	0.84)	0.0012
Pool result	0.22	(0.10	0.45)	0.0001

Fig. 16.3 Forest plot presenting particular and pool results of studies comparing diagnostic effectiveness of core- and fine-needle aspiration biopsies (FNAB) in lesions with one previous nondiagnostic result of FNAB. Adapted from: Wolinski K et al. Comparison of diagnostic yield of core-needle and fine-needle aspiration biopsies of thyroid lesions: Systematic review and meta-analysis. Eur Radiol. 2017; 27: 431–436

16.2.4 Discussion

The study aimed to evaluate the risk of nondiagnostic result using FNAB and CNB. According to the results, CNB brings significantly lower risk of such results with RR equal to 0.27. What is more, in case of the lesions with one previous nondiagnostic result of FNAB, the RR of repeating the result is even lower (0.22).

It is worth to notice that in fact the term "core needle biopsy" describes rather the family of similar techniques than one unified procedure; there is a great variety of equipment used in case of the technique—from quite simple needles which differ from conventional fine needles according to larger diameter and presence of removable inner stylet [7] to more sophisticated, but also invasive, automatic biopsy guns [13, 14]. Secondly, apart from the construction, core needles and also fine needles used in particular included studies differed regarding the diameter. For example, Stangierski et al. [7] used 22 G and 25 G needles, respectively, Samir et al. [16] used 20 G and 25 G needles respectively, and Lee et al. [14] used 18 G core needles; details about fine needles were not given. In consequence, the significant heterogeneity of the meta-analysis of all included studies is not surprising. Sub-analyses limited to studies performed with similar methodology brought more homogenous outcomes.

The amount of the available studies is at the moment not sufficient to perform the cost-effectiveness analysis and also to include the aspect of pain and patients' tolerability of the procedure in quantitative way. However, the meta-analysis presented above constitutes the proof that CNB is a more effective diagnostic method than FNAB and should be considered especially in case of thyroid lesions with previous nondiagnostic result of FNAB.

16.3 The Case Study 2: Sonographic Markers of Malignancy—Report on the Diagnostic Meta-Analysis

This chapter is based on the study "Usefulness of different ultrasound features of malignancy in predicting the type of thyroid lesions: a meta-analysis of prospective studies" [21].

16.3.1 Background

The problem addressed in this study is in fact one step before the issue of biopsy described above. Thyroid nodules constitute extremely common problem in everyday practice of endocrinologists as—according to different studies—they are present in 30–70% of the adult population [1]. What is more, numerous patients have multinodular goiter where the number of lesions can be high. Due to the relatively small risk of malignancy [1, 22], biopsy as—all in all—invasive procedure is not needed in every patient with thyroid lesions; on the other hand, in patients with multinodular goiter, biopsy of every nodule can be very difficult or just impossible, at least during the single visit [10, 23, 24]. Assessment if the biopsy is needed and—in case of patients with multinodular goiter—which lesions should underwent the biopsy and which should be single constitutes a vital issue. Thyroid ultrasonography (US) constitutes the most common and reliable method of preliminary diagnostics of thyroid lesions [21, 25]. Numerous sonographic features—so-called sonographic markers of malignancy—had been described as characteristic for the malignant lesions [21, 24]. The aim of the study was to assess which of the sonographic markers are increasing the risk of malignant character of the lesions and to assess the diagnostic value of particular features.

16.3.2 Materials and Methods

The PubMed/MEDLINE and Cochrane Library had been searched. The databases had been searched by two researchers independently. The search term was thyroid cancer *or* thyroid nodules and ultrasound *or* ultrasonography *or* elastography *or* "power Doppler" or "color Doppler." We have limited our search to studies written in English and published between January 2007 and February 2013.

16.3.2.1 Inclusion and Exclusion Criteria

Studies comparing the prevalence of sonographic features in benign and malignant thyroid nodules were included.

Exclusion criteria:

- Studies conducted before 2002 and performed with the use of a transducer with the frequency of less than 7.5 MHz have been excluded from the quantitative synthesis; the aim of these limitations was to avoid underestimation of the diagnostic value of US malignancy markers, which could result from taking into account older studies, performed with lower-quality equipment.
- Researches in which the diagnosis of malignant, or suspicious, nodules was based only on cytopathology, without further histopathological examination and final differentiation between malignant and benign ones.
- Studies focusing on particular subgroups of subjects (e.g., surgical or pediatric patients only), or particular kinds of nodules (e.g., subcentimeter, palpable, pure cystic or mixed, etc.)

16.3.2.2 The Data Synthesis

ORs and RRs were calculated using a random-effect model using Statistica v10 software with medical package. T^2 and i^2 values given in Sect. 16.3.3 are based on the odds ratio calculations. Quantitative synthesis was performed if at least free studies assessing particular marker of malignancy were available. Pooled sensitivities, specificities, positive (PPV) and negative predictive values (NPV) of particular markers of malignancy were calculated using a random-effect model according to the methodology described by Borenstein et al. [9].

16.3.3 Results

Fourteen studies had been included to meta-analysis. These studies encompassed 5439 thyroid lesions—4712 benign nodules and 727 cancers. Steps of literature selection are shown on Fig. 16.4. Included studies are summarized in Table 16.2.

16.3.3.1 Calculations for Particular Markers of Malignancy

Microcalcifications

Thirteen of fourteen meta-analyzed studies provided data on the frequency of microcalcifications, amounting to 5308 nodules (718 malignant, 13.5%). The pooled OR equalled 7.1 (95% confidence interval (CI) 4.3–11.9); RR, 3.8 (95% CI 3.0–5.0); sensitivity, 44.1% (95% CI, 37.9–51.3%); and specificity, 75.9% (95% CI, 70.3–82.0%). PPV is 42.3% (95% CI 33.6–53.3%). There was no evidence of significant heterogeneity (Q = 10.3, degrees of freedom (df) = 12, p-value = 0.59, i^2 = 0.0%) or publication bias (Kendall's tau = 0.15, two-tailed p-value = 0.46).

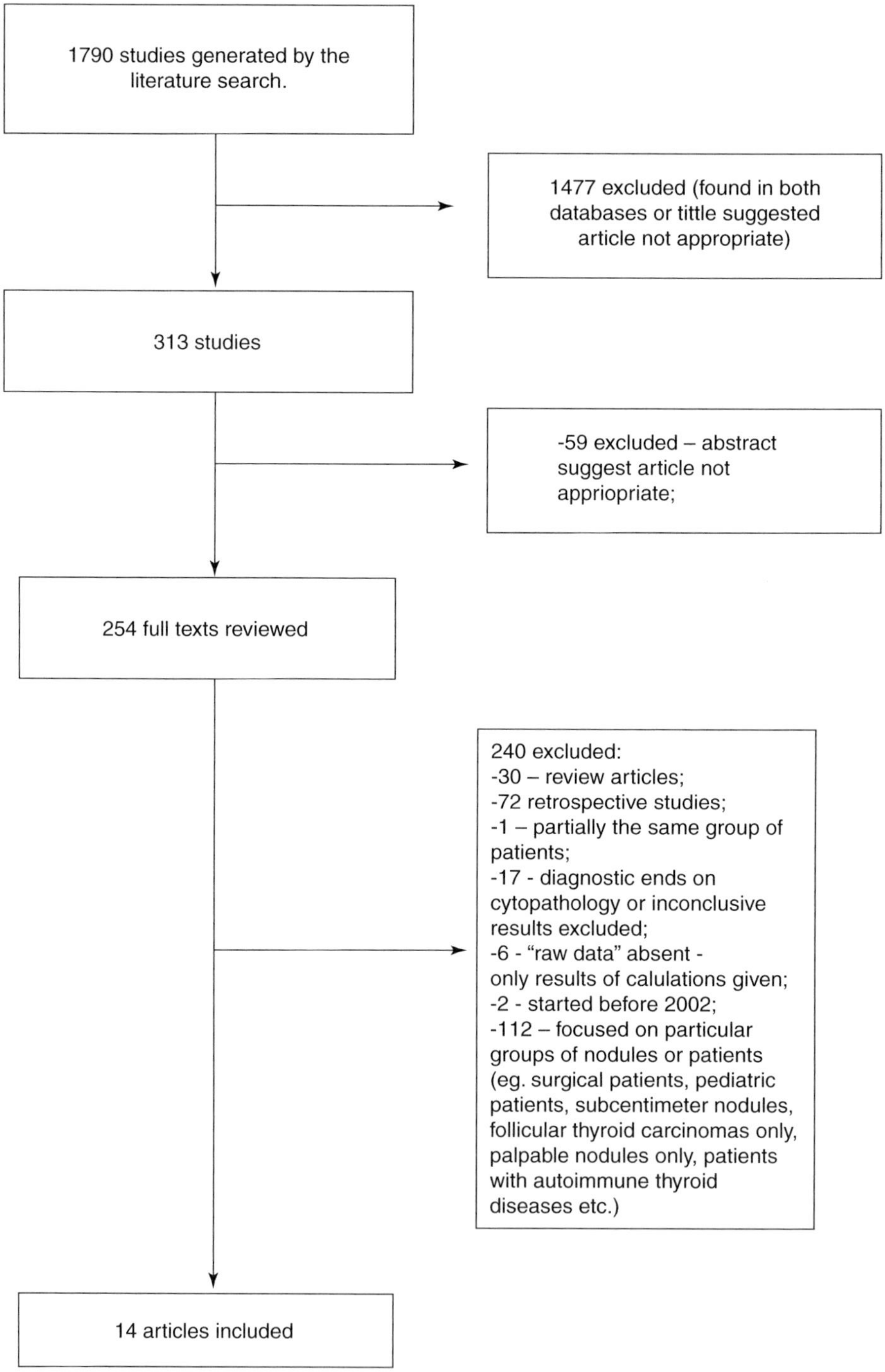

Fig. 16.4 Flowchart presenting steps of literature search and selection. Adapted from: Woliński K et al. Usefulness of different ultrasound features of malignancy in predicting the type of thyroid lesions: a meta-analysis of prospective studies. Pol Arch Med Wewn. 2014; 124: 97–104

Table 16.2 The main characteristics of studies included in meta-analysis

Author	Year	Patients	Mean age (years)	Nodules	Malignancies
Azizi et al. [31]	2012	706	Women, 48.5; men, 47.7	912	86
Bojunga et al. [32]	2012	99 women, 39 men	52.0	158	21
Rossi et al. [33]	2012	1439 women, 417 men	52	2421	233
Trimboli et al. [34]	2012	438 women, 138 men	53.0	498	126
Bhatia et al. [35]	2011	89 patients[a]	Not given	89	19
Merino et al. [36]	2011	89 women, 14 men	58	106	10
Ünlütürk et al. [37]	2011	157 women, 37 men	Women, 43.7; men, 47.5	237	58
D'Souza et al. [38]	2010	151 women, 49 men	Not given (range 8–74)	200	26
Friedrich-Rust et al. [39]	2010	37 women, 13 men	Women, 54; men, 52	53	7
Gietka-Czernel et al. [26]	2010	42 women, 10 men	45	71	22
Yunus et al. [40]	2010	58 women, 8 men	Not given (range 18–75)	78	25
Asteria et al. [27]	2008	54 women, 12 men	Women, 51.3; men, 60.5	86	17
Brunese et al. [41]	2008	264 women, 79 men	41.2	479	66
Rubaltelli et al. [42]	2008	25 women, 15 men	55	51	11

Adapted from: Woliński K et al. Usefulness of different ultrasound features of malignancy in predicting the type of thyroid lesions: a meta-analysis of prospective studies. Pol Arch Med Wewn. 2014; 124: 97–104

[a]After exclusion of metastases

Hypoechogenicity

Eleven studies provided data on the frequency of hypoechogenicity (5179 nodules including 682 malignant). The pooled OR was 3.2 (95% CI 2.3–4.5); RR, 2.5 (2.0–3.1); sensitivity, 68.7% (95% CI 58.8–82.6%); and specificity, 60.3% (95% CI 53.4–68.2%). PPV is 25.2% (95% CI 17.6–36.2%). There was no evidence of significant heterogeneity ($Q = 16.7$, df = 10, p-value = 0.08, $i^2 = 39.9\%$) or publication bias (Kendall's tau = 0.35, two-tailed p-value = 0.14).

16.3.3.2 Irregular Margins

Thirteen studies provided data on the frequency of irregular margins (5296 nodules, 707 malignant). The pooled OR is 7.2 (95% CI 4.5–11.5); RR, 4.1 (95% CI 3.1–5.5); sensitivity, 45.5% (95% CI 30.9–66.9%); and specificity, 79.6% (95% CI 71.9–88.2%). PPV is 40.4% (95% CI 29.9–54.7%). There was no evidence of significant heterogeneity ($Q = 12.9$, df = 12, p-value = 0.38, $i^2 = 7.1\%$) or publication bias (Kendall's tau = 0.03, two-tailed p-value = 0.90).

16.3.3.3 Elastography

Ten studies provided data on lesion stiffness graded according to elastography scores (2233 nodules, 367 malignant). The pooled OR is 10.5 (95% CI 6.4–17.2); RR, 6.0 (95% CI 4.2–8.6); sensitivity, 74.1% (95% CI 57.7–95.3%); and specificity, 69.7% (95% CI 62.8–77.2%). PPV is 37.2% (95% CI 28.4–48.7%). There was no evidence of significant heterogeneity ($Q = 13.4$, df = 9, p-value = 0.15, $i^2 = 32.9\%$). The publication bias turned out to be significant (Kendell's tau = 0.64, two-tailed p-value = 0.01). Apparently, two studies based on the smallest groups and presenting the highest study variances [26, 27] report outstanding results (OR 68.9 and 190, respectively). After the exclusion of these papers, the following results were obtained: OR 7.9 (95% CI 5.6–11.2), RR 5.4 (95% CI 3.8–7.5), sensitivity 73.3% (95% CI 56.6–95.0%), specificity 69.3% (95% CI 62.4–76.9%), and PPV 35.2% (26.5–46.7%). This step also eliminated the publication bias—Kendell's tau = 0.43, two-tailed p-value = 0.14.

16.3.3.4 "Taller than Wide"

Three studies provided data on the frequency of the "taller-than-wide" feature (665 nodules, 170 malignant). The pooled OR was 13.7 (95% CI 4.1–45.7); RR, 3.9 (95% CI 2.5–5.9); sensitivity, 25.9% (95% CI 12.1–55.3%); and specificity, 95.9% (95% CI 48.3–100.0%). PPV is 76.0% (95% CI 35.0–100.0%). There was no evidence of significant heterogeneity ($Q = 2.4$, df = 2, p-value = 0.30, $i^2 = 17.3\%$) or publication bias (Kendell's tau = 0.33, two-tailed p-value = 0.60).

16.3.3.5 Halo Absence

Four studies provided data on the halo absence frequency (648 nodules, 112 malignant). The pooled OR was 3.8 (95% CI 1.7–8.5); RR, 3.0 (95% CI 1.5–6.0); sensitivity, 63.8% (95% CI 38.1–100.0%); specificity, 47.5% (95% CI 33.4–67.8%); and PPV, 23.5% (95% CI 15.6–35.6%). There was no evidence of significant heterogeneity ($Q = 3.4$, df = 3, p-value = 0.33, $i^2 = 10.7\%$) or publication bias (Kendell's tau = −0.33, two-tailed p-value = 0.50).

16.3.3.6 Color Doppler Examination

Three studies provided data on the frequency of intranodular flow in color Doppler examination (1048 nodules, 214 malignant). The pooled OR was 4.3 (95% CI 3.1–6.1); RR, 2.6 (95% CI 1.6–4.0); sensitivity, 44.2% (95% CI 33.6–58.2%); specificity, 81.5% (95% CI 67.8–98.0%); and PPV, 41.3% (95% CI 28.4–60.2%). There was no evidence of significant heterogeneity ($Q = 1.8$, df = 2, p-value = 0.41, $i^2 = 0.0\%$) or publication bias (Kendell's tau with continuity correction = 0.0, two-tailed p-value = 1.0).

16.3.3.7 Power Doppler: Pattern 3 Flow (Intensive Central with Lower Peripheral Blood Flow)

Six studies provided data on the frequency of pattern 3 flow in power Doppler examination (1419 nodules, 204 malignant). The pooled OR was 2.6 (95% CI 0.8–8.3), and the result was statistically insignificant. There was no evidence for significant heterogeneity ($Q = 5.9$, df = 5, p-value = 0.32, $i^2 = 15.2\%$) or publication bias (Kendall's tau = 0.2, two-tailed p-value = 0.57).

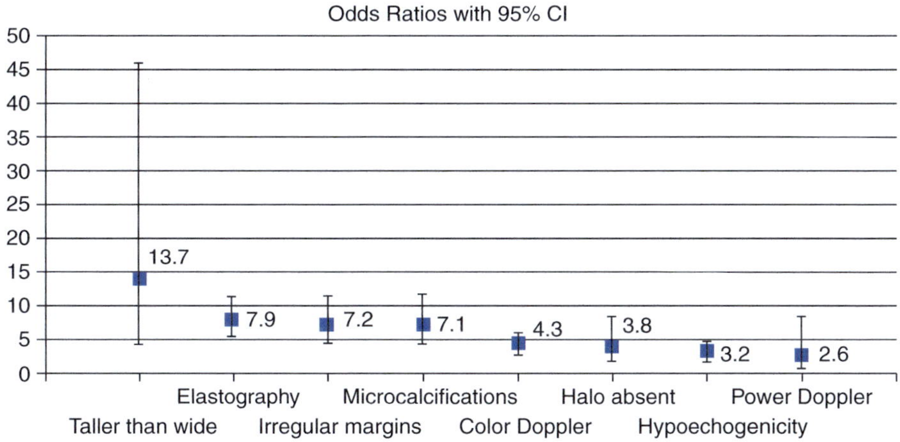

Fig. 16.5 Pooled odds ratios with 95% confidence intervals for analyzed sonographic markers of malignancy. Adapted from: Woliński K et al. Usefulness of different ultrasound features of malignancy in predicting the type of thyroid lesions: a meta-analysis of prospective studies. Pol Arch Med Wewn. 2014; 124: 97–104

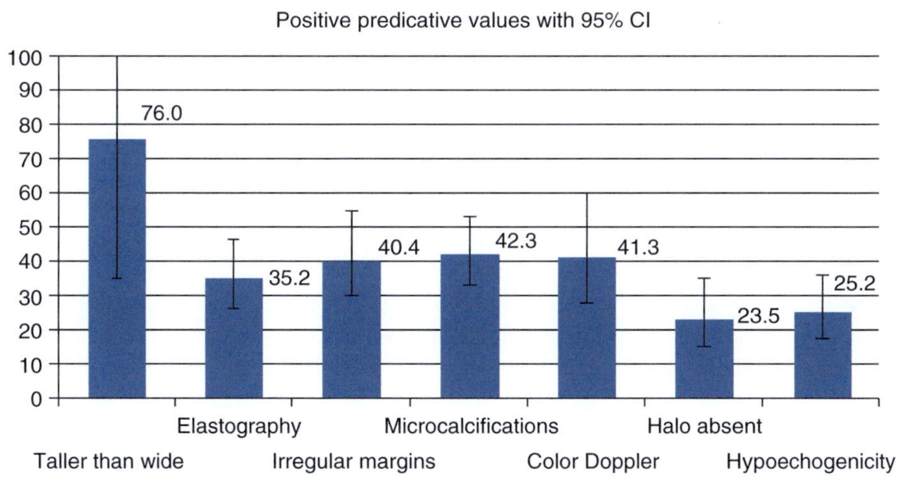

Fig. 16.6 Pooled positive predictive values of significant sonographic markers of malignancy with 95% confidence intervals. Adapted from: Woliński K et al. Usefulness of different ultrasound features of malignancy in predicting the type of thyroid lesions: a meta-analysis of prospective studies. Pol Arch Med Wewn. 2014; 124: 97–104

ORs and PPVs are summarized at Figs. 16.5 and 16.6.

16.3.4 Discussion

To our knowledge, the presented study comprised the first quantitative synthesis of the data on sonographic markers of malignancy. The study confirmed diagnostic value of most features considered as markers of malignancy; it also enabled to assess the clinical importance of particular features and to rank them or—at least—divide into categories depending on their clinical significance. Low elasticity of the lesions assessed in elastography, microcalcifications, irregular borders, and finally characteristic disproportion of the nodules' shape—anterior-posterior dimension visibly larger than lateral—so-called taller-than-wide feature can be interpreted as strong risk factors; central blood flow in color Doppler examination, hypoechogenicity, and lack of so-called halo (thin hypoechoic rim) could be interpreted as intermediate risk factors; type 3 flow in power Doppler examination is a doubtful marker without significantly increased risk in context of our results.

Particular markers of malignancy have different clinical characteristics; some of them are characterized with low sensitivity but very high specificity and extremely high positive prognostic value; such features—if present—should arise very high suspicion of malignancy and strong indication for further diagnostics. Other ones are more sensitive but less specific, quite common also in benign lesions. The aim of the study was to provide comprehensive characteristics of particular sonographic markers of malignancy—this is why not only ORs and RRs but also sensitivities, specificities, and positive predictive values had been meta-analyzed.

In this context the taller-than-wide feature turned out to be the most suggestive marker of malignancy; despite the low sensitivity, 76.0% of lesions possessing this feature turned out to be malignant. Oppositely, e.g., hypoechogenicity had relatively high sensitivity; however, the risk of malignancy in case of lesions possessing the feature was 25.2%.

The main limitation of the study was relatively small amount of included studies and—subsequently—quite broad confidence intervals. Partially it was the consequence of relatively strict inclusion and exclusion criteria. Another meta-analysis published at similar time by Brito et al. [28] had less strict exclusion criteria, and the number of included studies was much higher—31. The largest group of studies excluded from our meta-analysis were studies describing results of presurgical ultrasonography in patients referred for thyroidectomy. First methodological doubt is the fact that suspicious sonographic appearance can be one of reasons for the decision about the surgery; there can be some preselection of nodules with sonographic markers of malignancy. But what seems to be more important, the risk of malignancy in patients with nodular goiter is—according to most authors—about 5–10% [1]; in our meta-analysis, it was slightly higher than expected—about 13%. In studies concerning patients referred for the total thyroidectomy, the risk of malignancy is much higher—in most studies over 30% [29, 30]. These groups differ, and especially calculations of parameters strongly dependent on the prevalence of pathology (in this context—thyroid cancer) such as positive predictive value would not be reliable.

Another problem was that—probably due to large number of suggested sonographic markers—only few of the included studies described comprehensive panel of markers; most of them omitted some of them, also definitions and classification of particular markers were differed between studies (e.g., some studies described micro- and macrocalcifications separately, some of them just "calcifications"). In consequence, 13 studies contained data on the presence of microcalcifications, but only three assessed the taller-than-wide feature.

To conclude, however, the markers of malignancy cannot allow for fully reliable differentiation between benign and malignant thyroid lesions; they constitute valuable tool for the initial assessment of thyroid nodules and the decision for FNAB. As numerous studies on the topic are being published every year, it will be also interesting to perform similar meta-analysis after few years in order to achieve more reliable outcomes, based on larger numbers of included researches.

References

1. Tan GH, Gharib H. Thyroid incidentalomas: management approaches to nonpalpable nodules discovered incidentally on thyroid imaging. Ann Intern Med. 1997;126:226–31.
2. Wolinski K, Stangierski A, Ruchala M. Comparison of diagnostic yield of core-needle and fine-needle aspiration biopsies of thyroid lesions: systematic review and meta-analysis. Eur Radiol. 2017;27:431–6.
3. Cibas ES, Ali SZ, NCI Thyroid FNA State of the Science Conference. The Bethesda system for reporting thyroid cytopathology. Am J Clin Pathol. 2009;132:658–65.
4. Baier ND, Hahn PF, Gervais DA, et al. Fine-needle aspiration biopsy of thyroid nodules: experience in a cohort of 944 patients. AJR Am J Roentgenol. 2009;193:1175–9.
5. Zhong LC, Lu F, Ma F, et al. Ultrasound-guided fine-needle aspiration of thyroid nodules: does the size limit its efficiency? Int J Clin Exp Pathol. 2015;8:3155–9.
6. Seningen JL, Nassar A, Henry MR. Correlation of thyroid nodule fine-needle aspiration cytology with corresponding histology at Mayo Clinic, 2001–2007: an institutional experience of 1,945 cases. Diagn Cytopathol. 2012;40:E27–32.
7. Stangierski A, Wolinski K, Martin K, Leitgeber O, Ruchala M. Core needle biopsy of thyroid nodules—evaluation of diagnostic utility and pain experience. Neuro Endocrinol Lett. 2013;34:798–801.
8. Woliński K, Stangierski A, Szczepanek-Parulska E, Gurgul E, Wrotkowska E, Biczysko M, Ruchała M. Content of RNA originating from thyroid in washouts from fine-needle and core-needle aspiration biopsy—preliminary study. Endokrynol Pol. 2016;67:550–3.
9. Borenstein M, Hedges LV, Higgins JPT, Rothstein HR. Introduction to meta-analysis. Chichester: Wiley; 2009.
10. Haugen BR, Alexander EK, Bible KC, Doherty GM, Mandel SJ, Nikiforov YE, Pacini F, Randolph GW, Sawka AM, Schlumberger M, Schuff KG, Sherman SI, Sosa JA, Steward DL, Tuttle RM, Wartofsky L. 2015 American Thyroid Association management guidelines for adult patients with thyroid nodules and differentiated thyroid cancer: the American Thyroid Association guidelines task force on thyroid nodules and differentiated thyroid cancer. Thyroid. 2016;26:1–133.
11. Renshaw AA, Pinnar N. Comparison of thyroid fine-needle aspiration and core needle biopsy. Am J Clin Pathol. 2007;128:370–4.
12. Chen BT, Jain AB, Dagis A, et al. Comparison of efficacy and safety of ultrasound-guided core needle biopsy versus fine needle aspiration for evaluating thyroid nodules. Endocr Pract. 2015;21:128–35.
13. Choi SH, Baek JH, Lee JH, et al. Thyroid nodules with initially non-diagnostic, fine-needle aspiration results: comparison of core-needle biopsy and repeated fine-needle aspiration. Eur Radiol. 2014;24:2819–26.
14. Lee SH, Kim MH, Bae JS, et al. Clinical outcomes in patients with non-diagnostic thyroid fine needle aspiration cytology: usefulness of the thyroid core needle biopsy. Ann Surg Oncol. 2014;21:1870–7.

15. Na DG, Kim JH, Sung JY, et al. Core-needle biopsy is more useful than repeat fine-needle aspiration in thyroid nodules read as nondiagnostic or atypia of undetermined significance by the Bethesda system for reporting thyroid cytopathology. Thyroid. 2012;22:468–75.
16. Samir AE, Vij A, Seale MK, et al. Ultrasound-guided percutaneous thyroid nodule core biopsy: clinical utility in patients with prior nondiagnostic fine-needle aspirate. Thyroid. 2012;22:461–7.
17. Sung JY, Na DG, Kim KS, et al. Diagnostic accuracy of fine-needle aspiration versus core-needle biopsy for the diagnosis of thyroid malignancy in a clinical cohort. Eur Radiol. 2012;22:1564–72.
18. Park KT, Ahn SH, Mo JH, et al. Role of core needle biopsy and ultrasonographic finding in management of indeterminate thyroid nodules. Head Neck. 2011;33:160–5.
19. Strauss EB, Iovino A, Upender S. Simultaneous fine-needle aspiration and core biopsy of thyroid nodules and other superficial head and neck masses using sonographic guidance. AJR Am J Roentgenol. 2008;190:1697–9.
20. Karstrup S, Balslev E, Juul N, Eskildsen PC, Baumbach L. US-guided fine needle aspiration versus coarse needle biopsy of thyroid nodules. Eur J Ultrasound. 2001;13:1–5.
21. Woliński K, Szkudlarek M, Szczepanek-Parulska E, Ruchała M. Usefulness of different ultrasound features of malignancy in predicting the type of thyroid lesions: a meta-analysis of prospective studies. Pol Arch Med Wewn. 2014;124:97–104.
22. Pasqualetti G, Caraccio N, Basolo F, Miccoli P, Monzani F. Prevalence of thyroid cancer in multinodular goiter versus single nodule: iodine intake and cancer phenotypes. Thyroid. 2014;24:604–5.
23. Woliński K, Szczepanek-Parulska E, Stangierski A, Gurgul E, Rewaj-Łosyk M, Ruchała M. How to select nodules for fine-needle aspiration biopsy in multinodular goitre. Role of conventional ultrasonography and shear wave elastography—a preliminary study. Endokrynol Pol. 2014;65:114–8.
24. Szczepanek-Parulska E, Woliński K, Stangierski A, Gurgul E, Biczysko M, Majewski P, Rewaj-Łosyk M, Ruchała M. Comparison of diagnostic value of conventional ultrasonography and shear wave elastography in the prediction of thyroid lesions malignancy. PLoS One. 2013;8:e81532.
25. Ruchała M, Szczepanek E. Thyroid ultrasound—a piece of cake? Endokrynol Pol. 2010;61:330–44.
26. Gietka-Czernel M, Kochman M, Bujalska K, et al. Real-time ultrasound elastography—a new tool for diagnosing thyroid nodules. Endokrynol Pol. 2010;61:652–7.
27. Asteria C, Giovanardi A, Pizzocaro A, et al. US-elastography in the differential diagnosis of benign and malignant thyroid nodules. Thyroid. 2008;18:523–31.
28. Brito JP, Gionfriddo MR, Al Nofal A, Boehmer KR, Leppin AL, Reading C, Callstrom M, Elraiyah TA, Prokop LJ, Stan MN, Murad MH, Morris JC, Montori VM. The accuracy of thyroid nodule ultrasound to predict thyroid cancer: systematic review and meta-analysis. J Clin Endocrinol Metab. 2014;99:1253–63.
29. Salmaslioğlu A, Erbil Y, Dural C, Işsever H, Kapran Y, Ozarmağan S, Tezelman S. Predictive value of sonographic features in preoperative evaluation of malignant thyroid nodules in a multinodular goiter. World J Surg. 2008;32:1948–54.
30. Rago T, Santini F, Scutari M, Pinchera A, Vitti P. Elastography: new developments in ultrasound for predicting malignancy in thyroid nodules. J Clin Endocrinol Metab. 2007;92:2917–22.
31. Azizi G, Keller J, Lewis Pa M, et al. Performance of elastography for the evaluation of thyroid nodules: a prospective study. Thyroid. 2013;23:734–40.
32. Bojunga J, Dauth N, Berner C, et al. Acoustic radiation force impulse imaging for differentiation of thyroid nodules. PLoS One. 2012;7:e42735.
33. Rossi M, Buratto M, Bruni S, et al. Role of ultrasonographic/clinical profile, cytology, and BRAF V600E mutation evaluation in thyroid nodule screening for malignancy: a prospective study. J Clin Endocrinol Metab. 2012;97:2354–61.

34. Trimboli P, Guglielmi R, Monti S, et al. Ultrasound sensitivity for thyroid malignancy is increased by real-time elastography: a prospective multicenter study. J Clin Endocrinol Metab. 2012;97:4524–30.
35. Bhatia KS, Rasalkar DP, Lee YP, et al. Cystic change in thyroid nodules: a confounding factor for real-time qualitative thyroid ultrasound elastography. Clin Radiol. 2011;66:799–807.
36. Merino S, Arrazola J, Cárdenas A, et al. Utility and interobserver agreement of ultrasound elastography in the detection of malignant thyroid nodules in clinical care. AJNR Am J Neuroradiol. 2011;32:2142–8.
37. Unlütürk U, Erdoğan MF, Demir O, et al. Ultrasound elastography is not superior to grayscale ultrasound in predicting malignancy in thyroid nodules. Thyroid. 2012;22:1031–8.
38. D'Souza MM, Marwaha RK, Sharma R, et al. Prospective evaluation of solitary thyroid nodule on 18F-FDG PET/CT and high-resolution ultrasonography. Ann Nucl Med. 2010;24:345–55.
39. Friedrich-Rust M, Sperber A, Holzer K, et al. Real-time elastography and contrast enhanced ultrasound for the assessment of thyroid nodules. Exp Clin Endocrinol Diabetes. 2010;118:602–9.
40. Yunus M, Ahmed Z. Significance of ultrasound features in predicting malignant solid thyroid nodules: need for fine-needle aspiration. J Pak Med Assoc. 2010;60:848–53.
41. Brunese L, Romeo A, Iorio S, et al. A new marker for diagnosis of thyroid papillary cancer: B-flow twinkling sign. J Ultrasound Med. 2008;27:1187–94.
42. Rubaltelli L, Corradin S, Dorigo A, et al. Differential diagnosis of benign and malignant thyroid nodules at elastosonography. Ultraschall Med. 2009;30:175–9.

Diagnostic Meta-Analysis: Case Study in Gastroenterology

17

Bashar J. Qumseya and Michael Wallace

Abbreviations

AI	Advanced imaging
BE	Barrett's esophagus
CE	Chromoendoscopy
CI	Confidence interval
EAC	Esophageal adenocarcinoma
EMR	Endoscopic mucosal resection
EUS	Endoscopic ultrasound
HGD	High-grade dysplasia
LGD	Low-grade dysplasia
MA	Meta-analysis
QUADAS	Quality Assessment of Diagnostic Accuracy Studies
RD	Risk difference
RFA	Radiofrequency ablation
SR	Systematic review
VC	Virtual chromoendoscopy
WLE	White light endoscopy

B. J. Qumseya
Division of Gastroenterology and Hepatology, Archbold Medical Group/Florida State University, Thomasville, GA, USA
e-mail: bqumseya@archbold.org

M. Wallace (✉)
Division of Gastroenterology and Hepatology, Mayo Clinic, Jacksonville, FL, USA
e-mail: wallace.michael@mayo.edu

G. Biondi-Zoccai (ed.), *Diagnostic Meta-Analysis*,
https://doi.org/10.1007/978-3-319-78966-8_17

17.1 Introduction

As discussed in previous chapters, meta-analysis (MA) refers to the combination of results from different studies. The rationale for meta-analyses is simple. For many clinical outcomes, the effect of interest is uncertain when looking at multiple individual studies. Various studies may even show conflicting results leaving readers confused. It is common in medical literature to see the phrase, "results on this outcome are conflicting," or a similar phrase. With meta-analysis, we are able to gather existing results from various studies, compare the magnitude and direction of effect, and summarize the results in one number in many cases. This ability to look at the whole body of evidence is invaluable. Before meta-analyses, narrative reviews were common practice in medical literature. Such narrative reviews are still used today. In a narrative review, the authors use their best judgment and expertise to discuss the evidence on a particular outcome. MA, however, requires a systematic review of all available outcomes. This is then followed by careful synthesis and statistical analysis of the body of evidence across all studies. Clearly, the later approach is more superior and preferable.

If done correctly, meta-analysis can be a very powerful tool in synthesizing and presenting best evidence on a particular topic. Therefore, there has been a national trend toward evidence-based medicine. The Institute of Medicine and the National Guideline Clearinghouse now require all clinical guidelines to be evidence based. This includes a systematic review of evidence and meta-analysis of various clinical outcomes one possible. The three major GI societies in the USA are all moving toward evidence-based guidelines and away from narrative reviews.

As the influence of MA continues to grow, it is prudent for the average reader to be able to understand key concepts with regard to this type of studies. In this chapter we will try to shed light on some key issues related to meta-analyses. In doing so, we will use several recently published case studies of meta-analyses. The goal of this chapter is not to study every aspect of MA, but rather to focus on important challenges in conducting and understanding meta-analyses.

17.2 Background

The meta-analyses considered here are highly cited studies dealing with the several studies related to Barrett's esophagus (BE). Those studies were recently published and deal with various issues regarding this topic. BE is a change in the squamous epithelium of the esophagus columnar mucosa containing intestinal metaplasia (Fig. 17.1). BE is a major risk factor of esophageal adenocarcinoma (EAC). Studies have shown that BE appears to progress to EAC in a sequence events marked by low-grade dysplasia (LGD), high-grade dysplasia (HGD), and then EAC [1, 2]. While the risk of EAC is very low in patients with non-dysplastic BE (NDBE), the risk is significantly higher for patient with dysplasia [3, 4]. Dysplasia, however, is hard to detect on normal white light endoscopy (WLE) as it is often not very distinct. Therefore a standard biopsy protocol is recommended where four quadrants,

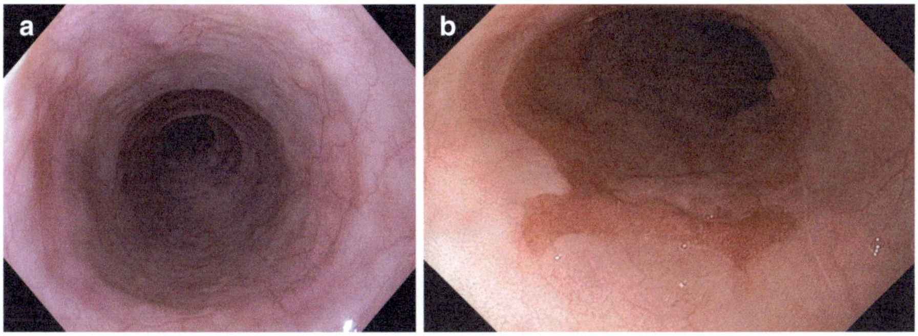

Fig. 17.1 (**a**) Normal view of the distal esophagus with pale/white epithelium typical of normal squamous cell lining; (**b**) Barrett's esophagus with salmon-colored mucosa extending into the distal esophagus. There is a sharp but irregular demarcation with the squamous cell lining

1–2 cm apart, are randomly biopsied throughout Barrett's segment (Seattle protocol). This method had been known to miss cases of dysplasia and neoplasia [5]. Hence, endoscopists have been trying to develop ways to detect dysplasia or early neoplasia, which can then be treated more effectively. Advanced imaging (AI) modalities offered a potential improvement to WLE. Chromoendoscopy (CE) refers to the use of various dyes to alter the surface color of the mucosa, which would allow better detection of dysplasia. Virtual chromoendoscopy (VC) achieves the same goal by employing light filters which are activated within the scope without the need to apply any dyes. The study by Qumseya et al. on AI for BE will be cited frequently in this chapter [6]. Another study will deal with the use of endoscopic ultrasound (EUS) for the detection of advanced disease in BE [7]. Similarly, we will also use the example of a study which focused on the use for radiofrequency ablation (RFA) for treatment of BE [8]. This study looked at rates and predictors of adverse outcomes after such treatment. Lastly, we will provide examples from the most recent study on low-grade dysplasia (LGD) in BE [9].

In this chapter, we will delve into some of the specifics of how these studies were done and the challenges of doing meta-analyses. Key features of those studies are included in Table 17.1. We hope that our examples will allow the reader to appreciate some of the key elements in meta-analyses and ways in which they have been addressed.

17.3 Inclusion and Exclusion Criteria

There are several key components of any MA. The process usually starts with a clinical outcome of interest. One of the most important next steps is to start with clear identification of the inclusion and exclusion criteria for studies to be included. These criteria will be described in the methods section of any MA and will detail the types of studies to be considered for the systematic review and specific criteria to be met for consideration. While most readers do not give much attention to these

Table 17.1 List of studies with key features

Topic	Author	Publication date	Meta-meter	Included retrospective studies	Included abstracts	Duplicate cohorts	Indirect comparisons
Advanced imaging in BE	Qumseya et al.	2013	Paired risk difference	No	No	3 with same author. Removed one at a time	No
EUS in BE	Qumseya et al.	2015	Proportion of patients with advanced disease on EUS	Yes	No	No	No
Adverse events post RFA	Qumseya et al.	2016	Risk of adverse outcomes (proportion)	Yes	Yes	US RFA registry (removed for sensitivity analysis)	Yes
LGD in BE	Qumseya et al.	2017	Relative risk of disease progression	Yes	Yes	Several studies removed for duplication	Yes

BE Barrett's esophagus, *RFA* radiofrequency ablation, *LGD* low-grade dysplasia, *EUS* endoscopic ultrasound

criteria, this is in fact one of the most consequential steps in a review. The decisions made at this point will have great effect on the results of the study. Additionally, these criteria will affect study quality and will likely alter decisions made downstream including choosing meta-meters of choice, heterogeneity, and publication bias.

As explained in previous chapters, before conducting a MA, one starts with a systematic review (SR). In a SR, the goal is to review all pertinent literature in a systematic and transparent method. The MA part then tries to summarize and compare effects between studies. Hence, the goal of the SR part is to be as inclusive as possible. Let us consider the example of the MA on advanced imaging. In this study, the authors decided to include prospective studies and clinical trials which are published in full text. This means that retrospective, observational studies were excluded from this analysis. The decision to include or exclude retrospective studies is to be considered in detail and should be done a priori. There are pros and cons to this decision. As the goal of a SR is to review all available literature on a particular topic, retrospective studies are part of the medical literature and should thus be reviewed in this context. For many clinical outcomes, retrospective reviews form a sizeable portion of available data. Consider the recent meta-analysis on adverse outcomes for treatments of Barrett's esophagus [8]. Of 37 studies included in this meta-analysis, 21 studies were retrospective in nature. The drawback of including such studies is that they are generally lower quality compared to clinical trials. For example, in the adverse outcomes study, retrospective studies showed lower rate of adverse outcomes compared to prospective studies. Thus, retrospective studies will likely lower the overall quality of the results and may also contribute to increasing heterogeneity.

To further illustrate that retrospective studies may lower study quality, consider the example of Grading of Recommendations, Assessment, Development, and Evaluation (GRADE) working group. This highly appraised system of assessing and grading clinical guidelines ranks meta-analyses of clinical trials as high quality and meta-analyses of retrospective or observational studies to be low quality. Those categories can then be rated up and down further based on the evidence. This illustrates that in the view of many experts, evidence from observational studies is lower in quality.

However, there are drawbacks to excluding such studies. Firstly there will be an increased chance of publication bias. That is, the included studies are mainly the positive studies, while all the negative data is being missed. There are statistical tools to help authors identify and quantify this issue. In the Qumseya et al. MA of advanced imaging, the risk of publication bias was assessed with funnel plot. There was some asymmetry noted and also some studies fell outside of the funnel plot. Both findings indicated the possibility of publication bias. To further quantify this possibility, the authors used the classic fail-safe test. The test measures the number of negative studies that would have to be missed in order for the p-value in the analysis to be >0.05. They found that more than 170 such studies would be needed. So in this case, excluding retrospective studies did not cause a significant concern for publication bias.

The second potential drawback in illuminating retrospective studies is that for many clinical outcomes, there are no, or limited, clinical trials. Within the field of gastroenterology, this is true for many clinical outcomes. Take the recent meta-analysis of disease progression in LGD. Of the 19 studies included, only 2 were clinical trials. One cannot do a meta-analysis of two studies. In such cases, researchers have to include retrospective and observational studies. One potential way to clarify the effect of retrospective studies on the overall results is to consider including retrospective studies but analyzing them separately. This was done by Qumseya et al. in their recent meta- analysis on LGD. This offers the reader the ability to compare results and make decisions on their own.

The issues discussed above are not unique to retrospective studies. Similar arguments can be made about including or excluding meeting abstracts. In the AI meta-analysis, the authors excluded abstracts. In the adverse outcomes and LGD studies, the authors did include meeting abstracts. The same trade-off applies here between publication bias and quality of data.

In this discussion, we have shown that choosing appropriate inclusion and exclusion criteria can be very consequential. In our experience, we have been involved in studies in which retrospective studies were included and the peer reviewers argued for excluding those. On the other hand, we have had reviewers ask to include such studies when we had decided to exclude them. We would advocate careful considerations of a particular outcome and available studies. Researchers need to make those decisions a priori with the understanding that such decision will have significant effect on study quality, heterogeneity, and publication bias.

17.4 Choosing the Best Meta-Meter

As discussed above, one of the first challenges in a MA is deciding on specific inclusion and exclusion criteria. Another very important aspect is choosing the best meta-meter of interest for a particular outcome. A meta-meter is the measurement of choice which will be the primary result of the meta-analysis. This is also referred to as *effect size* or *treatment effect*. This can be odds ratio (OR), relative risk (RR), risk difference (RD), or a proportion, to name a few metrics of choice. The meta-meter is of critical importance as it will be the number which will be most visible and will convey most of the results from a study.

There are several important factors to be considered when choosing the correct meta-meter or *effect size*. Most importantly is understandability and interpretability. That is, clinicians/readers within the field should be able to easily interpret the results of the analyses in a clinically meaningful way. Often, the *effect size* of choice is the main result of each of the individual studies included in the MA. However, this is not always the case, and authors have to be careful and thoughtful in their consideration of the most suitable meta-meter. We will try to use the case of the Qumseya et al. study on advanced imaging to illustrate this issue [6]. In the initial planning phase of this meta-analysis, the authors wanted to look at the diagnostic performance of AI in detection of dysplasia. Metrics like sensitivity, specificity, and accuracy of AI were reported in most of the studies to be included. Therefore, the natural inclination was to include one of those metrics as the primary meta-meter. This would have been straightforward. However, as the researchers studied this topic more carefully, they became concerned of using such metrics. When reporting specificity, for instance, one needs to have the true negative result. However, the only way to find out the true negativity of dysplasia in BE patients is to have an esophagectomy or complete resection of the Barrett's mucosa. Only then can we be sure that all cases with dysplasia can be detected. For example, a patient may have no dysplasia on WLE and also on AI. We would call this patient negative for dysplasia. But what if both modalities missed dysplasia?

This realization put the authors in a significant dilemma. Not reporting sensitivity and specificity would essentially mean that the authors believed that most published data on those measures were inaccurate. This may not be well received by the peer reviewers who would have likely contributed to such studies. Reporting such measures, on the other hand, would mean that the authors would report measures that are not accurate and may be misleading. Instead, the authors had to look for another measure to analyze. This would have to be a clinically meaningful measure. They decided to report the risk difference in the diagnostic yield in AI compared to WLE. Although this measure is not as intuitive as sensitivity and specificity, it is actually very useful. The measure simply tells the reader about the relative increase in the chances of finding dysplasia on AI compared to WLE. It made clinical sense and was more accurate.

A similar approach was done by Qumseya et al. in the meta-analysis on EUS for BE [7]. In this study, the primary meta-meter of interest was the proportion of patients with advanced disease who were correctly diagnosed by EUS. This outcome was not a primary outcome in any of the included studies. However, the authors were looking for the most clinically relevant clinical outcome.

Let us consider a more recent meta-analysis, which also illustrates the importance of selection of meta-meter. In the previously cited study, Qumseya et al. wanted to assess the usefulness in radiofrequency ablation (RFA) in treating patient with LGD [8]. This had been a highly controversial topic with conflicting society recommendations. However, there were only three studies with head-to-head comparison of RFA versus surveillance. None of those studies reported the same effect size. Additionally, there were another 16 studies which had indirect results on disease progression on either surveillance or in RFA patients. Many studies did report, however, disease progression in either of those two groups. Disease progression is not an *effect size* which can easily compare RFA to surveillance. However, dividing the two risks of disease progression between RFA and surveillance would result in a risk ratio (RR, also referred to as relative risk). Therefore, the authors chose to report risk ratio as the meta-meter of choice for the three studies that compared RFA to surveillance directly. They then calculated the indirect RR from the other studies to confirm the magnitude and direction of effect from the indirect studies.

Finding the proper meta-meter involves more research than just looking the published articles and using the same *effect size*s. As seen above, such strategy may not always be the most accurate. Rather, researchers need to have a clear understanding of the clinical question at hand and existing data on the outcome. This information can then be used to calculate the best meta-meter of interest.

17.5 Duplicate Cohorts

In the current case studies, we have reviewed the importance of selecting the proper inclusion/exclusion criteria and have illustrated the need for an accurate meta-meter. In our experience, another important challenge in meta-analyses is identifying and dealing with duplicate cohorts. This is especially relevant in the field of gastroenterology since randomized clinical trials are less common. Therefore, many meta-analyses rely on observational studies. In such a scenario, the potential for duplication in cohorts is increased. Finding and dealing with duplicate cohorts is, therefore, an important challenge which needs to be taken into consideration with designing, conducting, or reviewing any MA.

As with any statistical analyses, duplicate observations will bias the results of a MA. One of the important assumptions in conducting many statistical analyses is the assumption of independence. Having duplicate cohorts will violate the assumption of independence of observations which is critical to most statistical analyses. Essentially, using duplicate cohorts is like counting the same patient result multiple times.

As a result, each meta-analysis should have a clear plan to identify duplicate cohorts. Sometimes, duplicate studies will have similar names which will make identification easy. However, more often, the study names vary. Duplication could come in various forms. An update to a previous study is the most common form and is potentially the easiest to identify. However, using the same patients in various databases is common in retrospective studies. Consider the example of the US RFA registry [10]. This large dataset has over 5000 patients for various centers in the USA. When including this data, there may be some duplication with other patients from some of the centers which contribute this registry. This point was seen in the meta-analysis of adverse outcomes post RFA [6]. In this study, several of the centers which contributed studies included in the MA were also contributed to the US RFA registry.

In our studies, we start by extracting data on authors, institution, and country for each study. Any studies from the same group should be suspected for potential duplication. Based on reviewing the methods and number of patients, one can identify most duplicate cohorts. However, having the same lead author does not always mean duplication in cohorts. The author may simply be very interested in a particular topic. For instance, in the AI meta-analysis, there were three studies which had the same lead author. However, careful review of the studies revealed that they had varying co-investigators, study periods, and study centers. Therefore, the authors made the conclusion that they were different studies and all were included.

One approach to such studies is to contact the corresponding author. The corresponding author's email is usually listed in the study. However, depending on the study date and authors, this may not be successful. For example, authors may not respond to inquiries. In this case, we try to email the authors on two separate occasions. Though this is not based on any scientific guideline, we feel that two contacts are enough to establish that the team put in enough effort. This method was done by Qumseya et al. in the LGD study. If the authors do not respond, and one is still not sure, statistical methods can be employed to ensure that the potential duplication did not have a significant effect on the final results. For example, in the AI meta-analysis, the authors conducted a sensitivity where two of the three suspected studies were removed at a given time and the final outcome was assessed and compared. Similar approach was done within the adverse outcome; meta-analysis with the study from the RFA registry was removed from the analysis to ensure that potential duplication did not affect the final outcomes.

In summary, duplicate cohorts can bias the results of any MA. Careful review of methods, designs, patient numbers, authors, and study institutions will allow identification of most duplicates. However, contacting authors and using statistical methods may be needed to deal with this important challenge.

17.6 Direct Versus Indirect Comparisons

Having discussed the importance of duplicate cohorts, let us now turn our attention to another frequently encountered challenge in conducting and understanding meta-analyses. In clinical practice, many outcomes of interest are comparative in nature. We frequently need to analyze at the effects of an intervention versus no intervention, treatment versus no treatment, or a diagnostic test versus another. However, for many clinical outcomes of interest in the field of GI, such comparative studies may be scarce or lacking. Yet, in the era of evidence-based medicine, researcher may still be interested in comparing such outcomes despite the scarcity of published studies. Given such scenario, some methods can be used to compare data indirectly. We will discuss two such examples.

Firstly, consider the example of the meta-analysis on LGD in BE. As discussed earlier, the authors started with the direct comparison between RFA and surveillance as reported in three studies. The effect size was reported as relative risk (RR). Yet, there were another 16 studies which looked at RFA or surveillance alone. Rather than ignoring this valuable data, the authors decided to use this data and compared results to the direct evidence. To do so, authors calculated the risk of disease progression in RFA among studies that reported on RFA only. Similarly, they calculated the risk of disease progression among patients who had surveillance only. Those two risks were compared in a meta-analysis as a subgroup analysis. The results reported a frequency with 95% CI and a p-value. Additionally, dividing these two risks allowed for indirect comparison and resulted in an RR which was compared to the direct RR reported earlier. This served to confirm the magnitude and direction of the RR reported in the direct studies and supported the conclusions of this study. Indirect comparisons are not ideal and will lower the quality of the evidence. However, if employed correctly as above, such comparison can provide supportive evidence to the small number of comparative studies.

A similar approach was used in the MA of adverse events post RFA. In this analysis, the authors wanted to assess the effect of EMR on the risk of adverse outcomes. Based on clinical suspicion, the authors hypothesized that EMR increases the risk of adverse outcomes. However, no direct comparisons were available between the two groups. Three studies compared adverse outcomes between the RFA group and the EMR with RFA group. However, these studies were not clinical trials and were indirect comparisons of retrospective cohorts. When looking at those three studies alone, the authors reported a much higher rate of adverse outcomes in the EMR group compared to the non-EMR group with an RR of 4.4. This finding is very important and supports the fact that EMR is associated with increase in adverse outcomes in this patient population. This is another good example of how indirect comparisons can be very helpful in cases where direct comparisons are limited or lacking.

Hence, we have shown that MA does not always have to depend on direct comparative studies. While such studies provide the best and most direct evidence, indirect comparisons can be used to support direct evidence. On the other hand, indirect comparisons can be used to assess outcomes where comparative studies are lacking.

17.7 Other Considerations

There are various other considerations that we would like to briefly address at the end of this chapter.

17.7.1 Fixed Versus Random Effects

Using fixed versus random effects modeling is sometimes confusing to the researchers and readers.

In conducting a meta-analysis, we are trying to estimate the true effect size for a particular outcome. In our studies, this can be the relative risk of disease progression, the risk difference in dysplasia detection, or the prevalence of strictures post RFA. In fixed effects models, we assume that there is a true effect size. Under this assumption, any variability in the effect size among the studies is solely due to error in sampling between the different studies. In medical literature, this is unlikely to be the case. More commonly, studies have variation in population, intervention protocol, follow-up time, etc. In fact, it would be hard to find a clinical situation where the populations in the varying studies are the same. A good example of fixed effects modeling is a company which is testing a dosage of a drug in tandem animal populations. In such case, the animal population in each study is very similar with the exception of the drug being tested. It is reasonable in this case to use fixed effects models, as any variation in the result is likely due to random error. In the field of GI, the most commonly used modeling is random effects modeling. Under this model, we assume that the true effect size is different in different studies. This variation often comes from the differences in populations. Each of the studies cited in this chapter addresses this issue in the methods section. A priori sources of heterogeneity are hypothesized and stated in the protocol. Those are sources of differences among the included studies that will increase the variance between included studies. In such cases, using random effects modeling is most appropriate.

While many of the studies cited in this chapter will use the test of heterogeneity to inform the decision to use random versus fixed modeling, such strategy is now discouraged. Random effects modeling should be used when the baseline populations are different.

17.7.2 Search Strategy

This can be a challenging part of any MA, especially for the novice researcher. In the MA of advanced endoscopy, four researchers conducted the literature search with help from an expert librarian. In our experience, including an expert librarian in this process is crucial. With clear guidance from the research team, a librarian is more efficient and able to extract relevant studies and provide them to the team.

17.7.3 Screening Articles

This process has traditionally been the most laborious part of conducting a meta-analysis. Having to go through thousands of citations is very challenging and can be overwhelming. Initially, this process of reviewing articles is used to be done by hand, then using Excel (Microsoft Corporation, Redmond, WA), and later using EndNote (Thompson Reuters, Philadelphia, PA). For instance, in the case study of advanced imaging in BE, the authors used EndNote. This software allows the user to create subfolders within a library and move citations accordingly. While this is an appropriate way to do the search, there are newer methods. Other tools have become available which make the screening process easier and much faster. In the LGD study, the authors used the online tool *covidence.org*. This online tool allows researchers to import studies from various formats. Once imported, each citation appears in abstract form. Each step requires two reviewers who are blinded to the choices of each other. In our experience, we found this tool to be invaluable. Regardless of which method is used, researchers need to keep track of articles that are removed and reasons why they were excluded. As seen in the studies cited here, this process is usually reflected in Fig. 17.1 of each publication.

17.7.4 Quality Assessment

This is one of the most impactful topics to be addressed in MA. In combining different studies with varying populations and varying designs, the quality of studies will inevitably vary. Therefore, researchers need to assess the quality of each of the included studies. In the AI in BE and EUS in BE meta-analyses, the researchers used the Quality Assessment of Diagnostic Accuracy Studies (QUADAS) [11] tool. In the EUS study, they used Newcastle-Ottawa scale [12]. In the LGD study, quality assessment was done using the Downs and Black scale [13]. There are variable quality measures that have been developed depending on the study design and outcome. Choosing the right tool to assess study quality is essential.

Conclusions

In this chapter, we used several meta-analyses to illustrate some of the most common challenges and considerations when conducting or reviewing a meta-analysis (Tables 17.1 and 17.2). As we have pointed out, the field of meta-analysis is fast growing. The potential for high-quality, evidence-based results, using this method, is invaluable. In each of the subheadings, we were able to hone in on key issues. We started by detailing the significance of choosing the correct inclusion and exclusion criteria. We argued how this process should be carefully studied due to the important impactions on results and quality. We gave examples of how choosing the best meta-meter can be challenging but will have a huge impact in the final results. We assessed ways to deal with the critical issue of duplicate cohorts. We showed how indirect comparisons can be used to support direct comparisons or analyze outcomes that lack such comparative studies. As the scope of meta-analysis continues to grow, we will continue to do more such studies in the field of gastroenterology. Being able to understand some of the key issues presented here will be of great help to researchers and readers.

Table 17.2 Key topics and take-home messages

Topic	Take-home message
Inclusion/exclusion criteria	• Carefully consider retrospective studies and meeting abstract a priori • Trade-off between publication bias and quality of evidence • Consider sensitivity analyses to differentiate outcomes between different study designs
Choosing a meta-meter	• Consider options for most appropriate meta-meter • Does not have to be the same as published studies • Consider clinical relevance and understandability
Identifying and dealing with duplicate cohorts	• Can bias the results • Review of authorship, methods, designs, number of patients, and study institutions • Contacting authors or use statistical methods if needed
Indirect comparisons	• Comparative studies provide the best evidence, but are not mandatory for MA • Indirect comparisons can be used to support direct evidence • Indirect comparisons can assess outcomes where comparative studies are lacking

References

1. Oberg S, Wenner J, Johansson J, Walther B, Willen R. Barrett esophagus: risk factors for progression to dysplasia and adenocarcinoma. Ann Surg. 2005;242:49–54.
2. Menke-Pluymers MB, Hop WC, Dees J, van Blankenstein M, Tilanus HW. Risk factors for the development of an adenocarcinoma in columnar-lined (Barrett) esophagus. The Rotterdam Esophageal Tumor Study Group. Cancer. 1993;72:1155–8.
3. Desai TK, Krishnan K, Samala N, Singh J, Cluley J, Perla S, et al. The incidence of oesophageal adenocarcinoma in non-dysplastic Barrett's oesophagus: a meta-analysis. Gut. 2012;61:970–6.
4. Singh S, Manickam P, Amin AV, Samala N, Schouten LJ, Iyer PG, et al. Incidence of esophageal adenocarcinoma in Barrett's esophagus with low-grade dysplasia: a systematic review and meta-analysis. Gastrointest Endosc. 2014;79:897–909.
5. Kariv R, Plesec TP, Goldblum JR, Bronner M, Oldenburgh M, Rice TW, et al. The Seattle protocol does not more reliably predict the detection of cancer at the time of esophagectomy than a less intensive surveillance protocol. Clin Gastroenterol Hepatol. 2009;7:653–8.
6. Qumseya BJ, Wang H, Badie N, Uzomba RN, Parasa S, White DL, et al. Advanced imaging technologies increase detection of dysplasia and neoplasia in patients with Barrett's esophagus: a meta-analysis and systematic review. Clin Gastroenterol Hepatol. 2013;11:1562–70.e1–2.
7. Qumseya BJ, Brown J, Abraham M, White D, Wolfsen H, Gupta N, et al. Diagnostic performance of EUS in predicting advanced cancer among patients with Barrett's esophagus and high-grade dysplasia/early adenocarcinoma: systematic review and meta-analysis. Gastrointest Endosc. 2015;81:865–74.e2.
8. Qumseya BJ, Wani S, Desai M, Qumseya A, Bain P, Sharma P, et al. Adverse events after radiofrequency ablation in patients with Barrett's esophagus: a systematic review and meta-analysis. Clin Gastroenterol Hepatol. 2016;14:1086–95.e6.
9. Qumseya BJ, Wani S, Gendy S, Harnke B, Bergman JJ, Wolfsen H. Disease progression in Barrett's low-grade dysplasia with radiofrequency ablation compared to surveillance: systematic review and meta-analysis. Am J Gastroenterol. 2017;112:849–65.
10. Shaheen NJ, Kim HP, Bulsiewicz WJ, Lyday WD, Triadafilopoulos G, Wolfsen HC, et al. Prior fundoplication does not improve safety or efficacy outcomes of radiofrequency ablation: results from the U.S. RFA Registry. J Gastrointest Surg. 2013;17:21–8.
11. Whiting P, Rutjes AW, Reitsma JB, Bossuyt PM, Kleijnen J. The development of QUADAS: a tool for the quality assessment of studies of diagnostic accuracy included in systematic reviews. BMC Med Res Methodol. 2003;3:25.
12. Stang A. Critical evaluation of the Newcastle-Ottawa scale for the assessment of the quality of nonrandomized studies in meta-analyses. Eur J Epidemiol. 2010;25:603–5.
13. Downs SH, Black N. The feasibility of creating a checklist for the assessment of the methodological quality both of randomised and non-randomised studies of health care interventions. J Epidemiol Community Health. 1998;52:377–84.

Diagnostic Meta-Analysis: Case Study in Oncology

18

Sulbaran Marianny, Sousa Afonso,
and Bustamante-Lopez Leonardo

18.1 Cancer Epidemiology

Cancer is a major public health problem worldwide and is the second leading mortality cause in the United States [1].

The four most common cancers occurring worldwide are lung, female breast, colorectal, and prostate cancer, accounting for around 40% of oncologic diagnosis. Lung cancer represents 10% of cancers in men worldwide.

In the United States, prostate, lung/bronchus, and colorectal cancers account for 44% of all cases in men, with prostate cancer alone accounting for 1 in 5 new diagnoses. For women, the three most commonly diagnosed cancers are breast, lung/bronchus, and colorectum, representing one-half of all cases; breast cancer alone is expected to account for 29% of all new cancer diagnoses in women [1].

18.1.1 Cancer Mortality

In the United States, cancer is the second leading cause of death following heart disease, which accounted for 24% of total deaths in 2012. However, cancer is the leading cause of death among adults aged 40–79 years. It is also the leading cause of death in 21 states, primarily due to exceptional gains made in the progress against heart disease.

In addition, cancer is the leading cause of death among both Hispanics and Asian/Pacific Islanders, who combined comprise one-quarter of the US population [2].

S. Marianny (✉)
Gastrointestinal Endoscopy Service, Gastroenterology Department, Clinics Hospital, University of Sao Paulo School of Medicine, Sao Paulo, Brazil

S. Afonso · B.-L. Leonardo
Surgical Division, Gastroenterology Department, Clinics Hospital, University of Sao Paulo School of Medicine, Sao Paulo, Brazil

G. Biondi-Zoccai (ed.), *Diagnostic Meta-Analysis*,
https://doi.org/10.1007/978-3-319-78966-8_18

Breast cancer is the principal cause of death in women aged 20–59 years but is replaced by lung cancer in women aged 60 years or older. Among men, lung cancer is the leading cause of death for those aged 40 years or older.

The most common causes of cancer death are cancers of the lung/bronchus, prostate, and colorectum in men and lung/bronchus, breast, and colorectum in women. These four cancers account for 46% of all cancer deaths, with more than one-quarter (27%) due to lung cancer [1].

18.1.2 Cancer Survival

Although there has been an overall drop of 23% of cancer deaths during the last two decades, incidence and death rates are increasing for several cancer types, including liver and pancreas, which represent two of the most fatal cancers. Advances have been slow for lung and pancreatic cancers, for which the 5-year relative survival is currently 18% and 8%, respectively. These low rates are partly because more than one-half of cases are diagnosed at a distant stage, for which 5-year survival is 4% and 2%, respectively.

In contrast, progress has been most rapid for hematopoietic and lymphoid malignancies due to improvements in treatment protocols, including the discovery of targeted therapies. For example, the 5-year survival for acute lymphocytic leukemia increased from 41% during the mid-1970s to 70% during 2005 to 2011. The use of BCR-ABL tyrosine kinase inhibitors doubled survival for patients with chronic myeloid leukemia in less than two decades [3], from 31% in the early 1990s to 63% during 2005 to 2011.

18.2 Importance of Diagnostic Test Accuracy (DTA) Systematic Reviews and Meta-Analysis as a Methodological Tool for Improving Clinical Management in Oncology

Accurate diagnosis and staging are needed in order to optimize appropriate oncologic patient management. In this context, the internationally accepted TNM classification of cancer by anatomic disease extent (stage) is the major determinant of appropriate treatment and prognosis. Stage is an increasingly important component of cancer surveillance and cancer control and an endpoint for the evaluation of the population-based screening and early detection efforts.

Oncologic staging is universally expressed using the Union for International Cancer Control (UICC) TNM classification. This system represents an anatomically based classification that records the primary and regional nodal extent of the tumor and the absence or presence of metastases, including the following categories:

T category describes the primary tumor site.
N category describes the regional lymph node involvement.
M category describes the presence or otherwise of distant metastatic spread.

This system has been continuously updated and expanded for more than 50 years by the UICC TNM project group according to high-quality emerging clinical evidence [4].

However, summary and interpretation of quality and content of the overwhelming published material in oncology in order to make relevant updates may be challenging. In this context, well-designed DTA studies can help in making these decisions, provided that they transparently and fully report their participants, tests, methods, and results.

Diagnostic tests are a critical component of health care and clinicians. Whenever a new test is on the process of being incorporated in clinical practice, the physician needs to evaluate if testing improves outcome. It is important to objectively know what test to use, to purchase, or to recommend in practice guidelines and how to interpret test results [5].

DTA systematic reviews and meta-analysis represent an important methodological tool that enables efficient integration of current information, providing a basis for rational decision-making, thereby improving efficient evidence summary in oncologic diagnosis and staging [6].

As elsewhere in science, DTA systematic reviews and meta-analysis can be used to obtain more precise estimates when small studies addressing the same test and patients in the same setting are available. Reviews can also be useful to establish whether and how scientific findings vary by particular subgroups and achieve summary estimates with a stronger generalizability than estimates from a single study. Systematic reviews may help identify the risk of bias that may be present in the original studies and can be used to address questions that were not directly considered in the primary studies, such as comparisons between tests [5].

Additionally, whenever a policy decision is needed to promote use of a new index test, evidence is required that using the new test increases test accuracy over other testing options, including current practice, or has equivalent accuracy but offers other advantages [7–9]. As with the evaluation of interventions, systematic reviews need to include comparative analyses between alternative testing strategies and not focus solely on evaluating the performance of a test in isolation.

In relation to the existing situation, three possible roles for a new test can be defined: replacement, triage, and add-on [7]. If a new test is to replace an existing test, then comparing the accuracy of both tests on the same population and with the same reference standard provides the most direct evidence. In triage, the new test is used before the existing test or existing testing pathway, and only patients with a particular result on the triage test continue the testing pathway. When a test is needed to rule out disease in patients who then need no further testing, one will be looking for a test that gives a minimal proportion of false negatives and thus a relatively high sensitivity. Triage tests may be less accurate than existing ones, but they have other advantages, such as simplicity or low cost. A third possible role of a new test is add-on. The new test is then positioned after the existing testing pathway, to identify false positives or false negatives after the existing pathway. The review should provide data to assess the incremental change in accuracy made by adding the new test.

An example of a replacement question can be found in a systematic review of the diagnostic accuracy of urinary markers for primary bladder cancer [10]. Clinicians may use cytology to triage patients before they undergo invasive cystoscopy, the reference standard for bladder cancer. As cytology combines a high specificity with a low sensitivity [11], the goal of the review was to identify a tumor marker with sufficient accuracy to either replace cytology or to be used in addition to cytology. For a marker to replace cytology, it has to achieve equally high specificity with improved sensitivity. New markers, which are sensitive but not specific, may have roles as adjuncts to conventional testing. The review included studies in which the test under evaluation (several different tumor markers and cytology) was evaluated against cystoscopy or histopathology. Included studies compared one or more of the markers, cytology only, or a combination of markers and cytology.

Although information on accuracy can help clinicians in making decisions about tests, review authors and readers should realize that good diagnostic accuracy is a desirable but not a sufficient condition for the effectiveness of a test [8]. To show that using a new test does more good than harm to patients tested, randomized trials of test-and-treatment strategies and reviews of such trials may be necessary. In most cases, such randomized trials are rare, and systematic reviews of test accuracy may provide the most useful evidence to guide decision-making and provide key evidence to incorporate into decision models.

18.3 Current Quality Status of Diagnostic Systematic Reviews and Meta-Analysis in Oncology

Objective and transparent reporting is essential for reviews to be reliable and relevant. However, the methods used to conduct high-quality systematic reviews of diagnostic tests are developing and continuously being reviewed and updated.

Systematic reviews of diagnostic studies involve additional challenges to those of therapeutic studies [12, 13]. Studies are observational in nature, prone to various biases [14], and report two linked measures summarizing the performance in participants with disease (sensitivity) and without (specificity). In addition, there is more variation between studies in the methods, manufacturers, procedures, and outcome measurement scales used to assess test accuracy than in randomized controlled trials, which generally causes marked heterogeneity in results [15].

Systematic reviews need to report results from all included studies, with information on study design, methods, and characteristics that may affect clinical applicability, generalizability, and potential for bias.

Deficiencies in the reporting of research have been highlighted in several areas of clinical medicine [16]. Essential elements of study methods are often poorly described and sometimes completely omitted, making both critical appraisal and replication difficult, if not impossible. Sometimes study results are selectively reported, and other times, researchers cannot resist unwarranted optimism in interpretation of their findings [17, 18]. These practices limit the value of the research and impeding the identification, critical appraisal, and replication of studies.

A systematic review that aimed to assess the methods and reporting of systematic reviews of diagnostic tests in cancer identified specific limitations regarding different reporting steps of test accuracy studies in oncology [19].

1. Objectives, inclusion criteria, and search strategy
Objectives and inclusion criteria should be clearly stated in order to obtain a systematic approach [20]. Search strategies should also be clearly specified, in order for readers of the review appraise how well the review has avoided bias in locating studies. Additionally, report of the search strategy guarantees reproducibility of the results of the review.
Twenty-five percent of the 89 included reviews did not report inclusion criteria, and 49% (44) tabulated characteristics of included studies. Among total reviews that were assessed in detail [21], 64% used study inclusion criteria relating to sample size or study design, and 15 discussed the appropriateness of patient inclusion criteria used by the primary studies. Thirty-two percent of the reviews searched two or more electronic databases, 80% reported their search terms, and 84% searched bibliography lists or other nonelectronic sources.
2. Description of target condition, patients, and clinical setting
Clinical relevance and reliability require reporting of information on the target condition, patients, and clinical setting [22]. Fifty percent of the reviews did not report whether tumors were primary, recurrent, or metastatic. Only 17% (15/89) reported on the clinical setting, and 45% reported characteristics of patients for individual studies. Of 17 reviews of primary or recurrent tumors assessed in detail, 10 did not consider possible effects of tumor stage or grade on test performance. Reviews sometimes omitted information that had been collected, for example; 18% (16/89) of reviews collected information on the severity of disease but did not report it.
3. Study design
Consecutive prospective recruitment from a clinically relevant population of patients with masked assessment of index and reference tests is the recommended design to minimize bias and ensure clinical applicability of study results. Twenty of the 25 reviews assessed in detail did not report or were unclear on whether included studies used consecutive recruitment of patients. Few reviews limited inclusion to study designs less prone to bias, namely, consecutive (8%) or prospective (12%) studies. Sixty percent (15/25) discussed test masking. Poor reporting made it impossible to identify inclusion of case-control designs [23].
4. Description of index and reference tests
Both index and reference tests need to be clearly described for a review to be clinically relevant and transparent and to allow readers to judge the potential for verification and incorporation biases. Only 36% (9/25) of reviews reported the definition of a positive result for the index test. In 40% (10/25) it was unclear if the included studies used the same, or different, index tests or procedures. When index tests were reported to vary between included studies, 71% (10/14) reported the index test for each study and the compatibility of different tests was discussed in 86% (12/14) of reviews. Sixty-eight percent (17/25) of reviews assessed

in detail reported the reference tests used in the review; 40% reported reference tests for each included study. Six reviews reported whether reference tests were used on all, a random sample, or a select sample of patients.

5. Reporting of individual study results and graphical presentation
   We assessed the level of detail used to report the results of individual studies. Ideally reviews should report data from 2 × 2 tables.
   Graphs are efficient tools for reporting results and depicting variability between study results. Of the 89 reviews, 40% contained graphs of study findings, and 39% reported sensitivities and specificities, likelihoods ratios, or predictive values. Over half (56%, 14/25) of the reviews assessed in detail provided adequate information to derive 2 × 2 tables for all included studies. Four reviews included tests with continuous outcomes but presented only dichotomized results; three reported the cutoff used.
6. Meta-analysis, quality, and bias
   Appropriate use of meta-analysis can effectively summarize data across studies. Quality assessment is important to give readers an indication of the degree to which included studies are prone to bias. Sixty-one percent (54/89) of reviews presented a meta-analysis and 32% completed a formal assessment of quality. Twenty-three of the 25 reviews assessed in detail discussed the potential for bias. Spectrum bias was most commonly considered (80% of reviews), with verification bias and publication bias considered least (40%).
7. Procedures in review
   The reliability of a review depends partly on how it was done. Only 48% (12/25) of reviews provided information on review procedures, most reporting duplicate data extraction by two assessors (nine reviews), a method recommended to increase review reliability.
8. Abstracts
   In two recent literature surveys, abstracts of diagnostic accuracy studies published in high-impact journals or presented at an international scientific conference were found insufficiently informative, because key information about the research question, study methods, study results, and the implications of findings were frequently missing [24].

18.4 How to Overcome Limitations on Summary of Evidence of DTA Studies in Oncology

18.4.1 Quality Assessment of DTA Studies in Oncology

The Quality Assessment of Diagnostic Accuracy Studies (QUADAS-2) checklist is a valuable revised tool used to assess the quality of diagnostic test accuracy studies. It consists of four key domains that discuss patient selection, index test, reference standard, and flow of patients through the study and timing of the index tests and reference standard qualitatively. This checklist is useful in order to identify potential sources of bias and to take into consideration the effects of these biases on the estimates and the conclusions of the review. Additionally, authors should consider carefully whether specific items that reflect other sources of bias should be added to the QUADAS list [18].

It is important to consider that the use of different methods of weighting individual items from the same quality assessment tool can produce different quality scores. Criteria used to generate quality scores into the results of a review can lead to different conclusions regarding the effect of study quality on estimates of diagnostic accuracy [25].

Although there are clear limitations regarding the use of quality scores in diagnostic systematic reviews based on the subjectiveness of the weighting of items of key domains, the lack of a score may also potentially limit a clear comparison among studies. There is actually a lack of consensus on how to objectively report bias on diagnostic systematic reviews. We present two examples on how this limitation may be overcome:

> for example, stacked bars can be used for each QUADAS item. In the study: "Single-operator cholangioscopy and targeted biopsies in the diagnosis of indeterminate biliary strictures: a systematic review" [21] the risk for bias was described as follows: "In most studies, there was a low risk of bias regarding the selection of patients. There were no bias issues or concerns regarding applicability of the selection of patients. There was no risk of bias issues of the index test in any of the studies. In most studies there was a low risk of bias to determine whether an appropriate reference standard was used or its applicability. Ultimately, 10 studies with sufficient data that met our inclusion criteria were included in the final meta-analysis" [21] (Fig. 18.1).

The other option to evaluate the risk for bias within studies, using the QUADAS-2 tool, can be to define specific criteria for high-, moderate-, and low-quality studies. As an example in the study: "Overtube-assisted enteroscopy and capsule endoscopy for the diagnosis of small-bowel polyps and tumors: a systematic review and meta-analysis" [26] the risk for bias was described as follows: "The QUADAS-2 was applied to each of the studies. Studies of high quality were defined as those with low risk answers to at least three of four key items. Studies of poor quality were those

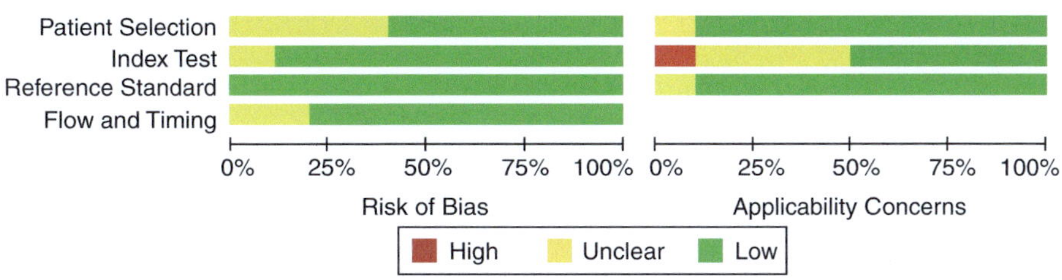

Fig. 18.1 Risk of bias report with the use of stacked bars in the study: "Single-operator cholangioscopy and targeted biopsies in the diagnosis of indeterminate biliary strictures: a systematic review"

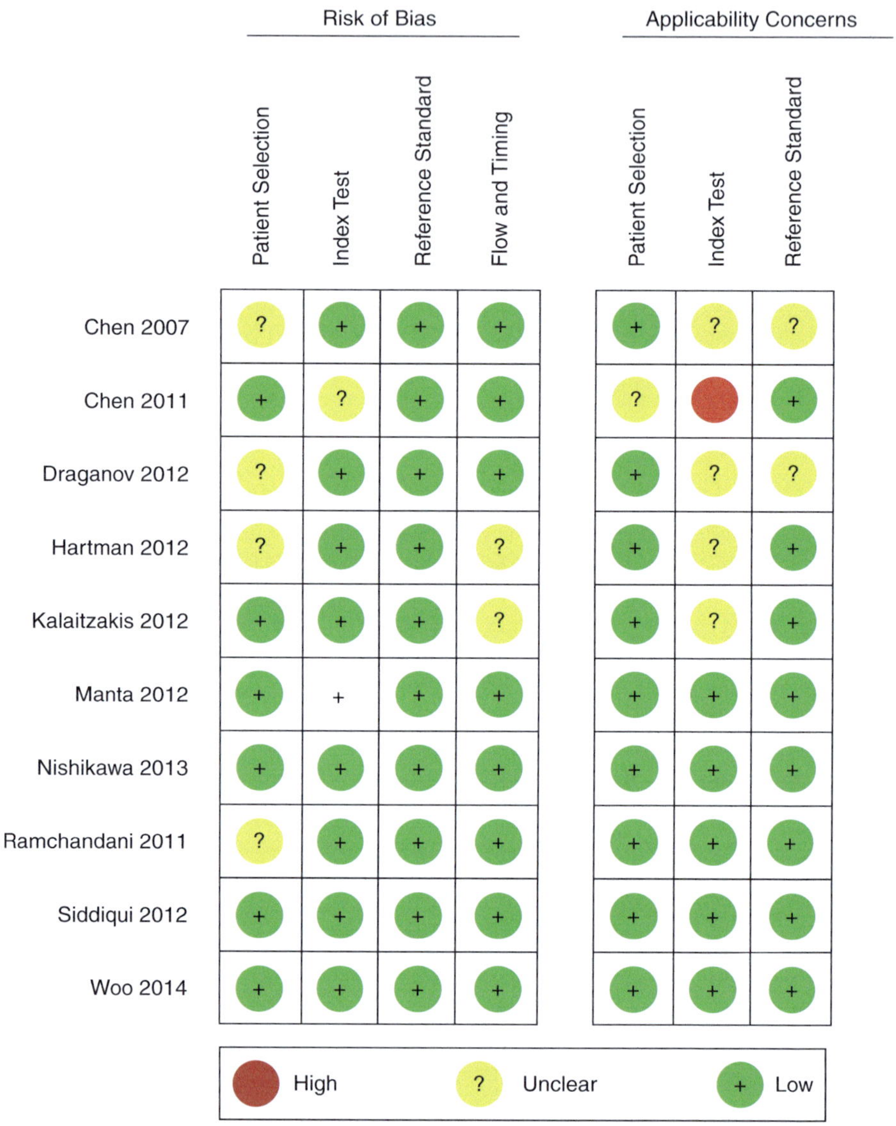

Fig 18.1 (continued)

that failed or had an unclear answer to three of the four items. Moderate quality was assigned for every other possibility" (Table 18.1) [26].

Another way of presenting the quality assessment results is by tabulating the results of the individual QUADAS items for each single study. In the analysis phase, the results of the quality appraisal may guide explorations of the sources of heterogeneity [42–44]. Possible methods to address quality differences are sensitivity

Table 18.1 Risk for bias according to QUADAS-2 (Quality Assessment of Diagnostic Accuracy Studies)

	Selection of patients	OAE	CE	Time and flow	Study quality
Arakawa [27]	L	U	L	L	Good
Buscaglia [28]	L	H	L	H	Moderate
Fry [29]	H	H	L	L	Moderate
Fujimori [30]	L	H	L	L	Good
Kamalaporn [31]	L	H	L	H	Moderate
Kameda [32]	L	L	L	U	Good
Lee [33]	H	H	L	U	Poor
Manno [34]	L	H	L	L	Good
Marmo [35]	L	L	L	L	Good
Matsumoto [36]	H	L	L	L	Good
Nakamura [37]	L	L	L	L	Good
Partridge [38]	L	H	L	U	Moderate
Sethi [39]	L	H	L	L	Good
Vere [40]	L	U	L	U	Moderate
Li [41]	L	H	L	L	Good

OAE overtube-assisted enteroscopy, *CE* capsule endoscopy, *L* low risk for bias, *U* unclear risk for bias, *H* high risk for bias

analysis, subgroup analysis, or meta-regression analysis, although the number of included studies may often be too low for meaningful investigations.

18.4.2 Strategies to Improve Quality of Reporting of DTA Studies in Oncology

The Standards for Reporting of Diagnostic Accuracy (STARD) statement was developed to improve the quality of reporting of diagnostic accuracy studies. Here we present a practical approach to some key items of STARD 2015 [24], including examples published in DTA reviews related to neoplastic diseases. We will refer specifically to the study "Overtube-assisted enteroscopy and capsule endoscopy for the diagnosis of small-bowel polyps and tumors: a systematic review and meta-analysis," in order to give some key examples.

Identification as a study of diagnostic accuracy using at least one measure of accuracy in title or abstract (such as sensitivity, specificity, predictive values, or AUC).

To facilitate retrieval of an article in electronic databases such as MEDLINE or Embase, authors can explicitly identify it as a report of a diagnostic accuracy study. This can be performed by using terms in the title and/or abstract that refer to measures of diagnostic accuracy, such as "sensitivity," "specificity," "positive predictive value," "negative predictive value," "area under the ROC curve (AUC)," or "likelihood ratio."

The specific keyword (MeSH heading) for indexing diagnostic studies, "sensitivity and specificity," has been introduced. However, the sensitivity of using this particular MeSH term to identify diagnostic accuracy studies can be as low as 51%. As of May 2015, Embase's thesaurus (Emtree) has 38 check tags for study types; "diagnostic test accuracy study" is one of them but was only introduced in 2011 [24].

Example Title. Overtube-assisted enteroscopy and capsule endoscopy for the diagnosis of small-bowel polyps and tumors: a systematic review and meta-analysis.

Abstract. "Patients and methods: The sensitivity, specificity, positive likelihood ratio, and negative likelihood ratio for the diagnosis of small-bowel polyps and tumors were analyzed. Secondarily, the rates of diagnostic concordance and discordance between OAE and CE were calculated" [26].

The abstract should represent a structured summary of study design, methods, results, and conclusions.

Readers use abstracts to decide whether they should retrieve the full study report and invest time in reading it. In cases where access to the full study report cannot be obtained or where time is limited, it is conceivable that clinical decisions are based on the information provided in abstracts only.

Informative abstracts help readers to quickly appraise critical elements of study validity (risk of bias) and applicability of study findings to their clinical setting (generalizability). Structured abstracts, with separate headings for objectives, methods, results, and interpretation, allow readers to find essential information more easily [45].

The introduction should state scientific and clinical background, including the intended use and clinical role of the index test and study aims.

In the introduction of scientific study reports, authors should describe the rationale for their study. In doing so, they can refer to previous work on the topic, remaining uncertainty, and the clinical implications of this knowledge gap. To help readers in evaluating the implications of the study, authors can clarify the intended use and the clinical role of the test under evaluation, which is referred to as the index test [24].

Example "Small-bowel tumors have been difficult to diagnose as a consequence of their nonspecific presentation and the poor accessibility of the distal small bowel.

Since the introduction of capsule endoscopy (CE) and overtube-assisted enteroscopy (OAE), the number of small-bowel polyps and tumors that are diagnosed has increased. Obscure gastrointestinal bleeding (OGIB) is the main indication for using these enteroscopic modalities. Importantly, the development of both double-balloon enteroscopy (DBE) and single-balloon enteroscopy (SBE) has made it possible to perform diagnostic and therapeutic procedures during a single examination.

Several studies have evaluated the utility of DBE and CE in the evaluation of patients with suspected small-intestinal disease, including OGIB. However, the studies have shown inconsistent results and are largely limited by their small sample size. Furthermore, these meta-analyses did not focus on small-bowel polyps and tumors. No systematic review has yet been conducted to evaluate OAE and CE for the diagnosis of small-bowel polyps and tumors" [26].

Defining Study Objectives and Hypotheses
Clinical studies may have a general aim (a long-term goal, such as "to improve the staging of esophageal cancer"), specific objectives (well-defined goals for this particular study), and testable hypotheses (statements than can be falsified by the study results).

In diagnostic accuracy studies, statistical hypotheses are typically defined in terms of acceptability criteria for single tests (minimum levels of sensitivity, specificity, or other measures). In those cases, hypotheses generally include a quantitative expression of the expected value of the diagnostic parameter. In other cases, statistical hypotheses are defined in terms of equality or non-inferiority in accuracy when comparing two or more index tests.

A priori specification of the study hypotheses limits the chances of post hoc data dredging with spurious findings, premature conclusions about the performance of tests, or subjective judgment about the accuracy of the test. Objectives and hypotheses also guide sample size calculations. An evaluation of 126 reports of diagnostic test accuracy studies published in high-impact journals in 2010 revealed that 88% did not state a clear hypothesis [46].

Methods: Whether data collection was planned before the index test and reference standard were performed (prospective study) or after (retrospective study).

There is great variability in the way the terms "prospective" and "retrospective" are defined and used in the literature. It is therefore necessary to describe clearly whether data collection was planned before the index test and reference standard were performed or afterward. If authors define the study question before index test and reference standards are performed, they can take appropriate actions for optimizing procedures according to the study protocol and for dedicated data collection [47].

Sometimes, the idea for a study originates when patients have already undergone the index test and the reference standard. If so, data collection relies on reviewing patient charts or extracting data from registries. Though such retrospective studies can sometimes reflect routine clinical practice better than prospective studies, they may fail to identify all eligible patients, and often result in data of lower quality, with more missing data points [47]. A reason for this could be, for example, that in daily clinical practice, not all patients undergoing the index test may proceed to have the reference standard.

Example Table 18.2 summarizes the characteristics of the studies of the systematic review, including the study and data collection design.

Eligibility criteria and on what basis potentially eligible participants were identified.

Since a diagnostic accuracy study describes the behavior of a test under particular circumstances, a report of the study must include a complete description of the criteria that were used to identify eligible participants. Eligibility criteria are usually related to the nature and stage of the target condition and the intended future use of

Table 18.2 Characteristics of studies included in a systematic review and meta-analysis of overtube-assisted enteroscopy and capsule endoscopy for the diagnosis of small-bowel polyps and tumors

Study	Population and study design	Indication	OAE approach and route of insertion, % (n/N)	CE model	Examination sequence	Time between tests	OAE mean procedure time, min	CE recording duration, min	OAE mean depth of insertion, cm	OAE complete examinations, % (n/N)	CE complete examinations, % (n/N)	OAE complications	CE complications
Arakawa [27]	Retrospective, 74 pts, Nagoya University Hospital, Japan, 2003–2007	OGIB	DBE; N/A	M2A PillCam	74 pts, DBE preceded by CE	Median 2 days (range 0–45)	N/A	N/A	N/A	70 (23/33)	68 (50/74)	1 perforation, 1 acute pancreatitis	Capsule retention in 4 pts: 2 in small bowel, 1 over jejunal lymphoma, 1 in ileal loop
Buscaglia [28]	Prospective, 56 pts, mean age 68 y, Stony Brook University, State University of New York, and Shands Hospital, University of Florida, USA, 2008–2009	OGIB, abnormal imaging, abnormal CE findings, suspected Crohn's disease	SE; antegrade, 56	N/A	56 pts, SE preceded by CE	87 days	42.1 ± 12.3	N/A	224.6 ± 68.7	N/A	N/A	No major complications; 6 minor lacerations of gastrointestinal mucosa, no interventions required	N/A
Fry [29]	Retrospective, 7 pts, mean age 51 years, University of Magdeburg Medical Center, Germany, 3.75-year period	OGIB, anemia, chronic diarrhea	DBE; N/A1	N/A	7 pts, DBE preceded by CE	N/A	75 (range 25–115)	N/A	300 (range 30–540)	N/A	N/A	1 transient oxygen desaturation, 1 post-procedural abdominal pain and bloating	Capsule retention in 2 pts, 1 extracted by DBE
Fujimori [30]	Prospective, 36 pts, mean age 60.2 ± 15.0 years, Nippon Medical School Hospital, Japan, 2004–2006	OGIB	DBE	PillCam TM	36 pts, DBE preceded by CE	72 h	N/A	N/A	N/A	N/A	N/A	Not reported	Not reported

Kamalaporn [31]	Retrospective, 51 pts, mean age 64.1 years (34–83), St. Michael's Hospital, University of Toronto, Canada, 2002–2007	OGIB	DBE; antegrade, 30; retrograde, 17; oral and anal, 12	M2A PillCam	51 pts, DBE preceded by CE	Mean 139 days (range 40–335)	Mean 179.8 (range 40–335)	Small intestine, 243.7 (0–465)	N/A	N/A	N/A	No significant complications	No capsule retention
Kameda [32]	Prospective, 32 pts, mean age 62.4 ± 14.8 years, male 13, female 19, Osaka City University Graduate School of Medicine, Japan, 2005–2006	OGIB	DBE; both antegrade and retrograde in attempt at total enteroscopy, 32	M2A PillCam	32 pts, DBE preceded by CE	1–7 days	N/A	Small Intestine, 245.3	N/A	50.0 (16/32)	73.3 (23/30)	Minor complications only, abdominal pain, nausea	Capsule retention (small bowel) in 2 pts, removed by DBE
Lee [33]	Retrospective, 183 pts, mean age 48.2 years (7–87), multicenter (8 Korean university hospitals), 2004–2009.	OGIB, chronic abdominal pain/ diarrhea, Peutz-Jehgers syndrome	DBE	CE	183 pts, DBE preceded by CE	N/A	N/A	N/A	N/A	43.90%	N/A	N/A	N/A
Manno [34]	Prospective, 75 pts, mean age 61 years (20–89), male 55.9%, multicenter (5 Italian tertiary care public hospitals or university-affiliated teaching hospitals), 2010–2011	OGIB, suspected tumor, Crohn's disease	SBE	CE	75 pts, DBE preceded by CE	Within 4 weeks	Antegrade, 61 ± 33; retrograde, 78 ± 41	N/A	Mean 254 ± 179; antegrade, 223 ± 93 beyond Treitz; retrograde, 96 ± 56 beyond ileocecal valve	47.06 (8/17)	N/A	1 transient oxygen desaturation	N/A

(continued)

Table 18.2 (continued)

Study	Population and study design	Indication	OAE approach and route of insertion, % (n/N)	CE model	Examination sequence	Time between tests	OAE mean procedure time, min	CE recording duration, min	OAE mean depth of insertion, cm	OAE complete examinations, % (n/N)	CE complete examinations, % (n/N)	OAE complications	CE complications
Marmo [35]	Prospective, 193 pts, median age 61.6 ± 16.2 years, multicenter (6 Italian institutions, tertiary care public hospitals, or university-affiliated teaching hospitals), 2004–2007	OGIB	DBE; antegrade, 56.4 (109/193); retrograde, 16.6 (32/193); oral and anal, 27 (52/193)	PillCam SB	193 pts, DBE preceded by CE	2 weeks in all cases	Antegrade, 88 ± 23; retrograde, 97 ± 36; oral and anal, N/A	Total, 470.21 ± 39.5; small bowel, 262.90 ± 90.80	Antegrade, 192.4 ± 89.7; retrograde, 103.5 ± 77; oral and anal, 321 ± 147.2	34.6 (18/52)	85.5 (165/193)	Minor complications only, 2 patients with transient oxygen desaturation	Capsule retention in 6 pts, 4 of them above neoplastic stricture
Matsumoto [36]	Prospective, 22 pts, 21–72 years, Kyushu University Hospital, Japan, 2004–2005	OGIB, gastrointestinal polyposis	DBE; antegrade, 50 (11/22); retrograde, 22.72 (5/22); oral and anal, 27.27 (6/22)	M2A PillCam	22 pts, CE preceded by DBE	1 week	Median 71 (range 25–112)	From ingestion until tattoo, median 103 (range 25–361) From tattoo to cecum, 260	N/A	N/A	90.9 (20/22)	No major complications	N/A

Nakamura [37]	Prospective. 28 pts, mean age 58.5 years (25–85), Nagoya University Graduate School of Medicine, 2004–2005	OGIB	DBE; antegrade or retrograde, 28.57 (8/28); oral and anal, 71.42 (20/28)	M2A PillCam	28 pts, DBE preceded by CE	2 days	N/A	Total, 510 ± 23.0; small bowel, 277 ± 105	N/A	62.5 (10/16)	90.6 (29/32)	N/A	N/A
Partridge [38]	Retrospective, 18 pts, mean age 65 ± 16 years, Fox Chase Cancer Center, USA, 2004–2009	OGIB, abnormal-cross sectional imaging	DBE and/or SE; initially antegrade unless distal source of bleeding suspected; oral and anal; N/A	N/A	18 pts, DBE/SE preceded by CE	N/A	N/A	N/A	N/A	N/A	N/A	N/A	1 capsule retention retrieved by DBE
Sethi [39]	Retrospective, 46 pts, mean age 63 years (17–92), Beth Israel Deaconess Center, Harvard Medical School, USA, 2011–2013	Anemia, OGIB, suspected mass	SBE	PillCam SB	113 pts, SBE preceded by CE		Overall, 47 ± 15 (range 14–114); antegrade, 46 ± 15 (range 14–114); retrograde, 55 ± 14 (range (27–78)	N/A	Distal jejunum/ proximal ileum reached in 67% of cases	16.7 (1/6)	N/A	1 esophageal perforation, managed conservatively; mild transient fever without infection	Capsule retention in 2 pts

(continued)

Table 18.2 (continued)

Study	Population and study design	Indication	OAE approach and route of insertion, % (n/N)	CE model	Examination sequence	Time between tests	OAE mean procedure time, min	CE recording duration, min	OAE mean depth of insertion, cm	OAE complete examinations, % (n/N)	CE complete examinations, % (n/N)	OAE complications	CE complications
Vere [40]	Retrospective, 21 pts, mean age 50.28 years (15–79), internal medicine and gastroenterology clinic at emergency county hospital of Craiova, Romania, 2008–2009.	Suspicion of tumors	SBE	N/A	21 pts, SBE preceded by CE	N/A	N/A	N/A	N/A	N/A	N/A	N/A	N/A
Li [41]	Prospective, 21 pts, Shanghai Institute of Digestive Diseases, China, 2004–2006	OGIB, abdominal pain, diarrhea	DBE; N/A1	M2A CE	18 pts with CE first, 3 pts with DBE first	12.9 days (range 2–50)	N/A1	Total, 487 (range 362–670); small intestine, 276 (range 19–498)	75 (range 55–120)	25.5	73.2		N/A1

OAE overtube-assisted enteroscopy, *CE* capsule endoscopy, *OGIB* obscure gastrointestinal bleeding, *N/A* not available

1 not available for the subgroup of patients who underwent both OAE and CE, *pts* patients, *DBE* double-balloon enteroscopy, *SE* spiral enteroscopy, *SBE* single-balloon enteroscopy

the index test; they often include the signs, symptoms, or previous test results that generate the suspicion about the target condition. Additional criteria can be used to exclude participants for reasons of safety, feasibility, and ethical arguments.

Differences in methods for identifying eligible patients can affect the spectrum and prevalence of the target condition in the study group, as well as the range and relative frequency of alternative conditions in patients without the target condition. These differences can influence the estimates of diagnostic accuracy [48].

Example "We included comparative studies in which OAE (including DBE, SBE, and SE) and CE were performed to diagnose small-bowel disease in patients with OGIB gastrointestinal polyposis, anemia, chronic abdominal pain, diarrhea, or suspected mass. Our search was applied to all databases through November 2014" [26].

In the example, participants were identified through searching a patient database if provided and were included if they underwent the index test and the reference standard.

Specify Where and when potentially eligible participants were identified (setting, location, and dates), whether participants formed a consecutive, random, or convenience series; index test, in sufficient detail to allow replication; and reference standard, in sufficient detail to allow replication.

Example Table 18.2 summarizes an example of these items.

Rationale for Choosing the Reference Standard (If Alternatives Exist)

In diagnostic accuracy studies, the reference standard is used for establishing the presence or absence of the target condition in study participants. Several reference standards may be available to define the same target condition. In such cases, authors are invited to provide their rationale for selecting the specific reference standard from the available alternatives. This may depend on the intended use of the index test, the clinical relevance, or practical and/or ethical reasons.

Alternative reference standards are not always in perfect agreement. Some reference standards are less accurate than others. In other cases, different reference standards reflect related but different manifestations or stages of the disease, as in confirmation by imaging (first reference standard) versus clinical events (second reference standard) [24].

Example "The sensitivity and specificity of OAE were calculated by establishing CE as the reference test for the diagnosis of small-bowel pathology. This was because of its ability to visualize the entire small bowel in a higher proportion of patients compared with OAE. When data for surgically resected specimens were available, OAE biopsy results were compared with the final surgical histopathological diagnosis" [26].

Whether clinical information and reference standard results were available to the performers or readers of the index test or whether clinical information and index test results were available to the assessors of the reference standard.

Medical tests require interpretation and judgement. These actions may be influenced by the information that is available to the reader [14, 16, 49]. This can lead to artificially high agreement between tests, or between the index test and the reference standard.

When the assessors of the reference standard may have had access to the index test results, the final classification may be guided by the index test result, and the reported accuracy estimates for the index test will be too high [16, 17, 50]. Tests that require subjective interpretation are particularly susceptible to this bias.

Withholding information from the readers of the test is commonly referred to as "blinding" or "masking." Blinding is neither desirable nor undesirable, but, rather, that readers of the study report need information about blinding for the index test and the reference standard to be able to interpret the study findings.

Example "Most studies used CE as an initial test, and its results served as a guide for the OAE route of insertion and localization of lesions. Indeed, OAE was frequently performed with an unblinded CE result, which introduced a higher risk for bias. However, this approach reflects the current standard of care, and it would not make sense to randomize patients to undergo OAE first when CE is a less invasive test" [26].

Methods for estimating or comparing measures of diagnostic accuracy.

Multiple measures of diagnostic accuracy exist to describe the performance of a medical test, and their calculation from the collected data is not always straightforward [51]. Authors should report the methods used for calculating the measures that they considered appropriate for their study objectives.

Example "Based on these data, the sensitivity, specificity, PLR, and NLR (with corresponding 95% confidence intervals [CIs]) of enteroscopy were calculated. Pooled results with corresponding 95% CIs were derived by using the random effects model. A summary receiver operating characteristic curve (SROC) was constructed based on the Moses-Shapiro-Littenberg method" [26].

Results: Baseline demographic and clinical characteristics of participants.

The diagnostic accuracy of a test may have variations according to the demographic and clinical characteristics of the population in which it is applied [17, 18]. These differences may reflect variability in the extent or severity of disease, which affects sensitivity, or in the alternative conditions that are able to generate false-positive findings, affecting specificity [52].

An adequate description of the demographic and clinical characteristics of study participants allows the reader to judge whether the study can adequately address the study question or whether the study findings apply to the reader's clinical question.

Example Table 18.2 summarizes characteristics of included studies, including population characteristics and main indication for reference and index test.

Time Interval and Any Clinical Interventions Between Index Test and Reference Standard

Studies of diagnostic accuracy are essentially cross-sectional investigations. In most cases, one wants to know how well the index test classified patients in the same way as the reference standard, when both tests are performed in the same patients, at the same time [53]. When a delay occurs between the index test and the reference standard, the target condition and alternative conditions can change; conditions may worsen, or improve in the meanwhile, due to the natural course of the disease or due to clinical interventions applied between the two tests. Such changes influence the agreement between the index test and the reference standard, which could lead to biased estimates of test performance.

The bias can be more severe if the delay differs systematically between test positives and test negatives or between those with a high prior suspicion of having the target condition and those with a low suspicion [16, 17].

Example Table 18.2 summarizes characteristics of included studies, including time interval between tests and examination sequence.

Estimates of diagnostic accuracy and their precision (such as 95% CIs).

Diagnostic accuracy studies never determine a test's "true" sensitivity and specificity; at best, the data collected in the study can be used to calculate valid estimates of sensitivity and specificity. The smaller the number of study participants, the less precise these estimates will be [54].

The most frequently used expression of imprecision is to report not just the estimates—sometimes referred to as point estimates—but also 95% CIs around the estimates. Results from studies with imprecise estimates of accuracy should be interpreted with caution, as overoptimism [46].

Example "The pooled sensitivity and specificity of OAE for the diagnosis of small-bowel polyps and tumors were 0.89 (95%CI 0.84–0.93), with heterogeneity $\chi 2 = 41.23$ ($P = 0.0002$) and inconsistency (I 2) = 66.0%, and 0.97 (95% CI 0.95–0.98), with heterogeneity $\chi 2 = 45.27$ ($P = 0.07$) and inconsistency (I 2) = 69.1%, respectively. The pooled PLR and NLR, random effects model, were 16.61 (95% CI 3.74–73.82), with heterogeneity Cochrane Q = 225.19 ($P < 0.01$) and inconsistency (I 2) = 93.8%, and 0.14 (95% CI 0.05–0.35), with heterogeneity Cochrane Q = 81.01($P < 0.01$) and inconsistency (I 2) = 82.7%, respectively" [26].

Any adverse events from performing the index test or the reference standard.

Not all medical tests are equally safe, and in this, they do not differ from many other medical interventions [55, 56]. The testing procedure can lead to complications, such as perforations with endoscopy, contrast allergic reactions in CT imaging, or claustrophobia with MRI scanning.

Measuring and reporting of adverse events in studies of diagnostic accuracy will provide additional information to clinicians, who may be reluctant to use them if they produce severe or frequent adverse events. Actual application of a test in clinical practice will not just be guided by the test's accuracy but by several other dimensions as well, including feasibility and safety. This also applies to the reference standard.

Example Table 18.2 summarizes characteristics of studies, including complications.

Discussion: Study limitations including sources of potential bias, statistical uncertainty, and generalizability.

In the discussion, authors should critically reflect on the validity of their findings, address potential limitations, and elaborate on why study findings may or may not be generalizable. As bias can come down to overestimation or underestimation of the accuracy of the index test under investigation, authors should discuss the direction of potential bias, along with its likely magnitude. Readers are then informed of the likelihood that the limitations jeopardize the study's results and conclusions [24].

Example "Our study has potential limitations. First, and important, is the limited number of comparison data with a gold standard method, such as intraoperative enteroscopy or surgery, found in most of the included studies. However, intraoperative enteroscopy is now rarely performed. Second, although histological confirmation is required for choosing the most adequate therapeutic option, histological confirmation by OAE may sometimes guide therapeutics other than surgery, such as chemotherapy. This is especially important in cases of malignant lymphoma or metastasis. Third, most studies had a relatively small sample size, and heterogeneity may also have limited the study" [26].

Implications for practice, including the intended use and clinical role of the index test.

To make the study findings relevant for practice, authors of diagnostic accuracy studies should elaborate on the consequences of their findings, taking into account the intended use (the purpose of testing) and clinical role of the test (how will the test be positioned in the existing clinical pathway) [24].

Example "Most studies used CE as an initial test, and its results served as a guide for the OAE route of insertion and localization of lesions. Indeed, OAE was frequently performed with an unblinded CE result, which introduced a higher risk for bias. However, this approach reflects the current standard of care, and it would not make sense to randomize patients to undergo OAE first when CE is a less invasive test" [26].

References

1. Siegel RL, Miller KD, Jemal A. Cancer statistics, 2016. CA Cancer J Clin. 2016;66:7–30.
2. Pew Research Center. Modern immigration wave brings 59 million to U.S., driving population growth and change through 2065: views of immigration's impact on U.S. society mixed. Washington, DC: Pew Research Center; 2015.
3. Ferdinand R, Mitchell SA, Batson S, Tumur I. Treatments for chronic myeloid leukemia: a qualitative systematic review. J Blood Med. 2012;3:51–76.
4. Amin MB, Greene FL, Edge SB, Compton CC, Gershenwald JE, Brookland RK, Meyer L, Gress DM, Byrd DR, Winchester DP. The eighth edition AJCC cancer staging manual: continuing to build a bridge from a population-based to a more "personalized" approach to cancer staging. CA Cancer J Clin. 2017;67:93–9.
5. Leeflang MM, Deeks JJ, Gatsonis C, Bossuyt PM, Group CDTAW. Systematic reviews of diagnostic test accuracy. Ann Intern Med. 2008;149:889–97.
6. Mulrow CD. Rationale for systematic reviews. BMJ. 1994;309:597–9.
7. Bossuyt PM, Irwig L, Craig J, Glasziou P. Comparative accuracy: assessing new tests against existing diagnostic pathways. BMJ. 2006;332:1089–92.
8. Lord SJ, Irwig L, Simes RJ. When is measuring sensitivity and specificity sufficient to evaluate a diagnostic test, and when do we need randomized trials? Ann Intern Med. 2006;144:850–5.
9. Thornbury JR. Eugene W. Caldwell Lecture. Clinical efficacy of diagnostic imaging: love it or leave it. AJR Am J Roentgenol. 1994;162:1–8.
10. Glas AS, Roos D, Deutekom M, Zwinderman AH, Bossuyt PM, Kurth KH. Tumor markers in the diagnosis of primary bladder cancer. A systematic review. J Urol. 2003;169:1975–82.
11. Lokeshwar VB, Selzer MG. Urinary bladder tumor markers. Urol Oncol. 2006;24:528–37.
12. Deeks JJ. Systematic reviews in health care: systematic reviews of evaluations of diagnostic and screening tests. BMJ. 2001;323:157–62.

13. Tatsioni A, Zarin DA, Aronson N, Samson DJ, Flamm CR, Schmid C, et al. Challenges in systematic reviews of diagnostic technologies. Ann Intern Med. 2005;142:1048–55.
14. Begg CB. Biases in the assessment of diagnostic tests. Stat Med. 1987;6:411–23.
15. Dinnes J, Deeks J, Kirby J, Roderick P. A methodological review of how heterogeneity has been examined in systematic reviews of diagnostic test accuracy. Health Technol Assess. 2005;9:1–113.
16. Whiting P, Rutjes AW, Reitsma JB, Glas AS, Bossuyt PM, Kleijnen J. Sources of variation and bias in studies of diagnostic accuracy: a systematic review. Ann Intern Med. 2004;140:189–202.
17. Whiting PF, Rutjes AW, Westwood ME, Mallett S, Group Q-S. A systematic review classifies sources of bias and variation in diagnostic test accuracy studies. J Clin Epidemiol. 2013;66:1093–104.
18. Whiting PF, Rutjes AW, Westwood ME, Mallett S, Deeks JJ, Reitsma JB, et al. QUADAS-2: a revised tool for the quality assessment of diagnostic accuracy studies. Ann Intern Med. 2011;155:529–36.
19. Mallett S, Deeks JJ, Halligan S, Hopewell S, Cornelius V, Altman DG. Systematic reviews of diagnostic tests in cancer: review of methods and reporting. BMJ. 2006;333:413.
20. Oxman AD, Guyatt GH. The science of reviewing research. Ann N Y Acad Sci. 1993;703:125–33.
21. Navaneethan U, Hasan MK, Lourdusamy V, Njei B, Varadarajulu S, Hawes RH. Single-operator cholangioscopy and targeted biopsies in the diagnosis of indeterminate biliary strictures: a systematic review. Gastrointest Endosc. 2015;82:608–14.e2.
22. Whiting P, Rutjes AW, Reitsma JB, Bossuyt PM, Kleijnen J. The development of QUADAS: a tool for the quality assessment of studies of diagnostic accuracy included in systematic reviews. BMC Med Res Methodol. 2003;3:25.
23. Lijmer JG, Mol BW, Heisterkamp S, Bonsel GJ, Prins MH, van der Meulen JH, et al. Empirical evidence of design-related bias in studies of diagnostic tests. JAMA. 1999;282:1061–6.
24. Cohen JF, Korevaar DA, Altman DG, Bruns DE, Gatsonis CA, Hooft L, et al. STARD 2015 guidelines for reporting diagnostic accuracy studies: explanation and elaboration. BMJ Open. 2016;6:e012799.
25. Whiting P, Harbord R, Kleijnen J. No role for quality scores in systematic reviews of diagnostic accuracy studies. BMC Med Res Methodol. 2005;5:19.
26. Sulbaran M, de Moura E, Bernardo W, Morais C, Oliveira J, Bustamante-Lopez L, et al. Overtube-assisted enteroscopy and capsule endoscopy for the diagnosis of small-bowel polyps and tumors: a systematic review and meta-analysis. Endosc Int Open. 2016;4:E151–63.
27. Arakawa D, Ohmiya N, Nakamura M, et al. Outcome after enteroscopy for patients with obscure GI bleeding: diagnostic comparison between double-balloon endoscopy and video-capsule endoscopy. Gastrointest Endosc. 2009;69:866–74.
28. Buscaglia JM, Richards R, Wilkinson MN, et al. Diagnostic yield of spiral enteroscopy when performed for the evaluation of abnormal capsule endoscopy findings. J Clin Gastroenterol. 2011;45:342–6.
29. Fry LC, Neumann H, Kuester D, et al. Small bowel polyps and tumours: endoscopic detection and treatment by double-balloon enteroscopy. Aliment Pharmacol Ther. 2009;29:135–42.
30. Fujimori S, Seo T, Gudis K, et al. Diagnosis and treatment of obscure gastrointestinal bleeding using combined capsule endoscopy and double balloon endoscopy: 1-year follow-up study. Endoscopy. 2007;39:1053–8.
31. Kamalaporn P, Cho S, Basset N, et al. Double-balloon enteroscopy following capsule endoscopy in the management of obscure gastrointestinal bleeding: outcome of a combined approach. Can J Gastroenterol. 2008;22:491–5.
32. Kameda N, Higuchi K, Shiba M, et al. A prospective, single-blind trial comparing wireless capsule endoscopy and double-balloon enteroscopy in patients with obscure gastrointestinal bleeding. J Gastroenterol. 2008;43:434–40.
33. Lee BI, Choi H, Choi KY, et al. Clinical characteristics of small bowel tumors diagnosed by double-balloon endoscopy: KASID multi-center study. Dig Dis Sci. 2011;56:2920–7.

34. Manno M, Riccioni ME, Cannizzaro R, et al. Diagnostic and therapeutic yield of single balloon enteroscopy in patients with suspected small-bowel disease: results of the Italian multicentre study. Dig Liver Dis. 2013;45:211–5.
35. Marmo R, Rotondano G, Casetti T, et al. Degree of concordance between double-balloon enteroscopy and capsule endoscopy in obscure gastrointestinal bleeding: a multicenter study. Endoscopy. 2009;41:587–92.
36. Matsumoto T, Esaki M, Moriyama T, et al. Comparison of capsule endoscopy and enteroscopy with the doubleballoon method in patients with obscure bleeding and polyposis. Endoscopy. 2005;37:827–32.
37. Nakamura M, Niwa Y, Ohmiya N, et al. Preliminary comparison of capsule endoscopy and double-balloon enteroscopy in patients with suspected small-bowel bleeding. Endoscopy. 2006;38:59–66.
38. Partridge BJ, Tokar JL, Haluszka O, et al. Small bowel cancers diagnosed by device-assisted enteroscopy at a U.S. referral center: a five-year experience. Dig Dis Sci. 2011;56:2701–5.
39. Sethi S, Cohen J, Thaker AM, et al. Prior capsule endoscopy improves the diagnostic and therapeutic yield of single-balloon enteroscopy. Dig Dis Sci. 2014;59:2497–502.
40. Vere CC, Foarfă C, Streba CT, et al. Videocapsule endoscopy and single balloon enteroscopy: novel diagnostic techniques in small bowel pathology. Rom J Morphol Embryol. 2009;50:467–74.
41. Li XB, Ge ZZ, Dai J, et al. The role of capsule endoscopy combined with double-balloon enteroscopy in diagnosis of small bowel diseases. Chin Med J (Engl). 2007;120:30–5.
42. Westwood ME, Whiting PF, Kleijnen J. How does study quality affect the results of a diagnostic meta-analysis? BMC Med Res Methodol. 2005;5:20.
43. Leeflang M, Reitsma J, Scholten R, Rutjes A, Di Nisio M, Deeks J, et al. Impact of adjustment for quality on results of metaanalyses of diagnostic accuracy. Clin Chem. 2007;53:164–72.
44. Jones CM, Athanasiou T. Diagnostic accuracy meta-analysis: review of an important tool in radiological research and decision making. Br J Radiol. 2009;82:441–6.
45. A proposal for more informative abstracts of clinical articles. Ad Hoc Working Group for Critical Appraisal of the Medical Literature. Ann Intern Med. 1987;106:598–604.
46. Ochodo EA, de Haan MC, Reitsma JB, Hooft L, Bossuyt PM, Leeflang MM. Overinterpretation and misreporting of diagnostic accuracy studies: evidence of "spin". Radiology. 2013;267:581–8.
47. Sorensen HT, Sabroe S, Olsen J. A framework for evaluation of secondary data sources for epidemiological research. Int J Epidemiol. 1996;25:435–42.
48. Leeflang MM, Bossuyt PM, Irwig L. Diagnostic test accuracy may vary with prevalence: implications for evidence-based diagnosis. J Clin Epidemiol. 2009;62:5–12.
49. Doubilet P, Herman PG. Interpretation of radiographs: effect of clinical history. AJR Am J Roentgenol. 1981;137:1055–8.
50. Philbrick JT, Horwitz RI, Feinstein AR. Methodologic problems of exercise testing for coronary artery disease: groups, analysis and bias. Am J Cardiol. 1980;46:807–12.
51. Knottnerus JA, Buntinx F. The evidence base of clinical diagnosis: theory and methods of diagnostic research. 2nd ed. London: BMJ Books; 2008.
52. Ransohoff DF, Feinstein AR. Problems of spectrum and bias in evaluating the efficacy of diagnostic tests. N Engl J Med. 1978;299:926–30.
53. Knottnerus JA, Muris JW. Assessment of the accuracy of diagnostic tests: the cross-sectional study. J Clin Epidemiol. 2003;56:1118–28.
54. Lang TA, Secic M. Generalizing from a sample to a population: reporting estimates and confidence intervals. Philadelphia: American College of Physicians; 1997.
55. Ioannidis JP, Evans SJ, Gøtzsche PC, O'Neill RT, Altman DG, Schulz K, et al. Better reporting of harms in randomized trials: an extension of the CONSORT statement. Ann Intern Med. 2004;141:781–8.
56. Ioannidis JP, Lau J. Completeness of safety reporting in randomized trials: an evaluation of 7 medical areas. JAMA. 2001;285:437–43.

19 Diagnostic Meta-Analysis: Case Study in Surgery

Eliana Al Haddad, Hutan Ashrafian, and Thanos Athanasiou

19.1 Introduction

It has been estimated that doctors should read ten peer-reviewed articles per day for 365 days a year to stay up to date with developments in their field [1]. Surgery is an ever-expanding, continuously evolving field and is subject to multiple streams of new knowledge. These include new evidence of (1) specific elements to the pre-, peri-, and postoperative period, (2) surgical and medical pathology, (3) advances in disease imaging and tissue guidance, and (4) awareness of new devices ranging from operative monitoring/diagnostic devices, stapling instruments, and robots. As a result, the evaluation of all of these elements requires substantiation with appropriate evidence. While several types of literature reviews attempt to merge this expansion of information, diagnostic meta-analysis seems to offer a particularly powerful role in combining pertinent quantitative study data from selected studies to develop a single conclusion with greater statistical power [2] that can supporting surgical decision-making.

Recent examples of diagnostic accuracy meta-analysis in surgery include intra-operative techniques for margin assessment in breast cancer surgery [3], assessing the diagnostic accuracy of percutaneous renal tumor biopsies [4], and a review of

E. Al Haddad
The Division of Cardiac Surgery, Department of Surgery, Columbia University, New York, NY, USA

H. Ashrafian
The Department of Surgery and Cancer, Imperial College London, London, UK
e-mail: h.ashrafian@imperial.ac.uk

T. Athanasiou (✉)
The Department of Surgery and Cancer, Imperial College London, London, UK

Department of Cardiac Surgery, Imperial College Healthcare NHS Trust, London, UK
e-mail: t.athanasiou@imperial.ac.uk

G. Biondi-Zoccai (ed.), *Diagnostic Meta-Analysis*,
https://doi.org/10.1007/978-3-319-78966-8_19

the diagnostic role of procalcitonin and C-reactive protein for the early diagnosis of intra-abdominal infection after elective colorectal surgery [5]. Broader topics include assessing different modalities for suspected acute appendicitis [6], evaluation of the effectiveness and risks of bariatric surgery outcomes [7], or even for the prenatal diagnosis of critical congenital heart disease and their effect on the reduction of death from cardiovascular compromise prior to planned neonatal cardiac surgery [8].

The aim of this chapter is to identify the principles, steps, and examples of diagnostic meta-analysis in the surgical setting.

19.2 Surgical Needs

Diagnostic accuracy meta-analysis in surgery can augment decision-making in the whole surgical pathway ranging from the pre-, intra-, and postoperative phases. It can affect the decision to undergo surgery when done preoperatively, can change the course of the operation when the diagnostic test is performed intraoperatively, or can evaluate the outcomes of certain surgical procedures on a long-term basis as illustrated below.

19.2.1 Preoperative Diagnosis

Diagnostic tests are usually performed preoperatively to determine the need and type of surgical procedure that will be done (Fig. 19.1). For example, accurate three-dimensional printing of hearts can now be undertaken preoperatively for children with congenital heart diseases to help physicians assess and visualize the precise cardiac anatomy of patients and plan the best surgical course of action [9]. Another common example includes the use of cardiac catheterization to determine the degree of diseased coronary arteries before deciding whether to undergo the placement of stents via percutaneous coronary intervention or to perform open-heart surgery. In terms of cancer, preoperative diagnostic tools such as imaging and biopsies determine the need and extent of surgery, and performing such studies could help in the formation of guidelines for preoperative diagnostic tools.

19.2.2 Intraoperative Diagnosis

In the study mentioned earlier, reviewers attempted to come to a conclusion for the best diagnostic measure to assess the margins for breast cancer intraoperatively using all different techniques available [3]. Having accurate information at hand about this topic can determine the course of the surgery as well as the prognosis of the patient. Another example would be attempting to establish whether using laparoscopic ultrasonography or intraoperative cholangiograms is the superior tool to be used intraoperatively for the detection of stones in the common bile duct [10].

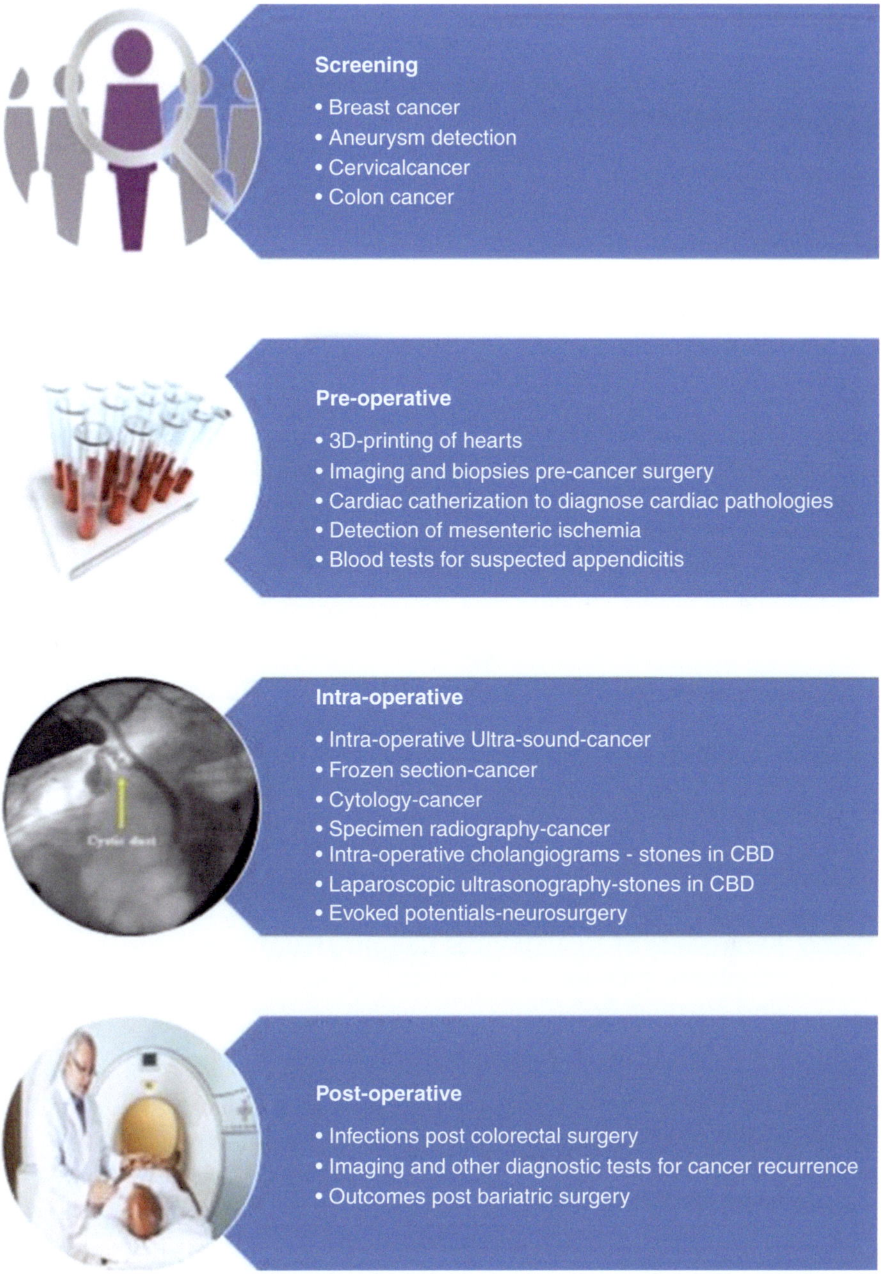

Fig. 19.1 The use of diagnostic tests in surgery

19.2.3 Postoperative Diagnosis

Diagnostic tests can also be performed postoperatively as to determine multiple important parameters pertaining to the outcomes of that specific surgery. Such examples include determining the outcomes of post-bariatric surgery such as weight loss on the long-term basis or the resolution of comorbidities, as well as the prompt and accurate diagnosis of complications such as leak or bleeding, and the best methods to deal with these complications.

19.2.4 Surgical and Medical Pathology

The diagnosis of underlying tissue pathology remains a core component of modern surgery. There are increased necessities of diagnosis pathological accuracy in precision surgery particularly in the identification of pathological tissue subgroups and their individual responses to treatment modalities. This can be illustrated in the evaluation of the pathological response to neoadjuvant chemotherapy in breast cancer patients [11] or the usage of fine needle aspiration for the detection of malignancy in pediatric thyroid nodules [12].

19.2.5 Advances in Disease Imaging and Tissue Guidance

Similarly, diagnostic radiology is also a fundamental component of precision surgery. Diagnostic surgical meta-analysis has recently identified [13] how F-FDG PET and PET-CT can assess the metabolic profile of cancers and aid in the diagnosis of colorectal liver metastasis [14].

19.2.6 Awareness of New Devices Ranging from Operative Monitoring/Diagnostic Devices, to Stapling Instruments, and Surgical Robots

All novel surgical devices ranging from surgical staplers to the newest robots have an impact in clinical outcomes, and diagnostic accuracy meta-analysis may offer an avenue into assessing how these may affect the results of established diagnostic and imaging modalities. Additionally, these techniques can be utilized to assess new surgical diagnostic platforms such as the use of novel intraoperative ultrasound for the detection of breast cancer margins [3].

One important area where diagnostic accuracy meta-analysis has an important role in surgery is its application in generating evidence for consensus statements and diagnostic tool, for example, which diagnostic tool is of most value for each step of disease diagnosis in various stages of the patient journey. Table 19.1 reveals some of the most prominent diagnostic meta-analytical studies performed in the surgery.

Table 19.1 Meta-analysis studies performed from 2012 to 2017, categorized by field of surgery and year of publication

Title	Authors	Field of surgery	Year	Time
Novel serological biomarkers to detect acute mesenteric ischemia [31]	Treskes N et al.	General surgery	2017	Preoperative
Fine needle aspiration biopsy for detection of malignancy in pediatric thyroid nodules [12]	Lai SW et al.	General surgery	2015	Preoperative
Detection of common bile duct stones during laparoscopic cholecystectomy [10]	Aziz O et al.	General surgery	2014	Intraoperative
Endoscopic ultrasound in pancreatic neuroendocrine tumors [32]	Puli SR et al.	General surgery	2013	Preoperative
Procalcitonin, C-reactive protein, and white blood cell count for suspected acute appendicitis [6]	Yu CW et al	General surgery	2013	Preoperative
Margin assessment in breast cancer surgery [3]	St John ER et al.	Cancer surgery	2017	Intraoperative
Ductoscopy in patients with pathological nipple discharge [33]	Waaijer L et al.	Cancer surgery	2016	Preoperative
Evaluation of pathologic response to neoadjuvant chemotherapy in patients with breast cancer [11]	Sheikhbahaei S et al.	Cancer surgery	2016	Preoperative
Evaluating PET-CT in the detection and management of recurrent cervical cancer [34]	Meads C et al.	Cancer surgery	2013	Postoperative
Evoked potential monitoring techniques during intracranial aneurysm surgery for predicting postoperative ischemic damage [35]	Thomas B et al.	Neurosurgery	2017	Intraoperative
Motor-evoked potentials to detect neurological deficit during idiopathic scoliosis correction [36]	Thirumala PD et al.	Neurosurgery	2017	Intraoperative
Brain microdialysis during surgery [37]	Bossers SM et al.	Neurosurgery	2013	Intraoperative
Dilemmas in the interpretation of diagnostic accuracy studies on presurgical work-up for epilepsy surgery [38]	Burch J et al.	Neurosurgery	2012	Preoperative
Early diagnosis of intra-abdominal infection after elective colorectal surgery [5]	Cousin F et al.	Colorectal Surgery	2016	Postoperative
Carcinoembryonic antigen to detect colorectal cancer recurrence [39]	Sørensen CG et al.	Colorectal Surgery	2016	Postoperative
(18)F-FDG PET and PET-CT in colorectal liver metastasis [14]	Maffione AM et al.	Colorectal Surgery	2015	Preoperative

(continued)

Table 19.1 (continued)

Title	Authors	Field of surgery	Year	Time
Risks of biopsy in the diagnosis of a renal mass suspicious for localized renal cell carcinoma [40]	Patel HD et al.	Urology	2016	Preoperative
18F-fluorodeoxyglucose positron emission tomography and computed tomography in staging bladder cancer [41]	Soubra A et al.	Urology	2016	Preoperative
Diagnostic accuracy of percutaneous renal tumor biopsy [4]	Marconi L et al.	Urology	2016	Preoperative
Prenatal diagnosis of critical congenital heart disease prior to planned neonatal cardiac surgery [8]	Holland BJ et al.	Cardiac surgery	2015	Preoperative
Transesophageal echocardiogram for the detection of patent foramen ovale [42]	Mojadidi MK et al.	Cardiac surgery	2014	Preoperative
Clinical tests for the diagnosis of hip femoroacetabular impingement/labral tear [43]	Reiman MP et al.	Orthopedic surgery	2015	Preoperative
CT angiography and MR angiography in the stenosis detection of autologous hemodialysis access [44]	Li B et al.	Vascular surgery	2013	Preoperative

19.3 Paper Selection

When undertaking a meta-analysis for the determination of the most accurate diagnostic tool, a certain design needs to be followed. In this step, we shall use multiple previously mentioned papers as references to illustrate each step.

19.3.1 Study Design Terms

Diagnostic accuracy is represented by two measures [15–17] that we apply with our example of surgical disease (breast cancer). The first being sensitivity, which asses the true positive proportion of disease diagnosis which and is calculated as $\frac{\text{true positives}}{\text{true positives} + \text{false negatives}}$. This reflects the probability that the person with the condition has a positive diagnostic test. The second measure is specificity, used to assess true negatives, and is calculated as $\frac{\text{true neagtives}}{\text{true negatives} + \text{false positives}}$ (Table 19.2).

The surgical test of interest is commonly known as the "index test," and it is the one that is being compared to the best currently available diagnostic test, also known

Table 19.2 Example for the classification of patient mammography test results

Index test outcome—mammography	Pathology for breast cancer positive	Pathology for breast cancer negative
Mammography positive	True positive	False positive
Mammography negative	False negative	True negative

as the "reference test." In St. John et al.'s study [3], the reference test used was permanent section histopathology, while the index tests included frozen section, cytology, specimen radiography, optical imaging, and intraoperative ultrasound. As shown by this example, multiple index tests can be compared to a common reference test to reach a consensus on which diagnostic tool is of best use.

19.3.2 Defining the Research Question

The review question includes the key elements of the inclusion criteria and establishes the objective and hypothesis. It should be structured as so: what is the diagnostic accuracy of (index test) compared with the (reference test) in (population) for the diagnosis of (disease) [18]. In our study [3], the research question was shown to be: the aim of this study was to perform a systematic review and meta-analysis to evaluate pooled diagnostic accuracy for intraoperative breast margin assessment (IMA) techniques that have been evaluated in clinical practice, as a benchmark against which the performance of emerging technologies can be compared.

19.3.3 Establishing the Study Selection Criteria

This step establishes the inclusion and exclusion criteria for identifying eligible studies. The PIRD mnemonic can be used for inclusion, and that includes population (important characteristics to define include the disease stage, symptoms, age, gender, race, and educational status), index test (there are multiple factors to consider here. Those include decision threshold, the expertise/qualification of the person doing or interpreting the test, the conditions under which the test was conducted, and details on how the test will be conducted), reference test (the "gold standard"), and diagnosis of interest (What exactly is being investigated? This needs to be specified when it comes to designing the search strategy) [13, 18].

In our study [3], the inclusion criteria included studies written in English that comprised margin assessment data and acquired from one or more IMA techniques used during breast cancer surgery (BCS) for breast cancer (invasive or in situ); only studies that stated sensitivity and specificity data compared with permanent section histopathology or in whom sensitivity and specificity data could be calculated from raw data were included. Study participants were adults (mean age >18 years).

19.3.4 Performing the Literature Search of the Topic

This step begins with the initial limited search that identifies relevant keywords and indexing forms. Secondly, a thorough search is performed using all included databases (Pubmed, Embase, CINAHL, SCOPUS, Cochrane Library). Subsequently, a review of the reference lists of the included studies is undertaken [13, 19]. After the search strategy is complete, the references need to be screened for duplicates, which can be done both on the search engine and also on referencing management software. Titles and abstracts are then reviewed for their relevance to be included, after which the full texts are reviewed. Studies that fit a preselected inclusion criteria are kept, whereas those that have elements listed in predefined exclusion criteria are rejected. It is important to note that, at each step, the studies that were included and excluded are kept track of, as well as the reasons behind why these articles were excluded.

The entire process needs to be reported, from the search to the selection. Afterwards, a flow chart that conforms to "Preferred Reporting Items for Systematic Reviews and Meta-Analyses" (PRISMA) would be created. Figure 19.2 illustrates this step.

19.3.5 Study Features, Outcomes, and Quality Assessment

This stage of the study assesses, firstly, the methodological quality of the diagnostic studies that were included, and secondly, critical appraisal is used to determine their quality. The best tool available at this instance to perform this step is the Quality Assessment of Diagnostic Accuracy Studies 2 (QUADAS-2) which is a set of critical appraisal checklist questions, answered as yes, no, unclear or N/A. This was developed in 2011 following the revision of the original QUADAS tool [20]. We recommended that reviewers use the QUADAS-2 tool when undertaking their critical appraisal and its "signaling questions," which are included in Table 19.3.

All studies need to be independently appraised by at least two reviewers, and if the questions are answered with a "yes," the study can be included. Disagreement regarding article inclusion would be resolved by consensus in discussion with a third senior author [21]. Figure 19.3 is an example of a QUADAS-2 questionnaire that would determine the quality of each paper to be included in the meta-analysis. A quantitative measure of reviewer agreement regarding study section is the Cronbach's tool. While there is no formal measure of the Cronbach's score for accepting adequate reviewer agreement before proceeding to the next stage of the analysis, a score of over 90% is generally considered adequate for this stage.

19.3.6 Data Extraction

The first step is to settle on a decision threshold for what value is positive/negative; this is unique for diagnostic test accuracy. A standardized data extraction tool is

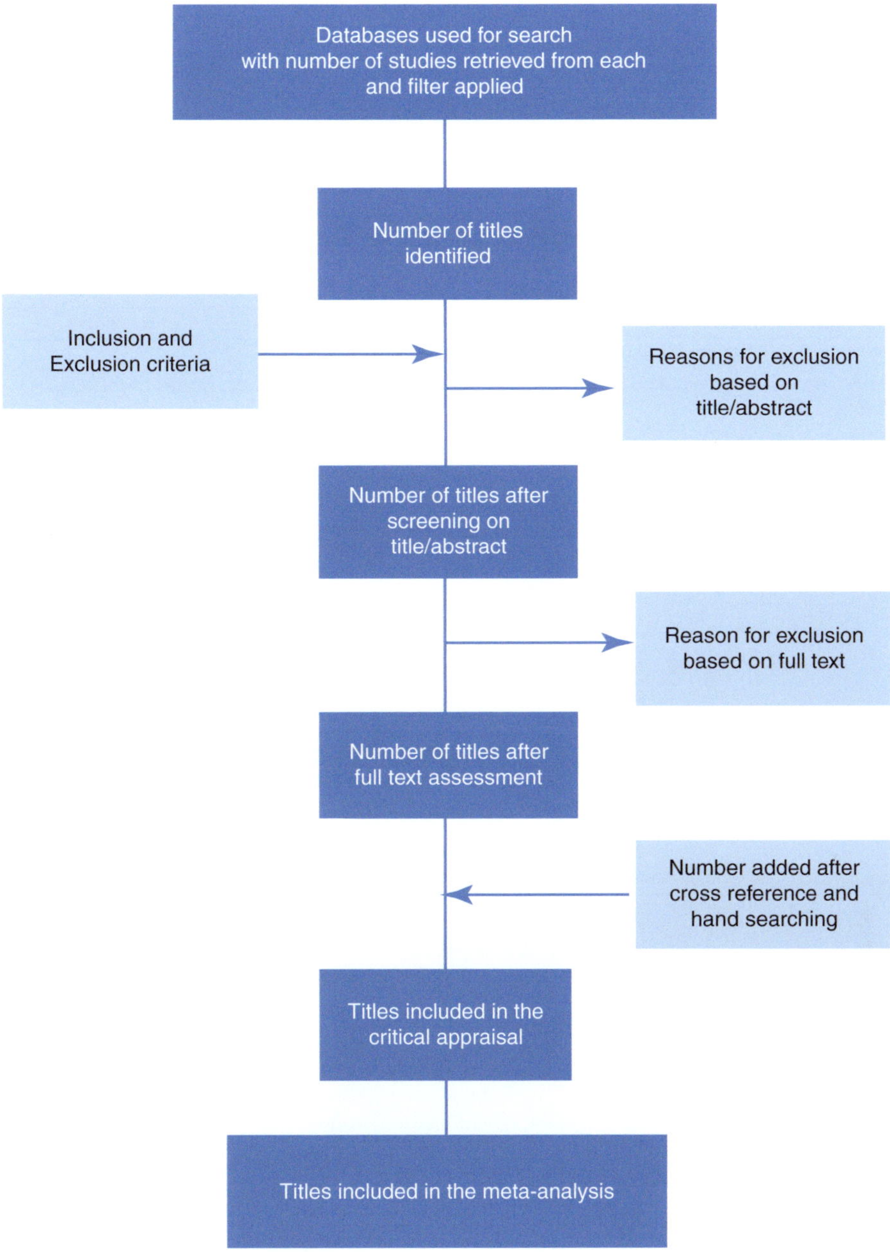

Fig. 19.2 PRISMA flow diagram

Table 19.3 QUADAS-2 signaling questions

Critical appraisal questions
Domain 1: patient selection
Was a consecutive or random sample of patients enrolled?
Was a case-control design avoided?
Did the study avoid inappropriate exclusions?
Domain 2: index test
Were the index test results interpreted without knowledge of the results of the reference standard?
If a threshold was used, was it prespecified?
Domain 3: reference test
Is the reference standard likely to correctly classify the target condition?
Were the reference standard results interpreted without knowledge of the results of the index test?
Flow and timing
Was there an appropriate interval between index test and reference standard?
Did all patients receive the same reference standard?
Were all patients included in the analysis?

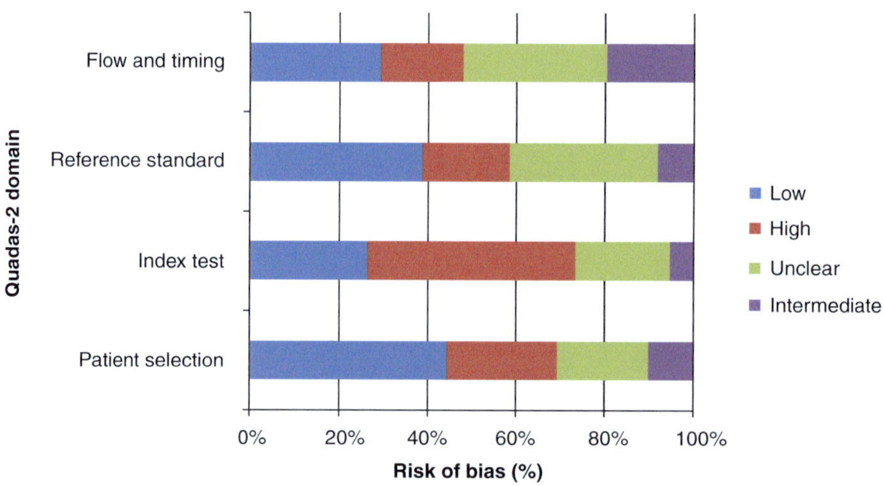

Fig. 19.3 Example of QUADAS-2 tool: risk of bias judgment

used. The Standards for Reporting Diagnostic accuracy studies (STARD) checklist and flow diagram (Table 19.4) provide a detailed guide on what should be reported. It includes a 2 × 2 table that classifies patients' test results and disease status. Subsequently a meta-analytical technique can be applied (see below) for combining data. This applies a weighted mean for results such that larger trials are given more weight since the results of smaller trials are more likely to be affected by chance [18, 21].

Table 19.4 STARD checklist

Section and topic	No.	Item	Reported on page #
Title or abstract			
	1	Identification as a study of diagnostic accuracy using at least one measure of accuracy (such as sensitivity, specificity, predictive values, or AUC)	
Abstract			
	2	Structured summary of study design, methods, results, and conclusions (for specific guidance, see STARD for abstracts)	
Introduction			
	3	Scientific and clinical background, including the intended use and clinical role of the index test	
	4	Study objectives and hypotheses	
Methods			
Study design	**5**	Whether data collection was planned before the index test and reference standard were performed (prospective study) or after (retrospective study)	
Participants	**6**	Eligibility criteria	
	7	On what basis potentially eligible participants were identified (such as symptoms, results from previous tests, inclusion in registry)	
	8	Where and when potentially eligible participants were identified (setting, location, and dates)	
	9	Whether participants formed a consecutive, random, or convenience series	
Test methods	**10a**	Index test, in sufficient detail to allow replication	
	10b	Reference standard, in sufficient detail to allow replication	
	11	Rationale for choosing the reference standard (if alternatives exist)	
	12a	Definition of and rationale for test positivity cutoffs or result categories of the index test, distinguishing prespecified from exploratory	
	12b	Definition of and rationale for test positivity cutoffs or result categories of the reference standard, distinguishing prespecified from exploratory	
	13a	Whether clinical information and reference standard results were available to the performers/readers of the index test	
	13b	Whether clinical information and index test results were available to the assessors of the reference standard	
Analysis	**14**	Methods for estimating or comparing measures of diagnostic accuracy	
	15	How indeterminate index test or reference standard results were handled	
	16	How missing data on the index test and reference standard were handled	
	17	Any analyses of variability in diagnostic accuracy, distinguishing prespecified from exploratory	
	18	Intended sample size and how it was determined	

(continued)

Table 19.4 (continued)

Section and topic	No.	Item	Reported on page #
Results			
Participants	**19**	Flow of participants, using a diagram	
	20	Baseline demographic and clinical characteristics of participants	
	21a	Distribution of severity of disease in those with the target condition	
	21b	Distribution of alternative diagnoses in those without the target condition	
	22	Time interval and any clinical interventions between index test and reference standard	
Test results	**23**	Cross-tabulation of the index test results (or their distribution) by the results of the reference standard	
	24	Estimates of diagnostic accuracy and their precision (such as 95% confidence intervals)	
	25	Any adverse events from performing the index test or the reference standard	
Discussion			
	26	Study limitations, including sources of potential bias, statistical uncertainty, and generalizability	
	27	Implications for practice, including the intended use and clinical role of the index test	
Other information			
	28	Registration number and name of registry	
	29	Where the full study protocol can be accessed	
	30	Sources of funding and other support; role of funders	

19.4 Study Analysis

Initially, it is necessary to assess the heterogeneity between studies, which can be performed by various methods. These include Cochrane Q or Higgins' I^2 statistics. Typically in surgical studies, the results for these statistics tend to be high due to the variable nature of surgery (different techniques between surgeon even for the same procedures in addition to variations in patients, units, and pathologies). This needs to be clarified in any data interpretation as higher heterogeneity in data results in a lower confidence of accepting diagnostic analysis results [22].

The first level of analysis hinges on meta-analytical pooling of individual sensitivity and specificity results (Fig. 19.4); this can be done through fixed-effects models or random-effects models (most commonly the DerSimonian and Laird method). The inherent variability of most surgical results typically requires most caution so that random-effects analysis predominates. Here the random-effects analysis offers an estimate of the mean effect of diagnostic test accuracy through the assumptions that (1) heterogeneity between studies is not purely random and that (2) it also stems from tau-squared, τ^2, or an intrinsic variability in test accuracy [23].

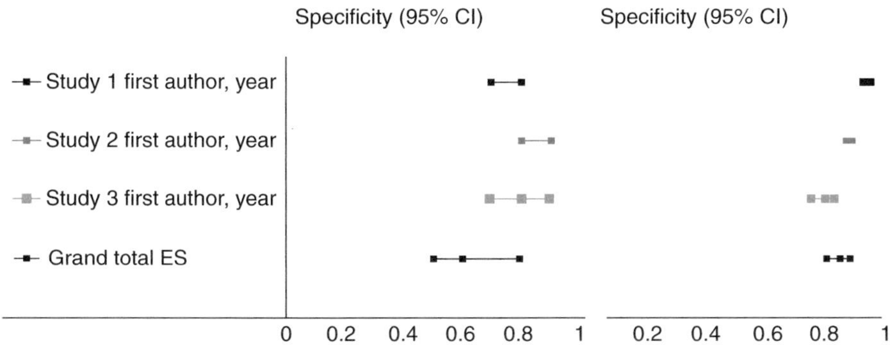

Fig. 19.4 Example of a pooled meta-analysis forest plots per group

Table 19.5 Additional methods for meta-analysis of diagnostic accuracy studies

Methods for meta-analysis of diagnostic accuracy studies	Description
Univariate pooling methods fixed effect versus random effects	Pool sensitivity and specificity separately, ignoring any correlation that may exist between the two measures Fixed = assume homogeneity Random = assume variability in test accuracy beyond sampling error
Summary receiver operating characteristic regression (SROC)	Account for possible heterogeneity in threshold by using a logistic transformation of true-positive (TPR) and false-positive rates (FPR) and linear regression It models the relationship between test accuracy and the proportion of test positive
Hierarchical models bivariate versus HSROC modelbivariate modelHSROC model	Take into account correlation between sensitivity and specificity across studies while also allowing for variation in test performance between studies through the inclusion of random effectsThis bivariate model is a linear mixed model that enables joint analysis of sensitivity and specificity. It assumes a bivariate normal distributionThe HSROC model can be viewed as an extension of the Moses SROC approach in which the TPR and FPR for each study are modeled directly. It is a nonlinear generalized mixed model

The next level of meta-analysis is based on pooling diagnostic odds ratios (DORs), and this is performed through two hierarchical approaches: (1) the Rutter and Gatsonis HSROC model and the (2) bivariate model (Table 19.5). Both approaches have the same primary level appraisal of inter-study variability through the assumption of a binomial distribution for the study factors of 1-specificity and sensitivity. However they differ in their second-level model in that the HSROC model utilizes a proxy threshold or theta "cutoff" and an alpha-natural logarithm of the study diagnostic odds ratio to quantify accuracy (derived from sensitivity and specificity). This requires a logit function with a dummy variable for subject disease standing [23].

The second level of the bivariate model also applies a logit function, but here it transforms sensitivity and specificity according to the assumption of a bivariate normal distribution. From the authors experience in surgical studies in diagnostic meta-analysis, both approaches offer similar results [24].

A graphical curve can now be derived from these meta-analytical results (Fig. 19.5). The Moses-Littenberg SROC method represents a fixed-effects model approach. Following a linear regression technique, a curve is generated of expected sensitivities across a range of specificities. Diagnostic accuracy is measured by the area under the curve (AUC) and Q^* values, where an AUC of 1 is a perfectly accurate test compared to a gold standard, whereas an AUC of 0.5 is indeterminate or representing random results with no accuracy. Alternatively the HSROC (hierarchical SROC) method can be applied as a representation of a random-effects approach [25]. This is favored in surgical studies due to its conservative nature of accommodating heterogeneity from within and between studies in addition to accommodating any correlations between specificity and sensitivity. Once again AUC is considered the primary measure of outcome.

Finally, meta-regression techniques can be utilized across of diagnostic variables to assess their role in overall diagnostic results. Here meta-regression assesses input study quality if variables of study quality (from quality questionnaires) have been included in the analysis. This will offer added value to overall diagnostic results as it can differentiate whether overall outcomes are derived from all studies or only the highest-quality studies.

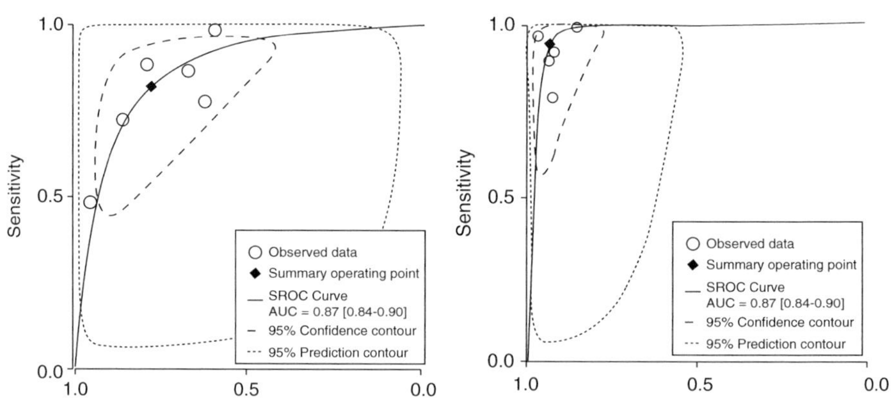

Fig. 19.5 (**a**) Example of meta-analysis SROC curves. The horizontal axis demonstrates specificity, while the vertical demonstrates sensitivity. The curve demonstrates the true-positive rate of each test at each true-negative value. The diagnostic accuracy of each modality is highest when the results of both axes tend closer to 100% (or 1) for both true positives and true negatives. Examples of an SROC curve with a smaller AUC (graph on the left) as compared to the graph on the right and, therefore, lower diagnostic accuracy

19.5 Typical Problems in Surgical Diagnostic Meta-Analysis

Surgical diagnostic meta-analysis studies can suffer from the biases of the underlying biases of surgical study data. Surgical studies are notoriously difficult to perform for multiple reasons that include the difficulties of surgeon equipoise, where surgeons typically have preference to their exact way of performing an operation compared to other techniques or other treatment modalities; this is typically due to the "craft" element of surgery where expert surgeons are archetypally trained as apprentices when on their surgical learning curve.

Randomized controlled trials (RCTs) are known to provide the highest level of evidence when used in meta-analyses studies due to the fact that they have the ability to reduce bias and deliver the most reliable results [26]. However, their conduction remains challenging for the majority of surgical studies [27, 28], and they remain predominantly applied for pharmacological interventions. Here surgical equipoise can be limited through the fundamental notion of selecting the appropriate operation for the appropriate patient. While this is classified as indication, and not necessarily bias, RCTs seek to erase this selection "bias" [26], and as a result surgical RCTs may not be instigated.

Patient equipoise issue also exists where patients typically can demonstrate a preference for or against surgical treatments, for example, a patient may feel that a robotic operation represents cutting-edge technology and would demonstrate more positivity to their outcomes from such an operation. Additionally there are the established problems of pooling nonhomogeneous data from different sources and biases from individual studies [29, 30]. The very nature of surgery results in the fact that no two operations are ever exactly the same, even when performed by the same individual. This renders direct comparisons tricky, as there are anatomical, pathological, and physiological differences in each case but also differences in operating environments, assistants, and even anesthetists. The subsequent interpretation of meta-analysis of this data is very complex, even when taken from a single surgical unit. Assessing surgical data from multiple surgeons and institutions leads to even greater data variation and nonhomogeneity that can afflict consequent diagnostic meta-analysis.

Additional sources of diagnostic accuracy meta-analysis bias revolve around the identification of studies because investigators familiar with the field often selectively choose familiar papers and who have individual opinions regarding specific operations and outcomes [26]. For example, an author who believes strongly in the benefits of the laparoscopic approach for colon cancer may unintentionally exclude studies that do not support their view. Language bias may exist when literature searches fail to include studies conducted in foreign languages, because some authors consider that significant results are more likely to be published in English [18, 19].

As each operation requires preoperative work-up, intraoperative staff and equipment factors, and postoperative care, the very nature of a surgical study (particularly in the setting of experimental and expensive devices) adds further difficulties in the execution of surgical studies. This is because of logistical, financial, and technical reasons. For this reason surgical studies are typically smaller than their medical and pharmacological counterparts. This smaller data sample size results in poorly powered trials such that the subsequent diagnostic meta-analytical studies can be limited by the limitations of the underlying data. Together these surgical study characteristics can augment the "rubbish-in rubbish-out" effect in surgical diagnostic meta-analytical study and should be considered strongly when interpreting results from surgical diagnostic accuracy meta-analyses.

Conclusion

Surgical diagnostic meta-analysis offers a mechanism to address the increasing need for accurate, time-effective diagnostic surgical questions. This includes the appraisal of (1) surgical pathology, (2) disease imaging and tissue guidance, (3) specific elements to the pre-, peri-, and postoperative period, and (4) assessment of the broad range of novel new devices ranging from operative monitoring/ diagnostic instruments, stapling instruments, and robots. While several limitations exist that stem from the underlying difficulties of executing surgical clinical trials, these can be addressed with clear and transparent methodology and a balanced interpretation of results. Surgery remains a dynamic and continually expanding field positioned at the forefront of technological innovation. Diagnostic meta-analytical techniques can therefore offer a prime solution through which to process the ever-increasing volume of surgical outcome data into meaningful information for enhancing clinical outcomes, supporting safety and developing the next generation of cutting-edge surgical technology.

References

1. Sackett DL, Haynes RB. On the need for evidence-based medicine. EBM Notebook. 1995;1:5–6.
2. Glass GV. Primary, secondary and meta-analysis of research. Educ Res. 1976;5:3–8.
3. St John ER, Al-Khudairi R, Ashrafian H, Athanasiou T, Takats Z, Hadjiminas DJ, Darzi A, Leff DR. Diagnostic accuracy of intraoperative techniques for margin assessment in breast cancer surgery. Ann Surg. 2017;265:300–10.
4. Marconi L, Dabestani S, Lam TB, Hofmann F, Stewart F, Norrie J, Bex A, Bensalah K, Canfield SE, Hora M, Kuczyk MA, Merseburger AS, Mulders PF, Powles T, Staehler M, Ljungberg B, Volpe A. Systematic review and meta-analysis of diagnostic accuracy of percutaneous renal tumour biopsy. Eur Urol. 2016;69:660–73.
5. Cousin F, Ortega-Deballon P, Bourredjem A, Doussot A, Giaccaglia V, Fournel I. Diagnostic accuracy of procalcitonin and C-reactive protein for the early diagnosis of intra-abdominal infection after elective colorectal surgery. Ann Surg. 2016;264:252–6.
6. Yu C-W, Juan L-I, Wu M-H, Shen C-J, Wu J-Y, Lee C-C. Systematic review and meta-analysis of the diagnostic accuracy of procalcitonin, C-reactive protein and white blood cell count for suspected acute appendicitis. Br J Surg. 2012;100:322–9.
7. Chang S-H, Stoll CRT, Song J, Varela JE, Eagon CJ, Colditz GA. The effectiveness and risks of bariatric surgery. JAMA Surg. 2014;149:275.
8. Holland BJ, Myers JA, Woods CR. Prenatal diagnosis of critical congenital heart disease reduces risk of death from cardiovascular compromise prior to planned neonatal cardiac surgery: a meta-analysis. Ultrasound Obstet Gynecol. 2015;45:631–8.

9. Tack P, Victor J, Gemmel P, Annemans L. 3D-printing techniques in a medical setting: a systematic literature review. Biomed Eng Online. 2016;15:115.
10. Aziz O, Ashrafian H, Jones C, Harling L, Kumar S, Garas G, Holme T, Darzi A, Zacharakis E, Athanasiou T. Laparoscopic ultrasonography versus intra-operative cholangiogram for the detection of common bile duct stones during laparoscopic cholecystectomy: a meta-analysis of diagnostic accuracy. Int J Surg. 2014;12:712–9.
11. Sheikhbahaei S, Trahan TJ, Xiao J, Taghipour M, Mena E, Connolly RM, Subramaniam RM. FDG-PET/CT and MRI for evaluation of pathologic response to neoadjuvant chemotherapy in patients with breast cancer: a meta-analysis of diagnostic accuracy studies. Oncologist. 2016;21:931–9.
12. Lai SW, Roberts DJ, Rabi DM, Winston KY. Diagnostic accuracy of fine needle aspiration biopsy for detection of malignancy in pediatric thyroid nodules: protocol for a systematic review and meta-analysis. Syst Rev. 2015;4:120.
13. Kelly GA. Meta-analysis: an introduction. http://www.pitt.edu/~super1/lecture/lec3221/index.htm. Accessed 2 July 2018.
14. Maffione AM, Lopci E, Bluemel C, Giammarile F, Herrmann K, Rubello D. Diagnostic accuracy and impact on management of 18F-FDG PET and PET/CT in colorectal liver metastasis: a meta-analysis and systematic review. Eur J Nucl Med Mol Imaging. 2014;42:152–63.
15. Leeflang MM, Deeks JJ, Takwoingi Y, Macaskill P. Cochrane diagnostic test accuracy reviews. Syst Rev. 2013;2:82.
16. Leeflang MM. Systematic reviews and meta-analyses of diagnostic test accuracy. Clin Microbiol Infect. 2014;20:105–13.
17. Habbema J, Eijkemans R, Krijnen P, Knottnerus J. Analysis of data on the accuracy of diagnostic tests. In: Knottnerus J, Buntinx F, editors. The evidence base of clinical diagnosis: theory and methods of diagnostic research. 2nd ed. London: BMJ Publishing Group; 2009. p. 118–45.
18. Wolf FM. Introduction to systematic reviews and meta analysis. http://depts.washington.edu/k30/Meta-analysis/Meta-analysis%20clinical%20research%200603_files/frame.htm. Accessed 2 July 2018.
19. Egger M, Smith GD. Potentials and promise. BMJ. 1997;315:1371–4.
20. Whiting P, Rutjes AWS, Westwood ME, et al., QUADAS-2 Group. QUADAS-2: a revised tool for the quality assessment of diagnostic accuracy studies. Ann Intern Med. 2011;155:529–36.
21. Meade MO. Selecting and appraising studies for a systematic review. Ann Intern Med. 1997;127:531–7.
22. LeLorier J, Grégoire G, Benhaddad A, Lapierre J, Derderian F. Discrepancies between meta-analyses and subsequent large randomized, controlled trials. N Engl J Med. 1997;337:536–42.
23. Performance of methods for meta-analysis of diagnostic test accuracy with few studies or sparse data. (n.d.). http://journals.sagepub.com/doi/full/10.1177/0962280215592269. Accessed 2 July 2018.
24. Reitsma JB, Glas AS, Rutjes AW, Scholten RJ, Bossuyt PM, Zwinderman AH. Bivariate analysis of sensitivity and specificity produces informative summary measures in diagnostic reviews. J Clin Epidemiol. 2005;58:982–90.
25. Rutter CM, Gatsonis C. A hierarchical regression approach to meta-analysis of diagnostic test accuracy evaluations. Stat Med. 2001;20:2865–84.
26. Garas G, Ibrahim A, Ashrafian H, Ahmed K, Patel V, Okabayashi K, Skapinakis P, Darzi A, Athanasiou T. Evidence-based surgery: barriers, solutions, and the role of evidence synthesis. World J Surg. 2012;36:1723–31.
27. Centre for Evidence Based Medicine. Levels of evidence. Oxford: University of Oxford; 2011.
28. Solomon MJ, McLeod RS. Clinical studies in surgical journals–have we improved? Dis Colon Rectum. 1993;36:43–8.
29. Egger M, Smith GD, Phillips AN. Meta-analysis: principles and procedures. BMJ. 1997;315:1533–7.
30. Egger M, Smith GD. Bias in location and selection of studies. BMJ. 1998;316:61–6.

31. Treskes N, Persoon AM, Van Zanten ARH. Diagnostic accuracy of novel serological biomarkers to detect acute mesenteric ischemia: a systematic review and meta-analysis. Intern Emerg Med. 2017;12:821–36.
32. Puli SR. Diagnostic accuracy of endoscopic ultrasound in pancreatic neuroendocrine tumors: a systematic review and meta analysis. World J Gastroenterol. 2013;19:3678.
33. Waaijer L, Simons JM, Borel Rinkes IHM, Van Diest PJ, Verkooijen HM, Witkamp AJ. Systematic review and meta-analysis of the diagnostic accuracy of ductoscopy in patients with pathological nipple discharge. Br J Surg. 2016;103:632–43.
34. Meads C, Davenport C, Małysiak S, Kowalska M, Zapalska A, Guest P, Martin-Hirsch P, Borowiack E, Auguste P, Barton P, Roberts T, Khan K, Sundar S. Evaluating PET-CT in the detection and management of recurrent cervical cancer: systematic reviews of diagnostic accuracy and subjective elicitation. BJOG Int J Obstet Gynaecol. 2013;121:398–407.
35. Thomas B, Guo D. The diagnostic accuracy of evoked potential monitoring techniques during intracranial aneurysm surgery for predicting postoperative ischaemic damage: a systematic review and meta-analysis. World Neurosurg. 2017;103:829–40.
36. Thirumala PD, Crammond DJ, Loke YK, Cheng HL, Huang J, Balzer JR. Diagnostic accuracy of motor evoked potentials to detect neurological deficit during idiopathic scoliosis correction: a systematic review. J Neurosurg Spine. 2017;26:374–83.
37. Bossers SM, De Boer RDH, Boer C, Peerdeman SM. The diagnostic accuracy of brain microdialysis during surgery: a qualitative systematic review. Acta Neurochir (Wien). 2012;155:345–53.
38. Burch J, Marson A, Beyer F, Soares M, Hinde S, Wieshmann U, Woolacott N. Dilemmas in the interpretation of diagnostic accuracy studies on presurgical workup for epilepsy surgery. Epilepsia. 2012;53:1294–302.
39. Sørensen CG, Karlsson WK, Pommergaard H-C, Burcharth J, Rosenberg J. The diagnostic accuracy of carcinoembryonic antigen to detect colorectal cancer recurrence—a systematic review. Int J Surg. 2016;25:134–44.
40. Patel HD, Johnson MH, Pierorazio PM, Sozio SM, Sharma R, Iyoha E, Bass EB, Allaf ME. Diagnostic accuracy and risks of biopsy in the diagnosis of a renal mass suspicious for localized renal cell carcinoma: systematic review of the literature. J Urol. 2016;195: 1340–7.
41. Soubra A, Hayward D, Dahm P, Goldfarb R, Froehlich J, Jha G, Konety BR. The diagnostic accuracy of 18F-fluorodeoxyglucose positron emission tomography and computed tomography in staging bladder cancer: a single-institution study and a systematic review with meta-analysis. World J Urol. 2016;34:1229–37.
42. Mojadidi MK, Bogush N, Caceres JD, Msaouel P, Tobis JM. Diagnostic accuracy of transesophageal echocardiogram for the detection of patent foramen ovale: a meta-analysis. Echocardiography. 2013;31:752–8.
43. Reiman MP, Goode AP, Cook CE, Hölmich P, Thorborg K. Diagnostic accuracy of clinical tests for the diagnosis of hip femoroacetabular impingement/labral tear: a systematic review with meta-analysis. Br J Sports Med. 2014;49:811.
44. Li B, Li Q, Chen C, Guan Y, Liu S. Diagnostic accuracy of computer tomography angiography and magnetic resonance angiography in the stenosis detection of autologous hemodialysis access: a meta-analysis. PLoS One. 2013;8:e78409.

Part IV

20 Avenues for Further Research

Yulun Liu and Yong Chen

Acronyms

GLMMs	Generalized linear mixed models
HSROC	Hierarchical summary receiver operating characteristic
IPD	Individual patient-level data
MRI	Magnetic resonance imaging
NPV	Negative predictive value
PPV	Positive predictive value
ROP	Retinopathy of prematurity
SROC	Summary receiver operating characteristic

20.1 Review of Existing Statistical Work on Diagnostic Meta-analysis

Systematic review of test performance is a rigorous approach for synthesizing evidence in the evaluation of diagnostic/screening tests performance. Previous chapters have been focusing on guiding the progress of diagnostic test assessments and discussing the major challenges during systematic reviews, such as small study

Y. Liu · Y. Chen (✉)
Department of Biostatistics, Epidemiology and Informatics, Perelman School of Medicine, University of Pennsylvania, Philadelphia, PA, USA
e-mail: yulunliu@pennmedicine.upenn.edu; ychen123@mail.med.upenn.edu, ychen123@upenn.edu, ychen123@pennmedicine.upenn.edu

G. Biondi-Zoccai (ed.), *Diagnostic Meta-Analysis*,
https://doi.org/10.1007/978-3-319-78966-8_20

effects, appraising inconsistency, and moderators. When the included studies meet the prespecified quality criteria, the results can be quantitatively summarized by a meta-analysis, providing the estimates for quantities of key interest while accounting for the possible heterogeneity.

To date, a variety of statistical methods for diagnostic meta-analysis have been developed in the presence and absence of a gold standard. Assume that the performance of a candidate test has been measured against a gold standard. The simplest method is to apply univariate fixed-effect or random-effects meta-analysis to estimate sensitivity and specificity separately, ignoring any correlations that may exist between the two measures. However, sensitivity and specificity are often negatively correlated across studies [1] due to the fact that different thresholds may have been used to define positive and negative test results. The current methods essentially can be classified into two categories. The first category includes the summary receiver operating characteristic (SROC) curve approach (or Moses-Littenberg model) [2, 3] and a hierarchical summary receiver operating characteristic (HSROC) model [2–5], which were based on modeling of accuracy and scale parameters while accounting for between-study heterogeneity. The second category includes models based on sensitivity and specificity, including the bivariate general mixed-effects models and bivariate generalized linear mixed models (GLMMs) [1, 5–9]. Interestingly, Harbord et al. [10] found that the bivariate GLMMs and HSROC models are closely related and even equivalent in the absence of covariates.

Despite that various statistical methods have been developed and available as guidance for investigators, it is time to consider future directions of diagnostic tests in meta-analysis. In fact, there remain many interesting and important topics in diagnostic meta-analysis that need to be investigated.

20.2 Advanced Methods of Diagnostic Meta-analysis

This subsection is an incomplete collection of topics that we believe are important for future research on meta-analysis of diagnostic test accuracy studies. These include (a) the robustness of model misspecifications and (b) the identifiability of models and the assumption of conditional independence for multiple diagnostic tests in the absence of a gold standard.

20.2.1 Model Robustness

Although the bivariate GLMMs and HSROC models take into consideration the correlation between sensitivity and specificity across studies, the standard likelihood-based inference sometimes suffers from computational issues, such as non-convergence or sensitivity to the choice of initial values due to the complexity of likelihood and the small number of studies; see Chen et al. [11]. To circumvent these difficulties, composite likelihood [12]-based inference of meta-analysis of diagnostic tests has been developed [13]. Such a procedure not only avoids the computational issues but also offers robustness to misspecification of joint distributions of sensitivity and specificity. In practice, many of diagnostic test accuracy studies involve not only case-control studies but also cohort studies. The bivariate GLMMs and HSROC models focus only on sensitivity and specificity and ignore the information on disease prevalence that is contained in cohort studies. As a consequence, such methods cannot provide estimates of measures related to disease prevalence, including positive and negative predictive values (PPV and NPV), which reflect the clinical utility of a diagnostic test. Additionally, due to possible clinical variability or artifactual variation, sensitivity and specificity may vary with disease prevalence [14, 15]. Chu et al. [16] proposed a trivariate model to jointly analyze sensitivity, specificity, and disease prevalence. Chen et al. [11] proposed a general framework of jointly analyzing case-control and cohort studies while producing robust inference on positive and negative predictive values. They also applied their method to the surveillance of melanoma patients where the goal was to detect the recurrence of melanoma in regional lymph nodes and/or distant sites at a point when it remains treatable. This method not only provided robust estimates of diagnostic accuracy for the four modern diagnostic imaging modalities but also produced patient-specific estimates of positive/negative predictive value of the recurrence of melanoma under various clinical settings, which directly supports clinical decision-making [11]. Ma et al. [17] developed Bayesian inference of this model. Although the composite likelihood-based inference can address the computational issues in standard likelihood-based inference and is robust to the misspecifications of correlations among sensitivity, specificity, and disease prevalence, more robust models are still warranted. For example, van Houwelingen et al. [6, 7] have relaxed the normality assumption of random effects to mixture distributions. Chen et al. [18] have developed beta-binomial distributions as an alternative to allow heavy-tailed distributions. More work along this line toward robust inference is needed.

20.2.2 Absence of Gold Standard Test: Identifiability and Conditional Dependence

In diagnostic meta-analysis, a common problem occurs when the selected reference test may not be a gold standard due to measurement error, high cost, or nonexistence [19]. Failure to account for the errors in reference test can lead to substantial bias in the evaluation of candidate test accuracy [20]. Several statistical methods have been proposed for dealing with such a situation in the literature. Among them, two models have been developed to account for an imperfect reference test, namely, a multivariate generalized linear mixed model [21] and a hierarchical summary receiver operating characteristic model [22]. In practice, investigators may have to choose between one of these two models. In order to provide a useful guideline for modeling with diagnostic meta-analysis, Liu et al. [23] provided a unification of these models and showed that these two models, although with very different formulations, are closely related and are mathematically equivalent in the absence of study-level covariates. Moreover, they have provided the exact relations between the parameters of these two models and assumptions under which two models can be reduced to equivalent sub-models. In other settings, studies may rely on two or more imperfect reference tests to verify the results of a candidate test, or studies may have multiple candidate tests with an imperfect reference. In the former case, the composite reference standard was developed by Alonzo and Pepe [24]; this method combines information from several imperfect reference tests to obtain a "pseudo-gold standard." Such a method is appealing because it provides a simple fixed rule to assign a final diagnosis to each subject in a study population, reducing the effect of misclassification of disease status [25]. For the latter case, the latent class models have been developed for estimating diagnostic accuracy [26, 27], among others. Nevertheless, some possible limitations of latent class approach have been discussed in the literature [28, 29].

It is worth noting that two important issues need to be carefully considered during the evaluating the accuracy of multiple candidate tests in the absence of a gold standard, namely, model identifiability and dependence of diagnostic tests. First, when two or more candidate tests in the absence of a gold standard are simultaneously applied to each subject of a population, the lack of identifiability may occur. For example, if two imperfect diagnostic tests are considered and the data is summarized as a 2×2 table with at most three degrees of freedom; yet, in fact, there are five unknown parameters (one disease prevalence, two sensitivities, and two specificities) in the probability distribution that characterizes these data. To overcome such non-identifiability, the Bayesian approach was conducted through the knowledge of unknown test characteristics as prior information [19]. Gustafson et al. [30] proposed to use nested models, i.e., model expansion and model contraction, to alleviate the identifiable issue, and concluded that non-identifiable models with moderate amount of prior information often outperform simpler but identifiable models. The second issue is the assumption of conditional independence. Some models and inferences for multiple tests rely critically on the assumption that the tests are independent conditional on disease status; see Hui and Walter [31], Pepe and Janes [32], and Chu et al. [21]. However, it is not always satisfied in practice. Dendukuri and Joseph [33] considered the conditional dependence between two tests by allowing pairwise correlation between two tests and random-effects model for correlation between more than two tests. In summary, the issue of model identifiability and conditional independence remains challenging, and further work in this direction is in great need.

20.3 Future Work and Direction

Traditional meta-analyses provide the results based on aggregated data (or study-level data) from published studies. Over the past few decades, although statistical methods relying on aggregated data have been well-studied, these procedures may be highly susceptible to ecological fallacy bias in the literature [34–37]. In contrast, individual patient-level data (IPD) meta-analysis, which synthesizes the evidence from patient-level data, is regarded as a gold standard. IPD meta-analysis offers several advantages compared with the traditional meta-analysis, including bias reduction, the ability to undertake updated analyses (e.g., follow-up data), and subgroup analyses [38]. More specifically, since IPD meta-analysis allows the results that are derived directly from each study, it has potential to substantially reduce the effects of publication and reporting biases [38]. Moreover, IPD meta-analysis collects more detailed information on individual-level characteristics/covariates; it therefore can increase statistical power to carry out subgroup analyses through meta-regression [34]. In particular, when the heterogeneity is present, the interpretation of overall summary results (e.g., study-level covariates) can be misleading, whereas IPD meta-analysis allows investigation on individual characteristic as potential sources of heterogeneity between studies [39]. Despite these benefits, however, IPD may not be always available from all relevant studies due to high cost or logistic reasons [38]. Additionally, in some situations, those studies with availability of IPD may represent a biased subset of the available studies [38, 40, 41].

Recently, incorporating IPD, if available, into aggregated data has received increasing attention, which offers opportunities to inform personalized medical decisions based on patient-level characteristics and produces results tailored to the individual patients or clinically relevant subgroups [42, 43]. In the following two subsections, we will discuss the future work efforts needed to address a set of statistical challenges in combining both IPD and aggregated data, development of diagnostic prediction research, and assessment of prediction models for further aiding of clinical decision-making. In addition, we will also discuss the opportunities and potential challenges when IPD is used alone.

20.3.1 Combination of Aggregated Data and Individual Patient-Level Data

IPD may be unavailable for all studies; the circumstance arises when IPD are accessible for a subset of studies and aggregated data alone are available for the remaining studies. To utilize all available data, several methods have been proposed to combine both IPD and aggregated data using treatment interventions or diagnostic studies [43–45]. Among them, only few published work focuses on how to synthesize both data from diagnostic tests, as well as to evaluate accuracy-by-covariate interactions; for example, see Riley et al. [45], where they have extended the standard bivariate random-effects meta-analysis.

When there is more than one diagnostic test simultaneously used to evaluate their accuracy, it is essential for patients and clinicians to select the most effective diagnostic test. In such case, the network meta-analysis, which is an extension of traditional pairwise meta-analysis, has been applied to compare multiple interventions for a combination of IPD and aggregated data. To our best knowledge, very few statistical methods on the synthesis of IPD and aggregated data for multiple diagnostic accuracy studies have been developed. Further research is needed on this topic. Additionally, for either pairwise meta-analyses or network meta-analyses, it is important to consider the case when there is no gold standard.

In clinical practice, patients and care providers often face decisional dilemmas when multiple diagnostic tests are available, and therefore, prediction models are essential tools in aiding decision-making. The diagnostic prediction model is useful to convert combinations of multiple predictors, such as individual characteristics (e.g., age and smoking status), test results, and biomarkers, with preassigned weights to an estimated absolute risk or probability of disease [46, 47]. By modeling these predictors, a commonly used statistical method is through the multivariable regression framework, such as logistic or Cox regression [48]. In fact, many prediction models are constructed from a single dataset. However, with the availability of IPD, the prediction models based on IPD has become increasingly appealing for improving the development and validation of prediction models [49]. For example, several authors [50–52] incorporated previously published univariable predictor-outcome association to construct a novel prediction model through univariate meta-analysis. When the multivariable associations are available from the literature, it will be difficult to incorporate them due to inclusion of different predictors, model overfitting, and other practical factors. These potential challenges have been discussed in Debray et al. [53]. Before implementing a diagnostic prediction model in clinical practice, model validation is also required, particularly for two major factors—discrimination and calibration [54, 55]. Debray et al. [56] focused on investigating the generalizability of prediction model through the internal-external cross validation to combine model development with validation. A principle on IPD meta-analysis for prediction modeling can be found in Debray et al. [57]. Riley et al. [48] highlighted the importance of external validation of prediction modeling (e.g., discrimination and calibration) on IPD meta-analysis. Nevertheless, several important issues remain open, including novel methods of model development and validation, particularly for the case in the absence of a gold standard, combination of tests, missing predictors, and between-studies heterogeneity in predictor effects.

20.3.2 Partial Verification Bias/No Gold Standard for Individual Patient-Level Data

Despite IPD method offers many opportunities, it still poses many methodological challenges, such as partial verification bias and no gold standard. Next we give two case studies to illustrate the potential challenges using IPD alone.

Case study 1: An example on the issue of verification bias is the study of endometrial carcinoma reported by Rockall et al. [58]. The histology test is considered as a gold standard, but an invasive method, for the diagnosis of the myometrial and cervical invasion in endometrial carcinoma. As an alternative, the magnetic resonance imaging (MRI) with gadolinium enhancement has been used as a surrogate; it is a noninvasive, highly accurate, and less expensive diagnostic test for detecting lymph node metastases [59, 60]. This study includes 96 patients with endometrial carcinoma who had a MRI test performed between May 1995 and November 2004. Out of 96 patients, 68 had a negative MRI test and 28 had positive MRI. For those patients with positive results, 18% of them have been evaluated by the gold standard test of the endometrial carcinoma. For those patients with negative results, 66% of them have been evaluated by the gold standard test following the MRI testing. This design, only partially verifies the subjects with gold standard, is more cost-effective compared to the standard design where all subjects are evaluated by both tests.

Case study 2: An example on the imperfect reference test is the study of retinopathy of prematurity (ROP), which is an eye disease that occurs in premature infants. It is a leading cause of avoidable blindness in children worldwide [61]. When infants with ROP are diagnosed in early stage, they can often be effectively treated with laser retinal ablative surgery or other treatments [62, 63]. In this ROP study, the enrolled infants have undergone a sequential screening examinations on their paired eyes by study-certified ophthalmologists (hereafter referred as the ophthalmology test), which is often treated as a gold standard. Such screening process essentially tends to be time-intensive for the ophthalmologists, stressful for the infants, and related to medicolegal liability concerns [64–66]. The telemedicine-based digital retinal imaging test (hereafter referred as the imaging test) has been widely used in practice. In this ROP study, the preliminary findings suggest that the prevalence rates of ROP significantly differ among subpopulations; specifically, the prevalence rates of female and male groups are 21% and 31%, respectively. The sensitivity and specificity of both diagnostic tests (i.e., the ophthalmology test and the imaging tests) are approximately the same across subpopulations.

In case study 1, since the subjects were evaluated by the gold standard selectively, i.e., subjects with positive results from the candidate test were less likely to be evaluated by the gold standard compared to the subject with negative result from the candidate test, ignoring such selective verification can lead to bias in the estimate of diagnostic accuracy. Such a problem has been recognized by researchers [67, 68], and this type of bias is known as the partial verification bias. Statistical methods have been proposed to correct for the potential partial verification bias when using IPD data alone [68–72]. For multiple studies, Ma et al. [17] recently proposed a hybrid GLMM to correct bias in diagnostic meta-analyses. However, little work has been done in the setting of correlated data or longitudinal studies.

In case study 2, the evaluation from study-certified ophthalmologists is also error-prone. In fact, previous studies have suggested that the agreement between two independent ophthalmologists is poor, suggesting that the reference test is not a gold standard. This problem is related to the Hui-Walter framework [31]. Specifically, Hui and Walter proposed the model to estimate the accuracy of diagnostic tests when the accuracy of the gold standard is unknown [31]. In particular, their proposed approach requires that (1) two diagnostic tests are both applied to two populations with different disease prevalence rates and (2) the results of one diagnostic test are assumed to be independent of the other ones within the disease subpopulation and the disease-free subpopulation. Additionally, the accuracy of both diagnostic tests is assumed to be consistent among two different subpopulations. Compared to the Hui-Walter framework, the key difference is that the ROP study involves the correlated and clustered data. Such correlated or clustered data are common collected in medical research. Further work is required to deal with such problem.

In conclusion, significant efforts are underway to enhance statistical methods for diagnostic test accuracy studies. This chapter aims to provide an overview of the recent statistical advances on meta-analysis of diagnostic tests and suggest a few directions for future research. We believe that more advances in this important topic will have direct impacts to better clinical decision-making and more effective screening of diseases.

References

1. Reitsma JB, Glas AS, Rutjes AW, Scholten RJ, Bossuyt PM, Zwinderman AH. Bivariate analysis of sensitivity and specificity produces informative summary measures in diagnostic reviews. J Clin Epidemiol. 2005;58:982–90.
2. Littenberg B, Moses LE. Estimating diagnostic accuracy from multiple conflicting reports: a new meta-analytic method. Med Decis Mak. 1993;13:313–21.
3. Moses LE, Shapiro D, Littenberg B. Combining independent studies of a diagnostic test into a summary ROC curve: data-analytic approaches and some additional considerations. Stat Med. 1993;12:1293–316.
4. Walter S. Properties of the summary receiver operating characteristic (SROC) curve for diagnostic test data. Stat Med. 2002;21:1237–56.
5. Arends L, Hamza TH, van Houwelingen JC, Heijenbrok-Kal MH, Hunink MG, Stijnen T. Bivariate random effects meta-analysis of ROC curves. Med Decis Mak. 2008;28:621–38.
6. Van Houwelingen HC, Arends LR, Stijnen T. Advanced methods in meta-analysis: multivariate approach and meta-regression. Stat Med. 2002;21:589–624.
7. Van Houwelingen HC, Zwinderman KH, Stijnen T. A bivariate approach to meta-analysis. Stat Med. 1993;12:2273–84.
8. Chu H, Cole SR. Bivariate meta-analysis of sensitivity and specificity with sparse data: a generalized linear mixed model approach. J Clin Epidemiol. 2006;59:1331–2.
9. Hamza TH, van Houwelingen HC, Stijnen T. The binomial distribution of meta-analysis was preferred to model within-study variability. J Clin Epidemiol. 2008;61:41–51.
10. Harbord RM, Deeks JJ, Egger M, Whiting P, Sterne JA. A unification of models for meta-analysis of diagnostic accuracy studies. Biostatistics. 2007;8:239–51.
11. Chen Y, Liu Y, Ning J, Cormier J, Chu H. A hybrid model for combining case–control and cohort studies in systematic reviews of diagnostic tests. J R Stat Soc Ser C Appl Stat. 2015;64:469–89.
12. Lindsay BG. Composite likelihood methods. Contemp Math. 1988;80:221–39.
13. Chen Y, Liu Y, Ning J, Nie L, Zhu H, Chu H. A composite likelihood method for bivariate meta-analysis in diagnostic systematic reviews. Stat Methods Med Res. 2017;26:914–30.
14. Feinstein A. Misguided efforts and future challenges for research on "diagnostic tests". J Epidemiol Community Health. 2002;56:330–2.
15. Leeflang MM, Rutjes AW, Reitsma JB, Hooft L, Bossuyt PM. Variation of a test's sensitivity and specificity with disease prevalence. Can Med Assoc J. 2013;185:E537–44.
16. Chu H, Nie L, Cole SR, Poole C. Meta-analysis of diagnostic accuracy studies accounting for disease prevalence: alternative parameterizations and model selection. Stat Med. 2009;28:2384–99.
17. Ma X, Chen Y, Cole SR, Chu H. A hybrid Bayesian hierarchical model combining cohort and case–control studies for meta-analysis of diagnostic tests: accounting for partial verification bias. Stat Methods Med Res. 2016;25:3015–37.

18. Chen Y, Liu Y, Chu H, Ting Lee ML, Schmid CH. A simple and robust method for multivariate meta-analysis of diagnostic test accuracy. Stat Med. 2017;36:105–21.
19. Joseph L, Gyorkos TW, Coupal L. Bayesian estimation of disease prevalence and the parameters of diagnostic tests in the absence of a gold standard. Am J Epidemiol. 1995;141:263–72.
20. Rutjes AW, Reitsma JB, Di Nisio M, Smidt N, van Rijn JC, Bossuyt PM. Evidence of bias and variation in diagnostic accuracy studies. Can Med Assoc J. 2006;174:469–76.
21. Chu H, Chen S, Louis TA. Random effects models in a meta-analysis of the accuracy of two diagnostic tests without a gold standard. J Am Stat Assoc. 2009;104:512–23.
22. Dendukuri N, Schiller I, Joseph L, Pai M. Bayesian meta-analysis of the accuracy of a test for tuberculous pleuritis in the absence of a gold standard reference. Biometrics. 2012;68:1285–93.
23. Liu Y, Chen Y, Chu H. A unification of models for meta-analysis of diagnostic accuracy studies without a gold standard. Biometrics. 2015;71:538–47.
24. Alonzo TA, Pepe MS. Using a combination of reference tests to assess the accuracy of a new diagnostic test. Stat Med. 1999;18:2987–3003.
25. Naaktgeboren CA, Bertens LC, van Smeden M, de Groot JA, Moons KG, Reitsma JB. Value of composite reference standards in diagnostic research. BMJ. 2013;347:f5605.
26. Qu Y, Tan M, Kutner MH. Random effects models in latent class analysis for evaluating accuracy of diagnostic tests. Biometrics. 1996;52:797–810.
27. Hui SL, Zhou XH. Evaluation of diagnostic tests without gold standards. Stat Methods Med Res. 1998;7:354–70.
28. Pepe MS, Alonzo TA. Comparing disease screening tests when true disease status is ascertained only for screen positives. Biostatistics. 2001;2:249–60.
29. Albert PS, Dodd LE. A cautionary note on the robustness of latent class models for estimating diagnostic error without a gold standard. Biometrics. 2004;60:427–35.
30. Gustafson P, et al. On model expansion, model contraction, identifiability and prior information: two illustrative scenarios involving mismeasured variables [with comments and rejoinder]. Stat Sci. 2005;20:111–40.
31. Hui SL, Walter SD. Estimating the error rates of diagnostic tests. Biometrics. 1980;36:167–71.
32. Pepe MS, Janes H. Insights into latent class analysis of diagnostic test performance. Biostatistics. 2006;8:474–84.
33. Dendukuri N, Joseph L. Bayesian approaches to modeling the conditional dependence between multiple diagnostic tests. Biometrics. 2001;57:158–67.
34. Lambert PC, et al. A comparison of summary patient-level covariates in meta-regression with individual patient data meta-analysis. J Clin Epidemiol. 2002;55:86–94.
35. Berlin JA, Santanna J, Schmid CH, Szczech LA, Feldman HI, Anti-Lymphocyte Antibody Induction Therapy Study Group. Individual patient-versus group-level data meta-regressions for the investigation of treatment effect modifiers: ecological bias rears its ugly head. Stat Med. 2002;21:371–87.
36. Thompson SG, Higgins J. How should meta-regression analyses be undertaken and interpreted? Stat Med. 2002;21:1559–73.
37. Schmid CH, Stark PC, Berlin JA, Landais P, Lau J. Meta-regression detected associations between heterogeneous treatment effects and study-level, but not patient-level, factors. J Clin Epidemiol. 2004;57:683–97.
38. Riley RD, Lambert PC, Abo-Zaid G. Meta-analysis of individual participant data: rationale, conduct, and reporting. BMJ. 2010;340:c221.
39. Smith CT, Williamson PR, Marson AG. Investigating heterogeneity in an individual patient data meta-analysis of time to event outcomes. Stat Med. 2005;24:1307–19.
40. Steinberg K, Smith SJ, Stroup DF, Olkin I, Lee NC, Williamson GD, Thacker SB. Comparison of effect estimates from a meta-analysis of summary data from published studies and from a meta-analysis using individual patient data for ovarian cancer studies. Am J Epidemiol. 1997;145:917–25.
41. Higgins JP, Green S. Cochrane handbook for systematic reviews of interventions, vol. 4. Chichester: John Wiley & Sons; 2011.
42. Thompson SG, Higgins JP. Can meta-analysis help target interventions at individuals most likely to benefit? Lancet. 2005;365:341–6.

43. Riley RD, Steyerberg EW. Meta-analysis of a binary outcome using individual participant data and aggregate data. Res Synth Methods. 2010;1:2–19.
44. Sutton AJ, Kendrick D, Coupland CA. Meta-analysis of individual-and aggregate-level data. Stat Med. 2008;27:651–69.
45. Riley RD, Dodd SR, Craig JV, Thompson JR, Williamson PR. Meta-analysis of diagnostic test studies using individual patient data and aggregate data. Stat Med. 2008;27:6111–36.
46. Steyerberg EW, Mushkudiani N, Perel P, Butcher I, Lu J, McHugh GS, Murray GD, Marmarou A, Roberts I, Habbema JD, Maas AI. Predicting outcome after traumatic brain injury: development and international validation of prognostic scores based on admission characteristics. PLoS Med. 2008;5:e165.
47. Collins GS, Reitsma JB, Altman DG, Moons KG. Transparent reporting of a multivariable prediction model for individual prognosis or diagnosis (TRIPOD): the TRIPOD statement. BMC Med. 2015;13:1.
48. Riley RD, Ensor J, Snell KI, Debray TP, Altman DG, Moons KG, Collins GS. External validation of clinical prediction models using big datasets from e-health records or IPD meta-analysis: opportunities and challenges. BMJ. 2016;353:i3140.
49. Ahmed I, Debray TP, Moons KG, Riley RD. Developing and validating risk prediction models in an individual participant data meta-analysis. BMC Med Res Methodol. 2014;14:3.
50. Steyerberg EW, Eijkemans MJ, Van Houwelingen JC, Lee KL, Habbema JD. Prognostic models based on literature and individual patient data in logistic regression analysis. Stat Med. 2000;19:141–60.
51. Debray TP, Koffijberg H, Lu D, Vergouwe Y, Steyerberg EW, Moons KG. Incorporating published univariable associations in diagnostic and prognostic modeling. BMC Med Res Methodol. 2012;12:121.
52. Greenland S. Quantitative methods in the review of epidemiologic literature. Epidemiol Rev. 1987;9:1–30.
53. Debray T, Koffijberg H, Vergouwe Y, Moons KG, Steyerberg EW. Aggregating published prediction models with individual participant data: a comparison of different approaches. Stat Med. 2012;31:2697–712.
54. Cook NR. Use and misuse of the receiver operating characteristic curve in risk prediction. Circulation. 2007;115:928–35.
55. Steyerberg EW, Vickers AJ, Cook NR, Gerds T, Gonen M, Obuchowski N, Pencina MJ, Kattan MW. Assessing the performance of prediction models: a framework for some traditional and novel measures. Epidemiology. 2010;21:128–38.
56. Debray T, Moons KG, Ahmed I, Koffijberg H, Riley RD. A framework for developing, implementing, and evaluating clinical prediction models in an individual participant data meta-analysis. Stat Med. 2013;32:3158–80.
57. Debray TP, Riley RD, Rovers MM, Reitsma JB, Moons KG, Cochrane IPD Meta-analysis Methods Group. Individual participant data (IPD) meta-analyses of diagnostic and prognostic modeling studies: guidance on their use. PLoS Med. 2015;12:e1001886.
58. Rockall A, Meroni R, Sohaib SA, Reynolds K, Alexander-Sefre F, Shepherd JH, Jacobs I, Reznek RH. Evaluation of endometrial carcinoma on magnetic resonance imaging. Int J Gynecol Cancer. 2007;17:188–96.
59. Saez F, Urresola A, Larena JA, Martín JI, Pijuán JI, Schneider J, Ibáñez E. Endometrial carcinoma: assessment of myometrial invasion with plain and gadolinium-enhanced MR imaging. J Magn Reson Imaging. 2000;12:460–6.
60. Nakao Y, Yokoyama M, Hara K, Koyamatsu Y, Yasunaga M, Araki Y, Watanabe Y, Iwasaka T. MR imaging in endometrial carcinoma as a diagnostic tool for the absence of myometrial invasion. Gynecol Oncol. 2006;102:343–7.
61. Gilbert C. Retinopathy of prematurity: a global perspective of the epidemics, population of babies at risk and implications for control. Early Hum Dev. 2008;84:77–82.
62. Schaffer DB, Palmer EA, Plotsky DF, Metz HS, Flynn JT, Tung B, Hardy RJ. Prognostic factors in the natural course of retinopathy of prematurity. The Cryotherapy for Retinopathy of Prematurity Cooperative Group. Ophthalmology. 1993;100:230–7.

63. Good WV, Hardy RJ, E.M.S. Group. The multicenter study of early treatment for retinopathy of prematurity (ETROP). New York: Elsevier; 2001.
64. Yen KG, Hess D, Burke B, Johnson RA, Feuer WJ, Flynn JT. The optimum time to employ telephotoscreening to detect retinopathy of prematurity. Trans Am Ophthalmol Soc. 2000;98:145.
65. Richter GM, Williams SL, Starren J, Flynn JT, Chiang MF. Telemedicine for retinopathy of prematurity diagnosis: evaluation and challenges. Surv Ophthalmol. 2009;54:671–85.
66. Ying G-S, Quinn GE, Wade KC, Repka MX, Baumritter A, Daniel E, e-ROP Cooperative Group. Predictors for the development of referral-warranted retinopathy of prematurity in the telemedicine approaches to evaluating acute-phase retinopathy of prematurity (e-ROP) study. JAMA Ophthalmol. 2015;133:304–11.
67. Ransohoff DF, Feinstein AR. Problems of spectrum and bias in evaluating the efficacy of diagnostic tests. N Engl J Med. 1978;299:926–30.
68. Begg CB, Greenes RA. Assessment of diagnostic tests when disease verification is subject to selection bias. Biometrics. 1983;39:207–15.
69. Zhou X-H. Maximum likelihood estimators of sensitivity and specificity corrected for verification bias. Commun Stat Theory Methods. 1993;22:3177–98.
70. Zhou X-H. Correcting for verification bias in studies of a diagnostic test's accuracy. Stat Methods Med Res. 1998;7:337–53.
71. Harel O, Zhou XH. Multiple imputation for correcting verification bias. Stat Med. 2006;25:3769–86.
72. De Groot J, Janssen KJ, Zwinderman AH, Moons KG, Reitsma JB. Multiple imputation to correct for partial verification bias revisited. Stat Med. 2008;27:5880–9.

Conclusion

21

Giuseppe Biondi-Zoccai

It is far more important to know what person the disease has than what disease the person has

Hippocrates

In the information era, it is naïve to believe that a single study, even if very well designed, conducted, and reported, with adequate precision and external validity, can provide a unifying and definitive answer to a clinical issue [1]. Accordingly, facing a plethora of similar studies, systematic reviews and meta-analyses remain the cornerstone of informed decision-making by pooling several disparate but similar studies and aiming at increasing precision and external validity [2, 3]. Diagnostic test accuracy studies represent a rule in this scenario, not an exception, as it is easy to perform such a type of study by, for instance, simply querying a sufficiently large administrative database and comparing the diagnostic accuracy of fasting blood glucose levels to serum levels of glycosylated hemoglobin levels for the diagnosis of diabetes mellitus [4].

Thanks to the seminal contributions provided in this book, we hope to guide clinicians and researchers dwelling into the subtleties of medical diagnosis with some useful guidance to correctly design, conduct, interpret, report, and apply a meta-analysis of diagnostic test accuracy studies. While the ultimate scientific test of any diagnostic tool remains a randomized controlled trial, such an effort may be often challenging, as well as occasionally futile, and thus decision-making rests in most cases on diagnostic accuracy features, such as sensitivity, specificity, predictive values, likelihood ratios, diagnostic odds ratios, and areas under the curve of the receiver operating curve. All of these dimensions can be easily and poignantly summarized by meta-analysis. In addition, novel meta-analytic methods for diagnostic test accuracy studies can highlight sources of inconsistency, moderators, and small study effects and also perform indirect and network analyses.

G. Biondi-Zoccai
Department of Medico-Surgical Sciences and Biotechnologies, Sapienza University of Rome, Latina, Italy

Department of AngioCardioNeurology, IRCCS Neuromed, Pozzilli, Italy
e-mail: giuseppe.biondizoccai@uniroma1.it

G. Biondi-Zoccai (ed.), *Diagnostic Meta-Analysis*,
https://doi.org/10.1007/978-3-319-78966-8_21

This textbook has made a compelling case of how careful application of established and reproducible methods can ensure high-quality reviews, with credible results. In particular, prospective registration, careful design, and thorough search are mandatory prerequisites. Rigorous selection, abstraction, and appraisal ensure that data fed into the chosen statistical package are reliable, yielding similarly reliable results. Several specific methods for data pooling are presented, encompassing frequentist as well as Bayesian frameworks. Additional analyses including consistency appraisal, small study effects, meta-regression, and network meta-analysis are also discussed. While most meta-analyses of diagnostic test accuracy studies will typically rest on a selection of such methods, it is important to become familiar with the more advanced methods, as they will likely become more and more common in the future, as evidence accrues and overlapping studies accumulate. Finally, several case studies in meta-analysis of diagnostic test accuracy hereby provided offer useful examples of best practices in this field, highlighting the strengths as well as the weaknesses of such endeavors.

In the continuum of evidence, from case studies to umbrella reviews, meta-analyses of diagnostic test accuracy studies maintain an important place and will continue to contribute important pieces of evidence to guide decision-making [5]. Nonetheless, meta-analyses of intervention studies (in particular randomized controlled trials) will continue to dominate the landscape of evidence synthesis. In addition, prognostic meta-analyses, while facing several challenges inherent to the primary studies included, are also an important piece of the puzzle, as are, at least to some extent, meta-analyses of prevalence and incidence studies.

We hope that this book will prove as a useful adjunct to the scholarly literature for practitioners aiming at better understanding and applying meta-analyses of diagnostic test accuracy studies, to clinician investigators aiming at conducting one on their own, and to researchers wishing to refine existing methods or devise new ones. As with any book devoted to clinical practice and research, it is likely it will become obsolete shortly. This should not be viewed pessimistically, as it will mean that novel and better methodological and applicative studies have broadened and deepened our shared understanding of evidence synthesis for clinical diagnosis.

In conclusion, the outstanding international team of contributors of this textbook should be congratulated for providing such a comprehensive, up to date, and pragmatic perspective on meta-analysis of diagnostic test accuracy studies.

Funding/Disclosure None

References

1. Guyatt GH, Mills EJ, Elbourne D. In the era of systematic reviews, does the size of an individual trial still matter. PLoS Med. 2008;5:e4.
2. Biondi-Zoccai G, editor. Network meta-analysis: evidence synthesis with mixed treatment comparison. Hauppauge: Nova Science Publishers; 2014.

3. Biondi-Zoccai G, editor. Umbrella reviews. Evidence synthesis with overviews of reviews and meta-epidemiologic studies. Springer International: Cham; 2016.
4. Gatsonis C, Paliwal P. Meta-analysis of diagnostic and screening test accuracy evaluations: methodologic primer. AJR Am J Roentgenol. 2006;187:271–81.
5. Biondi-Zoccai GG, Agostoni P, Abbate A. Parallel hierarchy of scientific studies in cardiovascular medicine. Ital Heart J. 2003;4:819–20.

MIX
Papier aus verantwortungsvollen Quellen
Paper from responsible sources
FSC® C105338

FSC
www.fsc.org

If you have any concerns about our products,
you can contact us on
ProductSafety@springernature.com

In case Publisher is established outside the EU,
the EU authorized representative is:
Springer Nature Customer Service Center GmbH
Europaplatz 3, 69115 Heidelberg, Germany

Printed by Libri Plureos GmbH
in Hamburg, Germany